Frontiers in Clinical Drug Research – Anti Allergy Agents
(Volume 1)

Editor

Atta-ur-Rahman, *FRS*
Kings College
University of Cambridge
Cambridge
UK

Bentham Science Publishers
Executive Suite Y - 2
PO Box 7917, Saif Zone
Sharjah, U.A.E.
subscriptions@benthamscience.org

Bentham Science Publishers
P.O. Box 446
Oak Park, IL 60301-0446
USA
subscriptions@benthamscience.org

Bentham Science Publishers
P.O. Box 294
1400 AG Bussum
THE NETHERLANDS
subscriptions@benthamscience.org

CONTENTS

Preface *i*

List of Contributors *iii*

CHAPTERS

1. **Topical Use of Calcineurin Inhibitors in Dermatology** **3**
Sedef Bayata and Aylin Türel Ermertcan

2. **New Therapies for Asthma. What Else Besides Steroids?** **24**
Jorge Sánchez and Javier Estarita

3. **Anti-Allergy Agents in Patients Practicing Sports** **50**
Mariana Couto, Diana Silva, Luís Delgado and André Moreira

4. **Omalizumab Therapy For Allergic Diseases** **118**
Juan Antonio Martinez-Tadeo, Eva Perez-Rodriguez and Zulay Almeida-Sanchez

5. **Therapeutics for Allergy Management** **162**
Sagar Laxman Kale, Naveen Arora

6. **Main Food Allergic Therapies (Promising Ongoing Projects)** **182**
Marina Pérez-Gordo, Carlos Pastor-Vargas and Bárbara Cases

7. **Vitamins in the Therapy of Inflammatory and Oxidative Diseases** **240**
Neena Philips, Mathew Samuel, Harit Parakandi, Halyna Siomyk, Michael Ret, Sesha Gopal, Hui Jia and Hossam Shahin

8. **A Novel Therapeutic Anti-allergy Approach: The Nontraditional Signaling Pathways of Adiponectin and Estrogen** **265**
Jianli Zhao, Wayne Bond Lau and Yajing Wang

9. Indications for Adrenaline: Use by Patients and Emergency Departments **330**
Miguel A. Tejedor-Alonso, Maria V. Mugica-Garcia and Mar Moro-Moro

Index **364**

PREFACE

Frontiers in Clinical Drug Research - Anti-Allergy Agents is an exciting eBook series comprising a selection of chapters relevant to the development of pharmacological agents used for the treatment of allergies. The contributions by leading researchers in the field shed light on new therapies for allergic reactions, nutrition based therapies and the use of substances such as omalizumab and adrenaline to counter inflammatory response and anaphylaxis in patients. The scope of the chapters includes clinical trials of anti-inflammatory and anti-allergic drugs, drug delivery strategies used to treat specific allergies (such as inflammation, asthma and dermatological allergies), lifestyle dependent modes of therapies and the immunological or metabolic mechanisms that are of interest to researchers as targets for new drugs.

In the first chapter, Sedef Bayata and Aylin Turel Ermertcan have discussed the mechanism of action, efficacy, safety, adverse effects of topical calcineurin inhibitors and their innovative use in dermatology. In chapter two, Jorge Sánchez and Javier Estarita present the biological agents available for the treatment of asthma and other allergic diseases such as omalizumab (Anti-IgE) and mepolizumab (Anti-IL5). The different monoclonal antibodies that are being studied in allergic disease with emphasis on the evidence of their use in asthma is also reviewed. Mariana Couto *et al.* demonstrate the hypersensitivity disorder problems for both recreational and competitive athletes such as asthma in the next chapter.

In chapter four Martinez-Tadeo *et al.* have discussed the use of omalizumab therapy for allergic diseases such as asthma of occupational origin, seasonal or perennial allergic rhinitis, and chronic urticaria. Sagar Laxman Kale and Naveen Arora provide a comprehensive overview of different therapeutic approaches for the management of allergic diseases which include allergen avoidance, pharmacotherapy and allergen specific immunotherapy (SIT) in chapter 5.

Food allergies have been increasing in prevalence over the last 10 years. In chapter six, Marina Pérez-Gordo *et al.* have discussed a number of promising emerging therapeutic modalities for food allergy, including allergen-specific and allergen non-specific immunotherapeutic approaches.

In chapter seven, Neena Philips *et al.* present the pathophysiology of several diseases, including allergy and asthma, which is linked to increased reactive oxygen or nitrogen species and inflammatory cytokines. They also discuss inflammatory and oxidative processes consisting of the breakdown of membrane lipids to generate important inflammatory mediators (prostaglandins, platelet activating factor) that activate immune cells, degranulate eosinophils, and mediate vascular alterations.

Jianli Zhao have reviewed the recent developments regarding adiponectin and estrogen in the context of allergic pathology, encompassing asthma, allergic rhinitis, and immune system components pertaining to inflammation in chapter eight. They have also discussed anti-inflammatory mechanisms underlying non-traditional pathways of these proteins, including adiponectin's AMPK-independent signaling pathway and estrogen's effects *via* its membrane receptor.

In the last chapter by Miguel A. Tejedor-Alonso *et al.* a comprehensive review is presented of the use of epinephrine in anaphylaxis episodes both by patients and by the emergency services.

I hope that the readers will find these reviews valuable and thought provoking so that they trigger further research in the quest for the development of pharmacological agents used for the treatment of allergies.

I am grateful for the timely efforts made by the editorial personnel, especially Mahmood Alam (Director Publications), Taimur A. Khan and Maria Baig at Bentham Science Publishers.

Atta-ur-Rahman, FRS
Kings College
University of Cambridge
Cambridge
UK

List of Contributors

André Moreira

Allergy, Asthma and Sports Unit, Immunoallergology Department, Centro Hospitalar São João, E.P.E., Porto, Portugal; Immunology Lab, Faculty of Medicine, University of Porto, Porto, Portugal

Aylin Türel Ermertcan

Celal Bayar University, Faculty of Medicine, Department of Dermatology, Manisa, Turkey

Bárbara Cases

Institute of Applied Molecular Medicine (IMMA) and San Pablo CEU University School of Medicine of Madrid, Jiménez Díaz Foundation (IIS-FJD) of Madrid, Research and Development Department of Inmunotek S.L, Madrid, Spain

Carlos Pastor-Vargas

Institute of Applied Molecular Medicine (IMMA) and San Pablo CEU University School of Medicine of Madrid, Jiménez Díaz Foundation (IIS-FJD) of Madrid, Research and Development Department of Inmunotek S.L, Madrid, Spain

Diana Silva

Allergy, Asthma and Sports Unit, Immunoallergology Department, Centro Hospitalar São João, E.P.E., Porto, Portugal

Eva Perez-Rodriguez

Hospital Universitario Ntra. Sra. De Candelaria, Allergy and Immunology Service, Canary Islands, Tenerife, Spain

Halyna Siomyk

School of Natural Sciences, Fairleigh Dickinson University, Teaneck, NJ 07666, USA

Harit Parakandi

School of Natural Sciences, Fairleigh Dickinson University, Teaneck, NJ 07666, USA

Hossam Shahin

School of Natural Sciences, Fairleigh Dickinson University, Teaneck, NJ 07666, USA

Hui Jia

School of Natural Sciences, Fairleigh Dickinson University, Teaneck, NJ 07666, USA

Javier Estarita

Internal Medicine Department, National University, Bogotá – Colombia

Jianli Zhao

Department of Anesthesiology, the First Affiliated Hospital and Department of Physiology, Shanxi Medical University, Shanxi, Taiyuan, China and Department of Emergency Medicine, Thomas Jefferson University, Philadelphia, PA, USA

Jorge Sánchez

GACE, Group of Clinical and Experimental Allergy, University of Antioquia, Medellín, Colombia

Juan Antonio Martinez-Tadeo

Hospital Universitario Ntra. Sra. De Candelaria, Allergy and Immunology Service, Canary Islands, Tenerife, Spain

Luís Delgado

Allergy, Asthma and Sports Unit, Immunoallergology Department, Centro Hospitalar São João, E.P.E., Porto, Portugal; Immunology Lab, Faculty of Medicine, University of Porto, Porto, Portugal

Mar Moro-Moro

Allergy Unit of University Hospital Fundacion Alcorcon, Spain

Maria V. Mugica-Garcia

Allergy Unit of University Hospital Fundacion Alcorcon, Spain

Mariana Couto

Immunology Lab, Faculty of Medicine, University of Porto, Alameda Prof. Hernani Monteiro, Portugal

Marina Pérez-Gordo

Institute of Applied Molecular Medicine (IMMA) and San Pablo CEU University School of Medicine of Madrid, Jiménez Díaz Foundation (IIS-FJD) of Madrid, Research and Development Department of Inmunotek S.L, Madrid, Spain

Mathew Samuel

School of Natural Sciences, Fairleigh Dickinson University, Teaneck, NJ 07666, USA

Michael Ret

School of Natural Sciences, Fairleigh Dickinson University, Teaneck, NJ 07666, USA

Miguel A. Tejedor-Alonso

Allergy Unit of University Hospital Fundacion Alcorcon, Spain

Naveen Arora

Allergy and Immunology Section, CSIR-Institute of Genomics and Integrative Biology, Delhi University Campus, India

Neena Philips

School of Natural Sciences, Fairleigh Dickinson University, Teaneck, NJ 07666, USA

Sagar Laxman Kale

Allergy and Immunology Section, CSIR-Institute of Genomics and Integrative Biology, Delhi University Campus, India

Sedef Bayata

Celal Bayar University, Faculty of Medicine, Department of Dermatology, Manisa, Turkey

Sesha Gopal

School of Natural Sciences, Fairleigh Dickinson University, Teaneck, NJ 07666, USA

Wayne Bond Lau

Department of Anesthesiology, the First Affiliated Hospital and Department of Physiology, Shanxi Medical University, Shanxi, Taiyuan, China and Department of Emergency Medicine, Thomas Jefferson University, Philadelphia, PA, USA

Yajing Wang

Department of Anesthesiology, the First Affiliated Hospital and Department of Physiology, Shanxi Medical University, Shanxi, Taiyuan, China and Department of Emergency Medicine, Thomas Jefferson University, Philadelphia, PA, USA

Zulay Almeida-Sanchez

Hospital Universitario Ntra. Sra. De Candelaria, Allergy and Immunology Service, Canary Islands, Tenerife, Spain

Send Orders for Reprints on reprints@benthamscience.net
Frontiers in Clinical Drug Research-Anti-Allergy Agents, Vol. 1, **2013, 3-23**

CHAPTER 1

Topical Use of Calcineurin Inhibitors in Dermatology

Sedef Bayata and Aylin Türel Ermertcan*

Celal Bayar University, Faculty of Medicine, Department of Dermatology, Manisa, Turkey

Abstract: Emollients have long been used to maintain the skin barrier function in patients with atopic dermatitis. For many years, topical corticosteroids have been mainstay for atopic dermatitis (AD) treatment. The introduction of topical calcineurin inhibitors represented the first new class of medication approved for the treatment of AD since topical corticosteroids. Topical calcineurin inhibitors, pimecrolimus and tacrolimus, were developed to provide an effective and safe alternative therapy for long-term control of the disease. They provide targeted anti-inflammatory activity without local or systemic side-effects seen with topical corticosteroids. They have been used not only in AD, but also in other inflammatory skin diseases such as psoriasis, lichen planus, seborrheic dermatitis, contact dermatitis, alopecia areata, acne rosacea, pyoderma gangrenosum and vitiligo.

In this chapter, mechanism of action, the efficacy, safety, adverse effects of topical calcineurin inhibitors and their innovative use in dermatology will be reviewed.

Keywords: Topical therapy, topical macrolide immunomodulator, calcineurin inhibitor, pimecrolimus, tacrolimus, atopic dermatitis, mechanism of calcineurin inhibitors, immunology of the skin.

INTRODUCTION

In 1976, during search for novitious antibiotics, a fungus, *Tolypocladeium inflatium*, from Norwegian soil sample, was isolated. This fungus, under certain conditions, produced an undecapeptide containing one unique amino acid, today known as cyclosporin. It was later on discovered to be a powerful immunosuppressive agent and had a major impact on transplant medicine. Subsequently its therapeutic effects in inflammatory skin diseases came to light.

***Address correspondence to Aylin Türel Ermertcan:** Celal Bayar University, Faculty of Medicine, Department of Dermatology, Manisa, Turkey; Tel: +905322243384; E-mail: draylinturel@hotmail.com

In 1984, a macrolide lactone antibiotic was isolated from an actinobacteria, *Streptomyces tsukubaensis*, named tacrolimus, also known as FK506. This new drug was 50-100 times more potent than cyclosporin as an immunosuppressive. Cyclosporin and tacrolimus both work by blocking intracellular signalling pathways that are crucial for the production of cytokines by lymphocytes. Although for the same purpose, they have different molecular structures and they bind to distinct intracellular proteins, cyclophilins and FK506 binding proteins (FKBPs) respectively [1].

Pimecrolimus is one of the new class of novel ascomycin immunomodulating macrolactams. Ascomycin, first isolated as a fermantation product of *Streptomyces hygroscopicus* var. *ascomycetus* in the early 1960's, was initially researched for its antifungal properties. It was 20 years later that ascomycin was investigated for its immunomodulatory functions in inflammatory skin diseases. Pimecrolimus is similar to tacrolimus in structure and binds specifically to the cytosolic receptor, immunophilin macrophilin-12, inhibiting calcineurin activity [2].

Also isolated from a fungus in 1965, sirolimus, was 20 years later developed as an immunosuppressant drug. Even though it binds to the same receptor with pimecrolimus, it does not inhibit calcineurin. Instead it inhibits a multifunctional serine-threonine kinase and is involved in a different pathway of T cell activation [1]. This chapter will focus on tacrolimus and pimecrolimus, as topical immunosuppressive agents that have opened a new era in the management of inflammatory skin disorders, mainly atopic dermatitis. As an introduction it is important to remember how inflammation is caused and how T cells are activated, in order to apprehend the mechanism of action of these drugs. Thereafter their applications in dermatology, future perspectives and long term safety will be discussed.

Mechanism of Action

The skin is a major defense organ, since it serves as a barrier against the outside environment. Constant confrontation with microbial, chemical and physical insults, generates an immune response in the skin. Classical immune response, also known as the adaptive immune response has a spesificity due to immunologic memory. Adaptive immune reactions can be in some conditions, rather harmful in nature, causing allergic and autoimmune reactions. The forerunner of these reactions is the T lymphocyte. A less specific, more primitive defense mechanism also exists, referred to as the innate immune response, which lacks memory. The skin can generate both types of responses. The main components of the latter immune system are neutrophils, eosinophils, natural killer cells, mast cells, cytokines, complement and antimicrobial peptides [3].

Excluding infections and tumors, most skin diseases are either allergic or autoimmune, both generated by adaptive immune mechanisms. The crutial event in this type of response is the antigen presentation, which can be done by various cells in the body. The most effective antigen-presenting cells (APCs) are located on the T cell region of the spleen and lymph nodes, whereas in the skin, Langerhans cells (LCs) of the epidermis are the relevant APCs. LCs in their housekeeping role, take up antigens from the epidermis and migrate to the draining lymph nodes where they present the antigen to the lymphocytes [3]. Lymphocytes are activated by binding of antigens to lymphocyte surface receptors. Engagement of the T-cell receptor (TCR) with a major histocompatibility complex (MHC) peptide ligand on APCs is followed by numerous bonds between adhesion molecules on one cell and their ligands on the other cell, which in turn stabilizes the T-cell APC interaction. The co-aggregation of TCRs activates a series of tyrosine kinases, which initiate downstream signalling pathways by phosphorylating tyrosine residues. One of the major activated molecules is the phospholipase C (PLC), which hydrolyses phosphoinositol-containing lipids in the plasma membrane, resulting in the release of 1,4,5 inositol triphosphate (IP_3) [1]. IP_3 stimulates the release of calcium from endoplasmic reticulum, by binding to its receptor. Increased intracellular calcium stimulates activation of the calmodulin complex, which binds calcineurin [4]. Calcineurin is a heterodimer composed of a 57-59 kDa catalytic A subunit (CaNA) and 19 kDa regulatory B subunit (CaNB). Activation of calcineurin dephosphorylates cytoplasmic NFAT (nuclear factor of activated T cells) proteins and NFAT is then translocated into the nucleus, together with calcineurin which is required to keep NFAT in a dephosphorylated state, preventing nuclear export. NFAT has a relatively low affinity for DNA and combination with other transcription factors is required for the activation of promoters such as interleukin (IL)-2 which are required for T cell activation [1]. NFAT conclusionally regulates mRNA transcription of a number of inflammatory cytokins (IL-2, IL-3, IL-4, IL-5, IFN-gamma, TNF-alpha, GM-CSF) [2]. Although this is a complex process, the major role player is the intercellular calcium. Furthermore, studies have shown that calcineurin is involved in controlling the expression of most Ca^{2+} regulated genes. This is directly related to the mechanism of action of cyclosporin, tacrolimus and pimecrolimus [1]. They selectively inhibit the activation of T cells by inhibiting calcineurin (Fig. **1**). This was demonstrated in a study using T cell clones isolated from the skin of atopic dermatitis patients. Pimecrolimus potently inhibited the proliferation of antigen spesific stimulated T cells and the production of inflammatory cytokines. Furthermore it inhibited the expression of cell surface co-receptor CD134 which appears in the activated T cells, inhibiting their apoptosis. By suppressing CD134, pimecrolimus also detained the survival of antigen activated T cells [5].

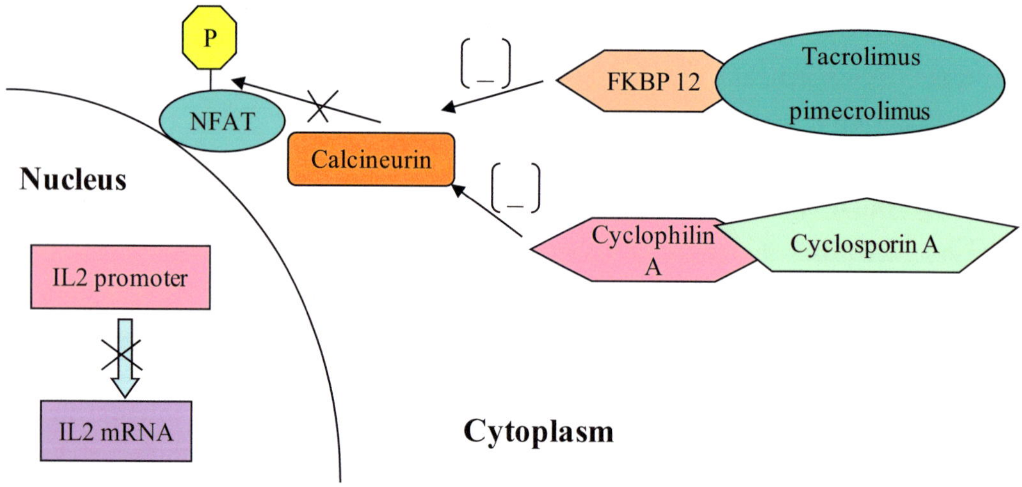

Figure 1: Mechanism of action of calcineurin inhibitors.

On cellular level, in contrast to corticosteroids, pimecrolimus does not suppress the viability and function of LCs. *In vitro* studies have shown that corticosteroids cause apoptosis of LCs and inhibit the expression of critical dendritic cell factors such as CD83, CD86, the synthesis of IL-12p70, and the ability of dendritic cells to activate primary CD4+ T cell proliferation. Topical corticosteroids also have an adverse effect on IL-12 expression, which is a major Th1-promoting cytokine. A lack of this cytokine may delay the maturation of the newborn's immune system. Taken together, topical calcineurin inhibitors act more selectively on the skin immune system and do not induce apoptosis in LCs. Therefore these agents have provided an innovation in the treatment of atopic dermatitis, especially in young children with a developing immune system [5]. Additionally tacrolimus inhibits cytokin production from eosinophils, mast cells and basophils, and reduces the capacity of LCs to activate T cells. Pimecrolimus decreases cytokine production from mast cells, but does not affect LCs. Lipophilic structure of pimecrolimus results in higher affinity for the skin and therefore lower penetration through the skin. Pimecrolimus is a weaker immunosuppressant, requiring higher concentrations for treatment [6]. An important advantage of topical calcineurin inhibitors, compared to corticosteroids is that they do not inhibit the activity of fibroblasts in the connective tissue, which spares the skin from atrophy, even after long term use [6, 7].

Over the last decade, both agents have been used widely and studied in clinical trials involving over 40,000 patients and have demonstrated their efficacy and safety for atopic dermatitis. More than 7 million patients, including over 3 million children, have been treated with either tacrolimus or pimecrolimus since their approval. They are effective in both adults and children and do not lead to tachyphylaxis [6].

Cyclosporin and tacrolimus were originally developed for the prevention of organ rejection in transplant patients and are widely used for this indication [7]. Open-label studies and case reports have shown cyclosporin and tacrolimus to be also effective in treating many inflammatory and non-inflammatory dermatoses, including Hailey-Hailey disease, which is not thought to be T cell mediated. However, long-term systemic use of these agents is limited by their side effects, especially renal toxicity. Topical use of cyclosporin was found to be ineffective in treating atopic dermatitis and psoriasis, whereas intralesional injections have resulted in local clearing of psoriatic plaques. This is due to the size of the cyclosporin molecule (1203Da) and ineffective absorption, even when the barrier function of the epidermis is compromised. On the other hand pimecrolimus

(809Da), specifically developed for the treatment of inflammatory skin diseases [7], and tacrolimus (804Da) molecules are absorbed effectively by human skin and are successful in treating atopic dermatitis when applied topically [1].

Atopic Dermatitis

Atopic dermatitis is a chronic relapsing dermatose, which primarily affects children. Approximately 15-20% of infants in Western countries suffer from this disease. Intractable itching causes sleep loss, affects appetite and mood of infants and young children. Its negative impact on quality of life extends to the patients' family, severely disrupting the lives of parents and the unaffected siblings [8]. Since late 1950s, topical corticosteroids have been an indispensable part of treatment for atopic dermatitis. Even though they provide excellent short term efficacy in the treatment of acute manifestations of the disease, topical corticosteroid usage is limited by potential adverse effects such as skin atropy, striae, telengiectasia, acneiform eruption and hypothalamic-pituitary-adrenal axis suppression in cases of increased systemic absorption [5]. Systemic side effects occur as a result of percutaneous absorption. The major risk factors for increased percutaneous absorption are disease extent and patient age. Young pediatric patients are at the highest risk because of their large skin surface area/body mass ratio [8]. Topical corticosteroids on molecular level, block the synthesis of inflammatory cytokines, by affecting the nuclear factor kappa B pathway. Even low potency corticosteroids, when applied topicaly, cause impairment of the function and viability of LCs in the skin. Calcineurin inhibitors however exhibit a more selective mechanism of action and do not affect LCs [5].

Tacrolimus ointment was launched in December 2000, while pimecrolimus was approved by the United States FDA in December 2001, for the treatment of atopic dermatitis [6]. Developed as a topical formulation of a systemic immunosuppressant, 0.03% and 0.1% tacrolimus ointment have been shown to be effective in the treatment of moderate to severe atopic dermatitis. Pimecrolimus 1% cream on the other hand was spesifically formulated for the treatment of mild to moderate atopic dermatitis. None of the topical calcineurin inhibitors have been associated with systemic immunosuppression, however preclinical and clinical data suggest a greater skin selectivity and larger safety margin for topical pimecrolimus [5]. Albeit both topical calcineurin inhibitors are indicated for the short term or intermittent treatment of atopic dermatitis in adults and children older than two years of age, they are off-labely used for certain cases of younger children aswell [9]. 1133 infants (age: 3-23 months) with mild to severe atopic dermatitis were treated intermittently with 1% pimecrolimus cream for up to 2 years. Results demonstrated rapid symptom relief, prevention of major flares, increased number of disease-free days and improved quality of life of patients and parents, while the cream was well tolerated [8]. However these agents are not to be used as first-line therapies. Aside from their low side effect profile, available data does not suggest an efficacy advantage for topical calcineurin inhibitors over topical steroids [10]. Patients who are appropriate to be treated with these agents are the ones unresponsive or intolerant of other conventional therapies or in whom these therapies are inadvisable because of potential risks. They should be taken as a part of an overall treatment strategy, addressing all aspects of atopic dermatitis, including treatment of secondary infections, an appropriate skin care regimen, topical steroids, anti-pruritic agents, and allergen identification and/or elimination [9].

A proactive treatment modality is recently being advised in the treatment of atopic dermatitis with topical tacrolimus ointment, to control residual disease with minimal use of the drug and no application of an active agent to non-affected skin [6]. In a multicentral study on a long term anti-inflammatory treatment for atopic dermatitis, Wollenberg *et al.* from Germany have treated 257 adults with atopic dermatitis, using tacrolimus 0.1% ointment, twice daily for six weeks. Later, as proactive administration, tacrolimus was applied twice weekly for 12 months. This has significantly decreased disease activation. It was proposed that even after treatment, normal looking skin in molecular basis still has subclinical inflammation and proactive treatment is important to suppress this subclinical inflammation [11]. Thaçi *et al.* have demonstrated in a similar study with 267 pediatric atopic dermatitis patients, that 0.03% tacrolimus ointment, twice weekly for 12 months has also significantly decreased disease activation, caused significantly less disease flares and increased the time until first relapse [6, 12]. Tacrolimus ointments are demonstrated to be more effective and equally safe when compared with 1% hydrocortisone in the treatment of moderate to severe atopic dermatitis [13]. Compared to pimecrolimus, a meta-analysis suggests that tacrolimus ointment has a higher efficacy and better tolerance rates [14]. Among all of the topical agents used, calcineurin inhibitors may be considered as a major breakthrough. However they should not be regarded as a candidate to replace all other medications, but they are highly valuable, effective and safe for the most demanding skin areas involved with atopic inflammation [6].

Off-Label Uses

Although topical calcineurin inhibitors are indicated for treatment of atopic dermatitis, they have also been studied in many off-label uses. Double-blind and open studies have shown favorable results in oral lichen planus. In one study of oral lichen planus, tacrolimus was detected in blood in 54% of patients, but no signs of systemic toxicity were observed.

Favorable results with tacrolimus, especially in combination with excimer laser in vitiligo patients have also been shown in double-blind and open studies. Similarly, in vitiligo, successful results were achieved with pimecrolimus, when combined with narrow-band UVB, especially for facial lesions.

Inverse psoriasis is another cutaneous disorder in which topical corticosteroids are effective but their use is limited due to their side effects, especially in flexural regions of the body. On the other hand topical tacrolimus and pimecrolimus have shown favorable results in the treatment of inverse psoriasis, in double-blind and open studies.

They have also been used in allergic contact dermatitis, seborrheic dermatitis, rosacea, cutaneous lupus erythematosus, alopecia areata, dermatomyositis, lichen sclerosus and pyoderma gangrenosum and have shown beneficial results [15, 16].

Vitiligo

One of the major off-label uses of topical calcineurin inhibitors is in the treatment of vitiligo. The etiology of vitiligo is still mainly unknown. Several theories have been proposed, among which the autoimmune hypothesis is the most important and popular one. To date, different treatment options are available in the treatment of vitiligo but a curative therapy does not exist. The aim of the treatment is the stabilization and/or repigmentation of the lesions. Nonsurgical therapeutic options include topical corticosteroids, topical calcipotriol, photochemotherapy or narrow band UV-B phototherapy. Surgical methods are based on autologous grafting of non-lesional epidermis or cultured melanocytes to depigmented areas. Cosmetic camouflage and antioxidants are adjuvant therapeutic options. Patients with extensive vitiligo can be further depigmented by hyroquinone. Due to the long duration of the treatment period, nearly all modalities are limited by adverse effects or poor efficacy. Recently tacrolimus ointment and pimecrolimus cream have been introduced in the treatment of this disease. The mode of action of these agents interfere with the autoimmune mediated destruction of melanocytes by activated T cells. However, lymphocytic infiltrate in the perilesional skin is not always present and recently *in vitro* evidence of a direct interaction between tacrolimus and keratinocytes, creating a favourable surrounding for melanocytic growth and migration has been obtained. Most trials on the treatment of vitiligo with tacrolimus have given successful results, especially in the head and neck region. This may be explained by greater density of hair follicules in these areas, and thus a greater melanocyte reservoir. One randomized, double blind, left-right comparative trial has shown tacrolimus to be almost as effective as clobetasol propionate in the treatment of vitiligo [17]. On the other hand it was reported that pimecrolimus was not effective on the body except for the face in childhood localized vitiligo [18]. Recently several studies in literature have described the use of excimer laser treatment and topical tacrolimus in patients with vitiligo to be more effective than tacrolimus or excimer laser monotherapy [19]. Results of pimecrolimus 1% cream in vitiligo was evaluated in an open study on 26 patients. Clinical assessment revealed repigmentation of the target lesion on the face or neck in 10 of 26 patients after 3 months and in 13 of 26 after 6 months. Reduction in the area of the target lesion was 26.2% and 72.9% after 3 and 6 months respectively. Compared to atopic dermatitis, in vitiligo, the barrier function of the skin is not disturbed. Therefore considering systemic absorbtion, the penetration of these agents is much lower. Also due to a higher lipophilicity, pimecrolimus has a more skin selective profile than tacrolimus, which theoratically results in a lower potential for systemic immunosupression in extended treatment periods. In vitiligo, both tacrolimus and pimecrolimus enable the physician to abstain side effects of the currently available therapies [17] and as mentioned above, they are effective and therefore good treatment alternatives, especially for facial lesions.

Allergic Contact Dermatitis

Topical calcineurin inhibitors are also good alternatives for corticosteroids in the treatment of allergic contact dermatitis. A study comparing the therapeutic ability of tacrolimus 0.1% ointment and mometasone furoate 0.1% ointment in patients with chronic hand eczema and positive patch tests revealed that tacrolimus is a promising alternative therapy for contact dermatitis patients as it is effective from the first month of treatment, well tolerated and offers similar therapeutic results to topical corticosteroids [20]. Their use is especially of great importance in areas where topical corticosteroids can be harmful, like periorbital region. In a patch test allergen challenge model, tacrolimus ointment has been shown to be effective in nickel sulphate related allergic contact dermatitis. In eyelid dermatitis, tacrolimus ointment has been well studied among atopic patients and is found to be effective and safe without causing skin atrophy, telengiectasia or increased intraocular pressure. In a study with twenty adult patients with allergic contact eyelid dermatitis, tacrolimus ointment was successfully used in the treatment. It was effective by the first month and was well tolerated. Although some reports have raised the possibility that topical macrolactams may, rarely, produce unusual manifestations of cutaneous infections, similar to those seen with topical corticosteroids, there were no infectious complications seen in these patients. Topical calcineurin inhibitors are also good alternatives for therapy for patients test positive to budesonide on patch testing. However it should also be taken into consideration that contact allergy to tacrolimus has also been reported and may coexist with allergy to other related calcineurin inhibitors, including pimecrolimus [21].

Seborrheic Dermatitis

These topical macrolactam immunomodulators have also been a safe alternative for topical corticosteroids, in the treatment of seborrheic dermatitis like other inflammatory dermatoses [22]. Seborrheic dermatitis is a common papulosquamous dermatose, affecting over 5% of the general population with male predominance. Both pimecrolimus and tacrolimus have been used in the treatment of this disorder. A brief review of the literature reveals that pimecrolimus 1% cream, when used twice a day, successfully treats seborrheic dermatitis on the facial region in approximately 10 days [23]. Interestingly tacrolimus and pimecrolimus have been shown to have antifungal activity against malessezia furfur *in vitro*. has been shown to have antifungal activity against malessezia furfur *in vitro* [4, 24]. The combination of potent anti-inflammatory activity and antifungal effects of these agents make them highly effective treatment alternatives for seborrheic dermatitis, specially when the many side effects of topical corticosteroids on the face is considered [4].

Psoriasis Vulgaris

It is already well known that oral cyclosporin is highly effective in treating psoriasis lesions. Although oral pimecrolimus has also been shown to be effective, topical treatment is restricted to mild disease due to limited effectiveness caused by thick scaling and limited penetration [2]. Neither tacrolimus ointment nor pimecrolimus cream appear to be effective for treating plaque type psoriasis when simply applied as commercially available. This is the case even though percutaneous absorbtion is higher in diseased skin. Occlusion on the other hand makes topical tacrolimus more effective in treating psoriasis. It decreases erythema and infiltration of the plaques. Changing the formulation of tacrolimus and pimecrolimus in attempt to increase penetration is a promising way to augment their effectiveness. Studies have shown that topical application of liposomal tacrolimus achieved nine times the concentration of tacrolimus at a target site. It appears to be most effective in treating psoriatic lesions on the face and intertriginous areas, where the skin is thin. In one study, tacrolimus 0,1% ointment was applied on facial lesions twice a day for 4 weeks without occlusion. A complete or good response was obtained in nearly half of the patients. The safety and efficacy of tacrolimus was evaluated in another trial of 21 patients, with psoriatic lesions on the face and intertriginous regions, 81% experienced total clearance at day 57, with only two reporting adverse events, limited to itching [25]. These calcineurin inhibitors appear to be beneficial especially in inverse psoriasis, where the use of topical corticosteroids is limited due to a variety of side effects.

Lichen Planus

Lichen planus is a chronic inflammatory mucocutaneous disease, affecting 0.5 to 1% of the adult population. Both cutaneous and oral involvement can be seen.

Clinical presentations of the oral form are varied, however the most common form is the reticular one. Erosive, atrophic and bullous forms are also reported. The latter ones are the most symptomatic and difficult to treat. Although the disease can affect all regions of the oral cavity, the buccal mucosa is the most common site. Cell mediated immunity seems to play a critical role in the pathogenesis of the disease, but the specific antigens responsible for the activation of the T cells have not been identified. Studies have shown the interaction of T cells and mast cells in a cyclic nature *via* the production of cytokins and TNF-α [26].

Treatment of oral lichen planus includes high potency corticosteroids, either topical or intralesional, retinoids, cyclosporin and most recently, topical tacrolimus. Studies have demostrated the efficacy of tacrolimus, specially in the erosive type of oral lichen planus. The 0.1% ointment formulation has been shown to be more effective compared to 0.03% ointment. Pimecrolimus on the other hand, due to its cream formulation, is difficult to use intraorally, because of its inability to adhere to moist oral tissues [26]. However there is evidence that its efficacy is equal to that of topical triamcinolone acetonide 0.1% paste. Both of the calcineurin inhibitors have also been shown to be effective in vulvovaginal lichen planus [27].

Cutaneous Lupus Erythematosus

In 23 studies, 15 of which are case reports, the efficacy of topical calcineurin inhibitors in the treatment of cutaneous lupus erythematosus have been evaluated. While both of the available agents showed favourable results with the cutaneous findings of systemic lupus erythematosus (SLE), only slight effects were demonstrated for subacute cutaneous lupus erythematosus (SCLE). As for discoid lupus erythematosus (DLE), even less convincing results were achieved due to low penetration of the compounds, caused by distinct hyperkeratosis. Monotherapy in highly active and disseminated cases does not seem promising, especially not in DLE, whereas SCLE and SLE lesions respond better. In more severe cases, combined systemic treatment with antimalarials is advised [16].

In a recent study, the effectiveness of topical calcineurin inhibitors as monotherapy, or in combination with hydroxychloroquine in cutaneous lupus erythematosus has been evaluated. Patients were diagnosed with discoid lupus erythematosus, cutaneous lupus erythematosus or lupus erythematosus tumidus. Size of the lesions were measured as 1 cm at most. Some of the patients were treated with either tacrolimus or pimecrolimus as monotherapy while others have used additional hydroxychloroquine. Edema, erythema and desquamation were clinically evaluated and desired results were achieved with both of the topical agents, especially significant improvement in edema was noted. With the combination therapy, improvement in all clinical parameters was achieved. The investigators suggest that both of the topical calcineurin inhibitors are effective in cutaneous lupus erythematosus as monotherapy as well as in combination with hydroxyxhloroquine. However comparison among the different clinical subtypes was not attempted [28]. Therefore it is more reasonable to use these agents as monotherapy in cutaneous lupus erythematosus lesions which fulfill the following criteria: acute or subacute type, small, localized lesion. For multiple, disseminated and large lesions, discoid lupus erythematosus and systemic lupus erythematosus with cutaneous involvement, combination therapy with hydroxychloroquine is advised.

Pyoderma Gangrenosum

Pyoderma gangrenosum is a neutrophilic dermatosis which present in either a classic ulcerative form or in atypical bullous, vegetative or pustular forms. It may be associated with several disorders or may also be idiopathic. Systemic immunosuppressants remain the choice of therapy for most patients, however in localized disease, topical treatments should be considered. In a study on five patients with localized, idiopathic, newly diagnosed pyoderrma gangrenosum, tacrolimus was used successfully and a complete remission was achieved within a mean time of six weeks. Thus it is suggested that topical tacrolimus monotherapy can be a good choice of treatment for pyoderma gangrenosum patients, who fulfill the following criteria: localized disease, idiopathic form, recent onset, negative microbiological tests [29].

Acne Rosacea

Acne rosacea is another dermatose in which topical calcineurin inhibitors have been used off-label for therapy. In 2005, Crawford *et al.* investigated the efficacy of pimecrolimus cream in 12 patients with erythematotelangiectatic or papulopustular rosacea and reported appreciable improvement of erythema in 10 patients and a decreased papulopustular component in five [30]. Cunha *et al.* reported dramatic clearing of a granulomatous rosacea with 4.5 months of pimecrolimus treatment [31]. Kim MB *et al.* demonstrated the efficacy of pimecrolimus cream in rosacea in a study with 26 patients. Approximately two-thirds experienced improvements in their clinical symptoms. The greatest response was observed in the first two weeks of the treatment, especially improvement of the severity of erythema was observed, while response to therapy plateaued in the following two weeks. These findings suggest that 1% topical pimecrolimus is a safe and effective therapeutic option for the treatment of rosacea [32]. In some patients, sudden aggravation occurs after applying topical agents. This might be due to the occlusive properties of topical medications and proliferation of Demodex folliculorum caused by local immunosuppression. Although only a few cases have been reported, continious topical use of immunomodulators has shown to cause rosaceiform dermatitis [33]. The subject remains to debate.

Alopecia Areata

Alopecia areata is a non-scarring type of localized hair loss. Topical or intralesional steroids are widely used for its treatment. Although very effective, there are always concers regarding their side effects. Topical calcineurin inhibitors have also been tried in the treatment of alopecia areata and even though there are conflicts on this topic, Ucak *et al.* have demostrated in a study that pimecrolimus 1% cream is as effective as clobetasol propionate 0.05% cream and even superior in terms of side effects, in the treatment of alopecia areata [34].

Dermatomyositis

Dermatomyositis, an inflammatory disease, characterized by well known cutaneous manifestations such as Gottron's sign and heliotrope rash, accompanied by proximal muscle weakness, usually requires the treatment of the underlying systemic disease such as an internal malignancy. However occasionally refractory skin lesions require further treatment with topical agents. Case reports have shown remarkable improvement in the cutaneous lesions of dermatomyositis with pimecrolimus and it is suggested as an efficacious treatment [35].

Systemic Absorption

Systemic immunnosuppression due to transepidermal absorption of calcineurin inhibitors have been a concern since their development. Pimecrolimus, due to its high lipophilicity, penetrates into the skin very well, however its absorption into the systemic circulation is very low. In fact lower than tacrolimus and much lower than corticosteroids. When compared to tacrolimus, pimecrolimus demonstrated a 9 to 10 fold lower permeation through skin *in vitro*. In pharmacokinetic studies of children with up to 92% body surface area affected, 67% had pimecrolimus blood concentrations below 0.5 ng/ml and 97% were below 2.0 ng/ml [5, 6].

Early studies with tacrolimus 0.1% ointment, in 49 adult atopic dermatitis patients, showed maximum blood concentrations ranging from undetectable to 20 ng/ml. However except for three, all other patients had a peek concentration below 5 ng/ml. This demonstrates an excessive systemic absorption in a few number of patients possibly due to severly impaired skin barrier function. Patients with Netherton syndrome for example represent a therapeutic challenge because of increased absorption of any topically applied treatment. Tacrolimus ointment 0.1%, when used in these patients, reach blood levels up to 37 ng/ml, within or even above the range of those orally administered calcineurin inhibitors for transplant patients [5]. Likewise significant systemic absorption of tacrolimus has been described in patients with other diseases such as erosive mucosal lichen planus, lamellar ichthyosis, generalized leukemic erythroderma and pyoderma gangrenosum [6]. Though in contrast, pimecrolimus cream was used in Netherton syndrome, where 99% of the body surface area was treated, observed blood levels were below 2.4 ng/ml over the whole treatment period [5]. Considering atopic dermatitis patients, even the ones with the largest extent of skin area involved, topical treatment with pimecrolimus 1% cream, consistently low blood concentrations were displayed. Therefore pimecrolimes is safe for long term use with no limitation in the extent of skin area treated and no restriction for the treatment of sensitive skin areas [36].

Common off-label use of pimecrolimus 1% cream for the treatment of atopic dermatitis in children younger than two years of age has raised concerns about systemic effects of the agent in infants. Pharmacokinetic studies conducted with infants with atopic dermatitis indicated that pimecrolimus blood concentrations after topical applications were consistently low, irrespective of the level of disease severity and percentage of total body surface area involved. The results were comparable to that observed in older patients, treated in the same way. This finding suggests that young pediatric patients are not at higher risk of significant percutaneous absorption after topical application of pimecrolimus cream, despite their large skin surface area/bady mass ratio [8].

On February 15, 2005, the Pediatric Advisory Committee of the FDA recommended "black box" warnings for pimecrolimus and tacrolimus when concerns of potential safety risks, including skin cancer and lymphomas came to light. Although these potential adverse effects were only shown in animal models, during search for the toxicity of the drugs, and routine therapeutic regimes used in humans are well below toxic levels, data from animal models should not be neglected. However for both agents, the European agency EMEA concluded on the basis of its safety review that the benefits of the treatment of atopic dermatitis with topical calcineurin inhibitors exceeded the risks [6].

Adverse Effects and Long-term Safety

One of the most common side effects of topical calcineurin inhibitors reported is transient skin burning at the site of drug application. It usually lasts around 10 minutes. Such discomfort is usually not a cause of treatment discontinuation. The pathomechanism of this burning symptom is not quite clear. Topical application of both pimecrolimus and tacrolimus have been shown to increase the release of substance P and calcitonin gene related peptide from primary afferent nerve fibers. In addition, mast cell degranulation, together with the release of inflammatory mediators such as histamine and tryptase may induce pruritus and burning by binding to the corresponding receptors on sensory nerve fibers. Oral acetylsalicylic acid taken 2 or 3 days prior to the treatment is an effective way in preventing burning sensation during topical treatment with tacrolimus. Other authors advise their patients to place the tube in the refrigerator for 15 to 20 minutes before application [6].

Like all other newly developed drugs, pimecrolimus and tacrolimus have been tested in numerous studies. A brief review of these studies have been summarized in an article published in 2005, titled *"Immunomodulation and safety of topical calcineurin inhibitors for the treatment of atopic dermatitis"*. In dermal toxicology studies, pimecrolimus was applied to mice topically for over 104 weeks, resulting in a mean daily exposure of 1.040 ng.h/ml. No drug related malignancies were observed and a non-observed adverse event level (NOAEL) was established. In a similar study, using a higher dose of 1.770 ng.h/ml, lymphoproliferative changes were observed after 13 weeks. In further research, an oral form of pimecrolimus was administered to monkeys in attempt to treat psoriasis. At a dose of 15 mg/kg/day, animals reached an average systemic exposure of 1.200 ng.h/ml. After 39 weeks, 1 of 8 monkeys developed lymphoproliferative disease. Similarly in monkeys, lymphoproliferative changes with tacrolimus, at a dose of 10 mg/kg/day, were observed after 90 days. These results confirm that prolonged exposure to high doses, 25 times the average exposure at the maximally recommended human dose (MRHD), can produce lymphoproliferative diseases. In adults the MRHD of tacrolimus is 20.4 ng.h/ml and 23 ng.h/ml for pimecrolimus. Compared to this baseline, the NOAEL for tacrolimus established in toxicity studies is 10 times the MRHD and 45 times the MRHD for pimecrolimus. These studies suggest a relatively larger safety margin for pimecrolimus compared with tacrolimus, which may be meaningful in cases of extensive, prolonged use in children [5].

To evaluate the immunosuppression with topical calcineurin inhibitors, 91 patients, who had been treated with pimecrolimus for up to 2 years were vaccinated against diphtheria, rubella, measles and tetanus. Seropositivity for these vaccinations did not differ from the control group. A similar study confirmed the same results for tacrolimus [5]. Application of ointments containing immunomodulators does not appear to adversely affect either immediate response to vaccination or generation of immune memory in childhood [6].

The delayed type hypersensitivity was used to asses immunocompetence. In patients using these agents for up to 1 year, no effect on the ability to develop a normal T cell mediated immune response was observed [5, 6].

Systemic absorption of topically applied tacrolimus and pimecrolimus in patients with atopic dermatitis appears to be low and well below the therapeutic range of organ transplant patients. However in patients with highly compromised skin barrier, such as Netherton syndrome, blood levels within this range have been documented [1].

Although poor in quality, there is data suggesting that DNA repair in keratinocytes is, *in vitro* conditions, inhibited by topical calcineurin inhibitors. If so, it would take years to observe the end point of increased rate of skin cancer in human subjects. Up to date, the risk being mentioned is not supported by enough evidence [9]. With these agents, there is also a concern about promotion of UV-induced carcinogenesis, due to the potentiation of UV-induced immunosuppression [1]. It is already known that systemic calcineurin inhibitors, as a part of an immunosuppressive therapy regime, increase the risk of sun-induced non-melanoma skin cancers as well as melanoma. The risk of cutaneous malignancies with topical calcineurin inhibitors is yet unknown [9]. The combination of UV exposure with these agents may be useful in treating various dermatoses, such as vitiligo. There is no evidence in humans that this combination is more carcinogenic than UV alone [6]. However, until further evidence is available, specialists agree that patients should be advised to avoid excessive UV exposure and apply a high protection factor sunblock daily to all exposed skin. This should especially be emphasized in patients at greater risk of developing skin cancer, including those with red hair and Fitzpatrick skin types I and II [9].

Today, in the treatment of several inflammatory skin disorders, topical calcineurin inhibitors pimecrolimus and tacrolimus serve as an alternative to topical corticosteroids by their significant, T cell selective anti-inflammatory activity, immunomodulatory capabilities and highly favourable adverse effects profile in long term use. Although momentarily approved only for the treatment of atopic dermatitis, aside from their noticeable success in the treatment of facial vitiligo, new roles are being assigned for topical calcineurin inhibitors every day in inflammatory dermatoses. However most are case reports or small series and replacing topical corticosteroids with calcineurin inhibitors in all inflammatory dermatoses does not neccessarily bring advantages. Therefore the topic is always open for new double blind, randomized, controlled trials to support the efficacy of topical calcineurin inhibitors in their newly assigned roles.

ACKNOWLEDGEMENTS

Declared none.

CONFLICT OF INTEREST

The author(s) confirm that this chapter content has no conflict of interest.

REFERENCES

[1] Reynolds NJ, Al-Daraji WI. Calcineurin inhibitors and sirolimus: mechanisms of action and applications in dermatology. Clin Exp Dermatol 2002; 27 (7): 555-61.
[2] Gupta AK, Chow M. Pimecrolimus: a review. J Eur Acad Dermatol Venereol 2003; 17 (5): 493-503.
[3] Schwarz T. Immunology. In:Bolognia JL, Jorizzo JL, Rapini RP, Schaffer JV, Eds. Dermatology. 2nd ed. Spain: Elsevier Limited 2008; pp.63-79.
[4] Ling MR. Topical tacrolimus and pimecrolimus: future directions. Semin Cutan Med Surg 2001; 20 (4): 268-74.
[5] Hultsch T, Kapp A, Spergel J. Immunomodulation and safety of topical calcineurin inhibitors for the treatment of atopic dermatitis. Dermatology 2005; 211 (2): 174-87.
[6] Czarnecka-Operacz M, Jenerowicz D. Topical calcineurin inhibitors in the treatment of atopic dermatitis – an update on safety issues. J Dtsch Dermatol Ges 2012; 10 (3): 167-72.
[7] Grassberger M, Steinhoff M, Schneider D, Luger TA. Pimecrolimus - an anti-inflammatory drug targeting the skin. Exp Dermatol 2004; 13 (12): 721-30.
[8] Paul C, Cork M, Rossi AB, Papp KA, Barbier N, de Prost Y. Safety and tolerability of 1% pimecrolimus cream among infants: experience with 1133 patients treated for up to 2 years. Pediatrics 2006; 117 (1): e118-28.
[9] Berger TG, Duvic M, Van Voorhees AS, VanBeek MJ, Frieden IJ. The use of topical calcineurin inhibitors in dermatology: safety concerns. J Am Acad Dermatol 2006; 54 (5): 818-23.
[10] Frankel HC, Qureshi AA. Comparative effectiveness of topical calcineurin inhibitors in adult patients with atopic dermatitis. Am J Clin Dermatol. 2012;13 (2): 113-23.
[11] Wollenberg A, Reitamo S, Girolomoni G, *et al.* Proactive treatment of atopic dermatitis in adults with 0.1% tacrolimus ointment. Allergy 2008; 63 (7): 742-50.
[12] Thaçi D, Reitamo S, Gonzalez Ensenat MA, *et al.* European Tacrolimus Ointment Study Group. Proactive disease management with 0.03% tacrolimus ointment for children with atopic dermatitis: results of a randomized, multicenter, comparative study. Br J Dermatol 2008; 159 (6): 1348-56.
[13] Reitamo S, Van Leent EJ, Ho V, *et al.* Efficacy and safety of tacrolimus ointment compared with that of hydrocortisone acetate ointment in children with atopic dermatitis. J Allergy Clin Immunol 2002; 109 (3): 539-46.
[14] Yin ZQ, Zhang WM, Song GX, Luo D. Meta-analysis on the comparison between two topical calcineurin inhibitors in atopic dermatitis. J Dermatol. 2012; 39 (6): 520-6.

[15] Lin AN. Innovative use of topical calcineurin inhibitors. Dermatol Clin 2010; 28 (3): 535-45.

[16] Sticherling M. Update on the use of topical calcineurin inhibitors in cutaneous lupus erythematosus. Biologics 2011; 5: 21-31.

[17] Boone B, Ongenae K, Van Geel N, Vernijns S, De Keyser S, Naeyaert JM. Topical pimecrolimus in the treatment of vitiligo. Eur J Dermatol 2007; 17 (1): 55-61.

[18] Köse O, Arca E, Kurumlu Z. Mometasone cream *vs.* pimecrolimus cream for the treatment of childhood localized vitiligo. J Dermatolog Treat 2010; 21 (3): 133-9.

[19] Tjioe M, Vissers WH, Gerritsen MJ. Topical macrolide immunomodulators: a role in the treatment of vitiligo? Am J Clin Dermatol 2006; 7 (1): 7-12.

[20] Katsarou A, Makris M, Papagiannaki K, Lagogianni E, Tagka A, Kalogeromitros D. Tacrolimus 0.1% *vs.* mometasone furoate topical treatment in allergic contact hand eczema: a prospective randomized clinical study. Eur J Dermatol 2012; 22 (2): 192-6.

[21] Katsarou A, Armenaka M, Vosynioti V, Lagogianni E, Kalogeromitros D, Katsambas A. Tacrolimus ointment 0.1% in the treatment of allergic contact eyelid dermatitis. J Eur Acad Dermatol Venereol 2009; 23 (4): 382-7.

[22] Brownell I, Quan LT, Hsu S. Topical pimecrolimus in the treatment of seborrheic dermatitis. Dermatol Online J 2003; 9 (3): 13.

[23] Kim BS, Kim SH, Kim MB, Oh CK, Jang HS, Kwon KS. Treatment of facial seborrheic dermatitis with pimecrolimus cream 1%: an open-label clinical study in Korean patients. J Korean Med Sci 2007; 22 (5): 868-72.

[24] Ang-Tiu CU, Meghrajani CF, Maano CC. Pimecrolimus 1% cream for the treatment of seborrheic dermatitis: a systematic review of randomized controlled trials. Expert Rev Clin Pharmacol 2012; 5 (1): 91-7.

[25] Scheinfeld N. The use of topical tacrolimus and pimecrolimus to treat psoriasis: A review. Dermatol Online J 2004; 10 (1): 3.

[26] Stoopler ET, Sollecito TP, DeRossi SS. Topical Tacrolimus for the Treatment of Oral Lichen Planus. The Internet Journal of Dermatology 2003 Volume 2 Number 1.

[27] Samycia M, Lin AN. Efficacy of topical calcineurin inhibitors in lichen planus. J Cutan Med Surg. 2012;16 (4): 221-9.

[28] Avgerinou G, Papafragkaki DK, Nasiopoulou A, Arapaki A, Katsambas A, Stavropoulos PG. Effectiveness of topical calcineurin inhibitors as monotherapy or in combination with hydroxychloroquine in cutaneous lupus erythematosus. J Eur Acad Dermatol Venereol 2012; 26 (6): 762-7.

[29] Marzano AV, Trevisan V, Lazzari R, Crosti C. Topical tacrolimus for the treatment of localized, idiopathic, newly diagnosed pyoderma gangrenosum. J Dermatolog Treat 2010; 21 (3): 140-3.

[30] Crawford KM, Russ B, BostromP. Pimecrolimus for treatment of acne rosacea. Skinmed, 2005; 4(3): 147-50.

[31] Cunha PR, Rossi AB. Pimecrolimus cream 1% is effective in a case of granulomatous rosacea. Acta Derm Venereol 2006; 86 (1): 71-2.

[32] Kim MB, Kim GW, Park HJ, *et al.* Pimecrolimus 1% cream for the treatment of rosacea. J Dermatol 2011; 38 (12): 1135-9.

[33] Fujiwara S, Okubo Y, Irisawa R, Tsuboi R. Rosaceiform dermatitis associated with topical tacrolimus treatment. J Am Acad Dermatol 2010; 62 (6): 1050-2.

[34] Ucak H, Kandi B, Cicek D, Halisdemir N, Dertlo SB. The comparison of treatment with clobetasol propionate 0.05% and topical pimecrolimus 1% treatment in the treatment of alopecia areata. J Dermatolog Treat 2012; 23(6): 410-20.

[35] Kim JE, Jeong MG, Lee He, Ko JY, Ro Ys. Successful treatment of cutaneous lesions of dermatomyositis with topical pimecrolimus. Ann Dermatol. 2011; 23 (3): 348-51.

[36] Van Leent EJ, Ebelin ME, Burtin P, Dorobek B, Spuls PI, Bos JD. Low systemic exposure after repeated topical application of Pimecrolimus (Elidel), SD Z ASM 981) in patients with atopic dermatitis. Dermatology 2002; 204 (1): 63-8.

CHAPTER 2

New Therapies for Asthma: What Else Besides Steroids?

Jorge Sánchez[1,2,3,*] and Javier Estarita[4]

[1]FUNDEMEB, Foundation for the Development of Medical and Biological Science, (Cartagena - Colombia); [2]Institute of Immunological Research, University of Cartagena (Cartagena – Colombia); [3]GACE, Group of Clinical and Experimental Allergy, University of Antioquia, (Medellín - Colombia) and [4]Internal Medicine Department, National University, (Bogotá – Colombia)

Abstract: Allergic disorders are a group of multifactorial diseases increasing in prevalence in recent years. Steroids remain the cornerstone of symptomatic treatment, but advances in molecular biology have led to a better understanding of the pathogenesis of allergic diseases and multiple medications; especially monoclonal antibodies have been developed with different therapeutic targets.

Omalizumab (Anti-IgE) and mepolizumab (Anti-IL5) are some of the biological agents already available for the treatment of asthma and other allergic diseases, but many other molecules are currently being studied in clinical trials. In this chapter we review the different monoclonal antibodies that are being studied in allergic diseases with emphasis on the evidence of their use in asthma.

Keywords: Asthma, allergy, allergen, immunotherapy, immunomodulation, monoclonal antibodies, mepolizumab, omalizumab, immunoglobulin, sensitization.

INTRODUCTION

Asthma is a chronic inflammatory disease of the airways, affecting around 10% of the global population, and 20% of children; it is considered childhood's most prevalent chronic disease [1-3].

Most asthma patients achieve proper symptom control through the use of steroids and beta-agonists, but because these medications are focused on symptom relief,

***Address correspondence to Jorge Sánchez:** GACE, Group of Clinical and Experimental Allergy, University of Antioquia, (Medellín - Colombia); Cell: +57 (300) 393 – 4000; Fax: 233 63 16; E-mail: jotamsc@yahoo.com

they don't modify the natural course of the disease. Currently in the management of chronic diseases "disease modifying drugs" are sought, which will allow to alter the disease's natural course or at least diminish it's progress [4].

In the last few decades important breakthroughs have been made in the understanding the pathogenesis of allergic diseases, which has drastically changed our point of view regarding diagnosis and management. Symptoms such as cough, wheezing and dyspnea upon exercise, suggest a diagnosis of asthma, however, asthma is a complex disease, with patients with different symptoms, severity and response to treatment. Due to the fact that these "phenotypes" don't reflect a single underlying mechanism, Anderson and colleagues suggested in 2008 the term "endotypes" to classify asthma in accordance to the different mechanisms involved, proposing that the signs and symptoms of the asthmatic patient are a manifestation of several inflammatory pathways, where multiple cytokines and cells are involved [5, 6] (Fig. **1**).

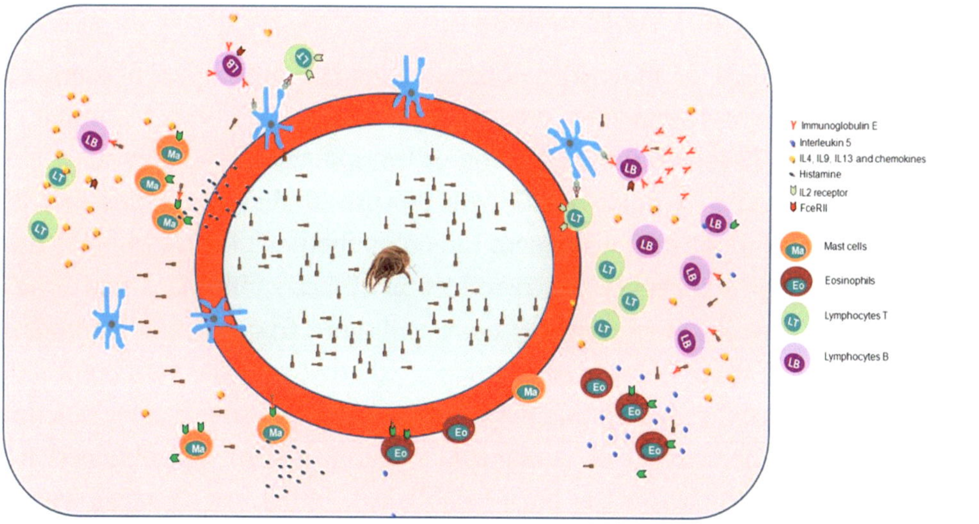

Figure 1: Inflammatory process in the lung. Different cells, quemoquines and interlequines have an active process during inflammation after exposition of allergen proteins. In this graphic we observed the inflammatory process after exposition with proteins from mites in the lung.

Along with a more thorough classification of asthma, advances in the understanding of its pathogenesis have allowed the identification of new therapeutic targets, especially through the use of monoclonal antibodies.

Advances in the development of new extracts and adjuvants for allergen specific immunotherapy have been made as well. The usage of these new immunomodulatory therapies will depend on the endotype present in each patient, making treatment more specific, and therefore more effective.

The better understanding of the pathophysiology of asthma has permitted some therapies utilized in other diseases to be used in asthma, such as certain oral hypoglycemic agents. Though this is an "off-label" indication, it certainly reflects the better understanding we now have of the underlying mechanisms.

In this chapter we will review some new therapies proposed for the management of asthma that seek to achieve symptom control through the modulation of the immune response. We will also discuss some monoclonal antibodies that even though have been in the market for several years now, are still subject to a great deal of scientific research.

Biologic Modifiers Approved in Asthma

Monoclonal antibodies are molecules obtained from B lymphocytes immortalized through fusion with myeloma cells, creating hybridomas. Antibody treatment was initially used in 1970 to avoid the rejection of transplanted organs, but ever since the 90´s it has taken a "second wind" with the use of fusion proteins that take advantage of the abilities of the segment joined antibodies that act as blockers or activators of specific signals [7]. The recollection of these antibodies was done on mice models at first, but it is currently more and more frequent that the constant fraction is obtained from "humanized" proteins and that only the variable fraction is obtained from mice, reducing this way the risks of triggering patient reactions. Depending on the percentage of humanized material and of that obtained from other sources a nomenclature has been established, but it has changed with the appearance of new proteins that don't fit the nomenclature [8].

Anti-IgE Monoclonals

Rationale. Two Anti-IgE molecules have been developed; however only one of them is currently available in the market. Omalizumab is a humanized monoclonal antibody that binds to the C3 dominion of unbound Immunoglobulin E, preventing the binding of this immunoglobulin to an allergen or its receptor [9]. Though multiple studies exist evaluating its utility in several allergic processes, currently in the United States it's only approved for use in asthmatic patients older than 12 years of age. Some studies have supported the efficacy and safety of this therapy in patients older than 6 years of age [10-12], and for this reason in some countries in Europe, Latin America and Asia its use is approved after the age of 6. The administration protocol (twice a month or once a month) and the dosage are weight and age dependent.

Efficacy. Several studies have been performed evaluating the safety and efficacy of this molecule in the management of asthma; the majority of them have been performed on patients with severe asthma. The clinical effect on most patients is appreciable after 3 months of treatment, however two hours after its application there is an IgE depletion of up to 90%. The difference observed between time of action and clinical effect may be due to the adherence of IgE to its membrane receptor on mast cells and basophiles which can last for several weeks, activating these cells when an allergen is recognized. Several parameters have been utilized to evaluate its clinical effect: Lin *et al.* [13] observed that two weeks after the administration of the first dose of omalizumab, patients tolerated greater exposure to the allergen causative of their respiratory symptoms. On patients receiving inhaled steroids in conjunction with other therapies or as single therapy, the addition of Omalizumab demonstrated a reduction in the number of exacerbations (>50%), the dose of inhaled steroids (>30%), use of salbutamol (>50%) and improvement in a 30% of patient pulmonary function, all of which results in an improved quality of life for patients. [14]. These clinical changes are accompanied by immunologic changes: 7 days after the administration of omalizumab the expression of FcεR1 is diminished in basophils, dendritic cells, and monocytes [15]; 16 weeks post treatment there's a significant reduction in the number of eosinophils present in serum and sputum, as well as Lymphocytes B and T CD4 and CD8+ in asthmatic patients [16].

Since IgE plays a crucial role in allergic asthma it's to be expected that its blockade should lead to an important improvement in afflicted patients, however even though this effects have been reproduced on several studies and don't seem to be limited by age, sex or patient origin, only around 60 to 80% of patients receiving omalizumab present such changes [17]. Among the multiple reasons that may be intervening in the lack of response in an important group of patients may be wrong patient selection (administration to non-allergic patients), which brings out the importance of knowing the endotype of every patient to know which therapy can provide the best response. Another potential reason is that most studies included patients with severe asthma, which means that many of them already had marked bronchial remodeling.

Some of the current questions regarding this treatment are for how long it should be administered and if the clinical effects will persist after its suspension. Some observational studies suggest that after 6 years of omalizumab administration over 80% of patients that had an initial favorable response, persisted with good symptom control after its suspension [17, 18], however studies with a more appropriate design are required to confirm this findings.

Other research have shown the utility of using omalizumab for 1 or 3 months prior to the use of immunotherapy in asthmatic patients with a background of or a high risk of developing a systemic reaction during immunotherapy [19, 20].

Significant adverse events. Anaphylaxis is seen in 0.1 to 0.2% of patients [21, 22], compromising skin and respiratory tract. Usually it isn't severe, and easily controlled through the use of adrenaline, however because of the high frequency of this reaction, omalizumab, like every other monoclonal must be applied in a health care center with a competent cardiopulmonary resuscitation team. A review of the adverse effects produced by omalizumab after the molecule was out in the market was published in the FDA (Food and Drug Administration) website; they observed that 20 patients out of 4127 treated with omalizumab (0.5%) presented neoplasms compared to 5 patients (0.2%) on the control group (Xolair®, **Omalizumab for Subcutaneous Use, Genentech Inc. July 2008 http: //www.xolair.com/ prescribing information.html**). These data don't show a causal relation between omalizumab and neoplasms, but the impact of the long term use of omalizumab on patients with high risk for neoplasms is currently unknown. On the particular case of patients that live in endemic zones for helminthic infections or with a high risk for cardiovascular diseases, even though a causal relation has not been shown with the use of omalizumab analysis can be undertaken to evaluate patient risk prior to the initiation of therapy, and every patient must be informed of the risks.

Anti-IL5 Monoclonals

Rationale. An important percentage of asthmatic patients have an increase in the eosinophil count in bronchoalveolar lavage [23, 24]. Because of this, eosinophils have for a long time been considered an important mediator of the inflammatory response on asthmatic patients: Two anti-IL5 antibodies have been created because this interleukin is necessary for eosinophil proliferation and maturation.

Efficacy. Using one of these monoclonals, mepolizumab, Leckie *et al.* observed a nearly complete reduction in the eosinophil count in sputum and in blood of asthmatic patients, however there were no changes in the challenge or in the forced expiratory volume in the first second (FEV1) [25]. Another study performed in 362 patients with moderate asthma evaluating pulmonary function, a symptom severity score and the frequency of use of beta-agonists, showed no change in any of these parameters with the use of mepolizumab [26, 27], they used another Anti-IL5 molecule to evaluate its safety and efficacy in patients with severe asthma. Just like with mepolizumab a reduction of eosinophils in blood and sputum, with a moderate improvement on FEV1 and no improvement in other clinical parameters was observed.

The lack of success of these molecules on asthma may be due to various reasons. On one hand not every asthmatic patient has an elevated eosinophil count [28, 29] and this point was not taken into account at the time of patient selection on previous studies. Another point is that even though these molecules reduce eosinophil levels in blood and sputum, only appear to reduce tissue levels in about 50% [30], which would suggest a lack of effect on the true effector cells that may be corrected by extending the treatment

Ballow and colleagues [4] suggest a third explanation for this lack of response, and that would be poor selection of evaluated results, because other than their presence in bronchoalveolar lavages there is scarce evidence supporting eosinophils as indispensable for airway obstruction [31], therefore the evaluation of outcomes such as bronchial hyperreactivity, daily symptoms, and bronchodilator use, that are directly linked to obstruction, would not be significantly modified with this therapy. These authors suggest that this molecule could show a relevant effect in those patients where eosinophils play a crucial role in airway obstruction, such as those with severe exacerbations associated to eosinophilic syndromes.

Following this line of thought, two articles with a limited number of patients, (one with 18, the other with 68) with asthma associated to severe exacerbations and peripheral eosinophilia have been conducted showing a reduction in both the use of steroids, inhaled and systemic as well as in crisis frequency on patients treated with Anti-IL5 [32, 33]. These results support that both mepolizumab and andrezlisumab may be useful in asthma associated to eosinophilic syndromes where the endotype supporting the disease's physiopathology is driven by eosinophils.

Significant adverse events. Side effects in these studies were reported as mild and temporary, and did not differ between the treatment and placebo groups. There were no type-I hypersensitivity reactions reported. However, since eosinophils are important for the protective response to parasites it's necessary to thoroughly evaluate the effect of this drug in patients in endemic countries.

Biological Modifiers Being Studied for the Management of Asthma

IL4 and IL3 Modulators

Rationale. Because in most asthmatic patients there's an allergic background, IgE and interleukins IL5, IL4 and IL13 have been broadly studied. IL4 and IL13 have a synergistic function, by acting on the same signaling pro-inflammatory pathways and binding to the same receptor. An alternative to achieve blockade of these molecules is the creation of soluble receptors that block these interleukins.

Efficacy. Blockade of IL4 by the use of this antibody demonstrated clinical efficacy when compared to a group of patients that received steroids in a study of 25 patients [34]. The variables evaluated were the number of exacerbations and the level of symptom control. In another study of 62 patients no relevant clinical changes were observed [34].

It's possible that the encountered lack of effect may be due to IL13 having a homologous function to IL4, which would cause a blockade of only one of these pathways to be insufficient. Because both interleukins bind to the same receptor, its blockade would impede the function of both. It was under this principle that the monoclonal pitrakinra was developed, a recombinant similar to IL4 that binds to the receptor without activating its function. So far on the studies conducted on this molecule or on others that function under the same principle no effect has been observed, or it has been only moderate, regarding immediate symptom improvement but has been significant on late symptoms as well as in diminishing exhaled nitric oxide levels [35, 36], which is a marker of inflammation specially on patients with elevated levels of periostin, another inflammatory marker [37, 38]. Most of these studies have been conducted on short time periods analyzing few patients, therefore the lack of efficacy and the lack of adverse events reports may be secondary to this factor.

Significant adverse events. Side effects such as type-I hypersensitivity reactions in these studies were not reported probably because of the short period of observation.

IL9 Modulators

Rationale. IL9 a recently described interleukin on *in vitro* models, has been strongly associated with the development of allergies through its effects on mast cells, by favoring their proliferation as well as the migration and formation of eosinophils and facilitating airway hyperreactivity [39].

Efficacy. So far no studies have been conducted evaluating its efficacy.

Significant adverse events. Up until now few clinical trials have been reported where the safety of this molecule in asthmatic patients with mild to moderate disease has been evaluated, however in such studies no greater risk of adverse events was observed when compared to the control group [40].

Chemokine Modifiers

Rationale. Because chemokines permit the migration of cells like lymphocytes, eosinophils, mast cells, *etc.* towards inflammatory sites a blockage of these molecules could prevent the migration of these cells, however currently there are few studies evaluating them on asthmatic patients and most of them are on preclinical phase [36, 41-43].

Efficacy. Prostaglandin D2 (PGD2) is a potent prostanoid produced by the activation of mast cells posterior to the exposure to an allergen and it's an important mediator of late response. The homologous molecule to the chemoattractant receptor expressed on Th2 lymphocytes (CRTh2) is the receptor for PGD2 and its metabolites [44]. Several CRTh2 antagonists are under development and some of them already have clinical trials. OC000459 is an oral CRTH2 antagonist, developed in the United Kingdom, and it was evaluated in 132 asthmatic patients on a randomized, controlled trial. During the 28 day treatment course, the active group had a significant improvement on FEV1 (7.4%). Likewise this molecule demonstrated an improvement on patient quality of life, a reduction on total IgE and sputum eosinophil levels [45]. Other CRTH2 antagonists like AMG 853, ACT-129,968, ARRY-005 and ARRY-006 are currently being studied, with some clinical trials already underway **("AMG 853 phase 2 study in subjects with inadequately controlled asthma." 2010. Available at: clinicaltrials.gov/ct2/show/NCT01018550.)**.

Significant adverse events. There were no type-I hypersensitivity reactions reported in these studies. Some of the clinical trials that are in development are evaluating for a long period of time the effect of these molecules.

Interleukin Modulators of Th2 Response

Rationale. Suplatast tosilate is an orally consumed molecule derived from dimethylsulfonium. Even though its effector mechanisms are not clear, suplatast tosilate has shown that it can significantly reduce the Th2 profile cytokines (Il4, IL5, IL13, eotaxina-1) levels as well as those of transforming growth factor (TGF-β) on asthmatic mice models [46-48].

Efficacy. On patients with mild or moderate asthma that receive suplatast a significant improvement on FEV1, peak expiratory flow, symptom control and a reduction on the use of inhaled steroids was reported [49, 50]. Other studies have demonstrated that suplatast can also reduce pulmonary eosinophilia and bronchial hyperreactivity [51-53]. Although this molecule has shown some promising results, currently it's only commercialized in Japan.

Significant adverse events. Several studies in Japan evaluating efficacy and safety of this molecule do not report severe adverse events.

T Lymphocyte Proliferation and Activation Modulators

Ratonale. Due to the central role of T lymphocytes on inflammatory responses, including that seen in allergies, the modulation of their proliferation to certain stimuli has been proposed through the blockage of some of their membrane receptors, however so far only two molecules have been tested in the management of asthma: Daclizumab and the humanized monoclonal antibody IgG1, that binds to the alpha subunit of IL2 and blocks the action of this molecule, required for lymphocyte maturation and is used on renal transplant patients. TNF-α is a pro-inflammatory cytokine with pleiotropic biological effects that may be important on refractory asthma, by maintaining the expression of chemokines and adhesion molecules that promote active neutrophil recruitment. Some molecules like eternacept have been produced to block TNF-α activity. Other molecules, such as CXCL8 are being evaluated on clinical trials, but the results have not been published.

Efficacy. One study with daclizumab on asthmatic patients have shown an improvement on symptom control on patients that didn't respond to conventional treatment with steroids [54].

Etanercept has been tested on some clinical trials with controversial results: Berry and colleagues observed an improvement on bronchial hyperreactivity and quality of life on a group of 10 patients with severe asthma when compared with 10 controls [55]. In another study with 132 patients a 4 month follow up was done, evaluating several outcomes, among them symptom control, medication doses, and changes on pulmonary function, without finding any significant results [56].

Significant adverse events. The side effects of dacrlzumab have been poorly studied. Eternacept has been significantly associated with respiratory infections in 30% of patients and with less frequency with recurrent skin and gastrointestinal tract infections, and infusion reactions [57].

CD23 Receptor Modulators

Rationale. CD23 is IgE low affinity receptor (FcεRII) and its expression on monocytes, alveolar macrophages and B lymphocytes is increased in allergic patients. *In vitro* studies have demonstrated that binding to this receptor reduces IgE synthesis.

Efficacy. Lumixilimab is an anti CD23 monoclonal that has shown a reduction on IgE levels on patients with asthma or rhinitis, however, no efficacy on symptom reduction has been seen so far [58].

Significant adverse events. In the few studies with this drug no adverse effects have been reported.

Phosphodiesterase 4 Modulators

Rationale. Phosphodiesterase (PDE) is an enzyme that intervenes in protein metabolism, and PDE-4 expression is increased on inflammatory cells on asthma and COPD (chronic obstructive pulmonary disease). Theophylline was the first molecule utilized on asthma several decades ago with a non-selective inhibition of PDEs but due to its narrow therapeutic window it has fallen out of use. Newer, more selective molecules have been tested, such as roflumilast, a PDE4 inhibitor approved for use on COPD.

Efficacy. A phase 2/3 study conducted on asthmatic patients for four months demonstrated a significant improvement with all doses tested [59]. Another study showed that roflumilast increased the allergen tolerance threshold in controlled challenges diminishing both immediate and late symptoms [60]. When comparing roflumilast with an inhaled steroid (beclomethasone dipropionate) in a study with 499 asthmatic patients, a similar response on symptom control and FEV1 improvement with the advantage of a reduction on steroid use was observed [61].

Significant adverse events. Although these studies show promising results, a group of COPD patients managed with this medication presented an increase on suicide rates, suicide attempts and malignant neoplasms, when compared to a control group, which has led to its withdrawal from the market in several countries including the United States [62].

Other Monoclonal Therapies

Several other molecules as Anakinra, an IL-1R antagonist [63]; Canakinumab, a monoclonal antibody to neutralize human IL-1β [64]; Rilonacept, a fusion protein of IL-1 receptor accessory protein and Fc fraction of IgG1 [65]; and VX-765, a caspase inhibitor [66] have been tried or used for other inflammatory diseases like cryopyrin associated periodic syndromes and macrophage activation syndrome. The application of these molecules in asthma is not know because there is not study about it; however in recent years the roll of IL1 in some studies demonstrates that the IL1 gene complex is involved in the regulation of IgE-mediated atopic reactions [67, 68]. These results require special attention and should be further evaluated in other clinical settings.

Advances on Allergen Immunotherapy

Currently immunotherapy is the only treatment that can modify the natural course of the disease on allergic asthma. Advances on this therapy are being made towards improving safety profiles and efficacy through modifications on the allergen extract, types of adjuvant, administration route and release mode.

Allergen Extract Modifications

Immunotherapy has traditionally been administered using the full extract of the allergic source the patient is allergic to. Though this therapy has proven to be effective, new approaches have been sought that maintain efficacy and reduce the risk of adverse events. The use of polymerized extracts seems to reduce the risk of adverse events maintaining protein immunogenicity [69]. The procedure consists on the administration of an extract grouped on a heavy molecular weight molecule which prevents its recognition by IgE, but can be processed by antigen presenting cells inducing the production of IgE. Several clinical trials have been done with these extracts demonstrating both efficacy and safety [70, 71]. Polymerized extract immunotherapy has shown to reduce steroid doses, increase the number of symptom free days and improve patient control. In a comparative study between adult and pediatric population, we observed that use of these extracts is effective on both populations, however monosensitized pediatric population showed a better response. To evaluate polymerized extracts we studied 575 patients that had received 7256 injections, finding a frequency of adverse reactions per number of injections of 0.1%, much lower than that reported on other studies with aqueous un modified extracts [72].

Another strategy currently under study is the construction of fusion proteins, containing both the allergen and immunomodulating peptides, as an example a fusion protein combining the *Fel d* 1 allergen with the crystallizable IgG fragment has been created. This bi-functional molecule prevents acute reactivity, diminishing the risk of reactions [73]. Also, a recombinant fusion protein has been tested, associating the *Phl p 1* with a rhinovirus derived protein [74]. The association between Bet v1 to the bacterial Wall protein SbpA has shown to form particles that facilitate the capture by antigen presenting cells with the subsequent induction of Th1 response and Treg cells [75]. So far the efficacy of these molecules has not been studied enough and currently only *in vitro* studies are available.

Extracts contain all of the proteins from an allergenic source, though effectiveness through both subcutaneous and sublingual application has been shown these extracts contain proteins to which the patient is sensitized as well as others he's not, so the risk of sensitizing the patient to new proteins exists. To avoid these sensitizations, the risk of adverse reactions and to increase immunotherapy efficacy, vaccination with the proteins the patient is sensitized by producing them through vectors or by purifying them has been proposed. The utilization of recombinants may also allow reaching a reduction on protein allergenicity through small changes, such as mutations contributing to the protein's conformational folding, resulting in epitopes that retain the capacity to be processed by T lymphocytes with a reduction on IgE reactivity [76-78]. The production of these recombinant molecules allows the selection of specific proteins and the formation of multi-allergenic hybrids [79-82]; currently some of these vaccines are already being tested on clinical trials and some of them are even in the market, but so far no studies comparing these therapies to the traditional approach exist. Jutel y colleagues [83] performed a phase 2/3 clinical trial. This study was conducted for two years, covering two summers, when pollen production is increased, and they observed significant changes in both symptom reduction and medications used after 18 months of treatment. Pauli and colleagues [84] did a multi-centric, randomized, double blind, placebo controlled study comparing the safety and efficacy of the Bet v 1a recombinant, the purified natural protein Bet v 1 and the standard Avedul pollen extract. Patients received treatment for a two year period and all three patient groups had a significant improvement on the evaluated parameters when compared to the control group, without any difference between them, however 3 of the 29 patients treated with the full extract displayed sensitization to new epitopes. Valenta and colleagues [85] constructed a trimer containing three Bet v 1 monomers, which showed changes on biologic markers as well as a significant reduction on both cutaneous sensitivity and patient symptoms [86].

New Adjuvants

The use of new adjuvants that potentiate Th1 response to improve the efficacy of immunotherapy have been proposed. The "Toll Like receptors" (TLR) and their ligands for example CpG sequences and bacterial membrane lipopolysaccharide, being innate response molecules, favor mainly Th1 immune activation, so presenting the allergen with these molecules would favor a deviating of the response several molecules have been tested on small clinical trial son asthmatic patients, among those a synthetic ligand of the TLR7 obtaining a modest improvement on symptoms [87, 88], however most research has been focused on TLR9 and lipopolysaccharide use as ligand for TLR4. Monophosphoril Lipid A is a lipopolysaccharide that is already being used as an adjuvant in pollen grain immunotherapy, showing great efficacy and a good safety profile with continuous or seasonal use, both through subcutaneous and sublingual administration [89-92]. Following the same principle of LPS, bacterial oligonucleotides with un-methylated CpG sequences are the specific ligands for TLR9, the administration of an allergenic extract with these sequences would preserve their immunogenicity but due to the immunomodulatory effect of the bacterial DNA the response induced would be Th1 [93, 94]. In a study performed on 20 patients, seeking to evaluate the safety and efficacy of dust mite extract with CpG sequences as coadjutants, adequate tolerance was observed during 10 weeks of treatment. Clinical improvement was significant on every patient and it persisted up to 38 weeks after suspension of therapy [95].

Other adjuvants, such as vitamin D [96], the Calmette-Guerin bacillus [97], cholera toxin [98, 99], and lactobacilli [100, 101] are being studied in animal models and in small groups of patients with promising results, therefore bigger clinical trials are required to evaluate the safety and effectiveness of these adjuvants.

Because parasites are capable of inducing a Th2 non allergic response, characterized by an increase in cytokine and immunoregulating cells, their effect as adjuvants or as extracts for the management of allergies is increasing, studies conducted on mice so far, have shown that this therapy may be effective and have no effect on the immune response against parasites, avoiding an increase in the frequency of infection by these organisms [102-104].

New Allergen Release Forms

Several vector systems have been used to mark allergens and assure a controlled release to dendritic cells. DNA plasmids or macroparticle absorbed DNA enhances the immune response after injection [105]. These particles have been constructed using different systems. Viral particles have been utilized to ensemble molecules similar to a capsid to present the antigen while taking advantage of its adjuvant characteristics and the release system provided by its form [106, 107]. Vehicles similar to liposomes utilizing cholesterol particles or phospholipid mixtures that incorporate the functions of the virosomes, increasing the production of IgG and IgA antibodies have also been used [108]. Polyglycolic acid based liposomes have been used to form nano-particles or micro-particles that allow antigen presentation facilitating its capture by the antigen presenting cells [109, 110].

Synthetic carbohydrate based particles that form polymers represent a tool to direct allergens towards antigen presenting cells. Vectors utilizing maxtrodextrin or chitosan polymers using the sublingual route have been tested in mice with variable results, so more studies are required before human testing [111-113].

New Administration Routes

Along with traditional administration routes for immunotherapy (subcutaneous and sublingual route) new routes have been proposed in an attempt to diminish the number of doses required in order to achieve greater patient comfort and adherence as well as a better safety profile [114, 115]. Taking into account that only a small fraction of the allergen administered *via* the subcutaneous route reaches lymph nodes [116, 117], a direct intra-lymphatic shot may be a better strategy to increase immunotherapy efficacy [118].

Even though lymph nodes are widely distributed throughout all the body, their size and location requires that intra-lymphatic injections be sonography guided, and makes the inguinal zone the preferred area, due to its ease of Access, node size and lesser innervation [119].

Several clinical trials are evaluating the efficacy of intra-lymphatic immunotherapy (ILIT) for the management of patients with grass pollen allergy, hymenopterans poison hypersensitivity and cat dandruff allergy. For asthmatic patients with grasses pollen allergy, a significant increase in allergen tolerance was observed 4 months after the administration of just 3 intra-lymphatic injections, whereas a year of continuous subcutaneous injections were necessary to obtain the same result. It is of note, that ILIT was safe, without the induction of grade III or IV systemic secondary allergic effects when compared with SCIT, however the fact that this study was conducted with few patients must be kept in mind (ClinicalTrials.gov Identifier NCT00470457) [119].

Even though the administration of epidermal or intraepidermal immunotherapy (IDIT) is as old as immunotherapy itself, because few years after the reports done by Philips with 29 patients en 1926, allergen application on a similar manner to that used during prick testing to achieve a therapeutic effect was reported, it has fallen out of use. Although this administration route is no longer commonly used, new advances have evaluated patch application and other systems that lead to a controlled release of allergens. Blamoutier and colleagues utilized a patch that works by removing the stratum corneum and facilitating a controlled penetration into the epidermis [120]. Along with a reduction in some proinflammatory cytokines such as IL-1, IL-6, IL-8, TNF-a, and INF-g [121, 122], this system has proven to be effective on a group of 28 patients, by reducing respiratory symptoms by 70% on average, compared to 20% for placebo. Although no systemic adverse reactions were observed, eczematous reactions on the site of application were frequently observed. New trials are underway to validate these results.

Other Therapies

Some medications, initially used on other diseases have been utilized on asthma. PPARs (peroxisome proliferator activated receptor) can block the transcription factor GATA-3, required for the activation of several Th2 response cytokines [123]. Hypoglycemic agents, agonists of PPAR-gamma (thiazolidinediones, rosiglitazone, *etc.*) have been utilized in patients with asthma, and have demonstrated an effect on inhibition of eosinophilic migration, [124-126], improving the pulmonary tolerance threshold upon allergen exposure as well as bronchodilator properties [123]. These studies have involved few patients, so an increase in sample size is necessary to confirm these results.

Other therapies, such as acupuncture [127], natural herbs [128, 129] and diet modifications [130-132] that have been proposed as strategies for the management of asthma have been discarded for a long time, due to the lack of scientific evidence sustaining their effects, however on last few years, new interest for this therapies has emerged, and the number of controlled trials is rising with results that are controversial, but promising.

CONCLUSIONS

As the number of studies permitting a better understanding of the pathogenesis of asthma increase, a better characterization of the underlying endotypes for the disease is achieved, this in turn facilitates the creation of more efficacious therapeutic strategies, such as those presented on this chapter (Fig. **2**). Currently many immunomodulators are being developed and evaluated on preclinical trials with interesting results, however, most of these molecules don't display in humans the effectiveness observed in such trials. One of the greatest difficulties for the use of these therapies is the elevated costs they carry, which makes their popularization and the performance of a larger number of studies harder. However advances regarding heath care policies are being made worldwide, that in the medium term, may permit easier access to these medications for all patients. In the United States changes on the regulatory systems enforced by the FDA, focused on reducing the time required for the approval of these medications would help achieve these goals. Over the next few years a greater number of trials will appear, using these therapies, which will separate those therapies that are truly effective and safe, from those that are not, which in turn will lead to a greater number of tool for the management of the asthmatic patient.

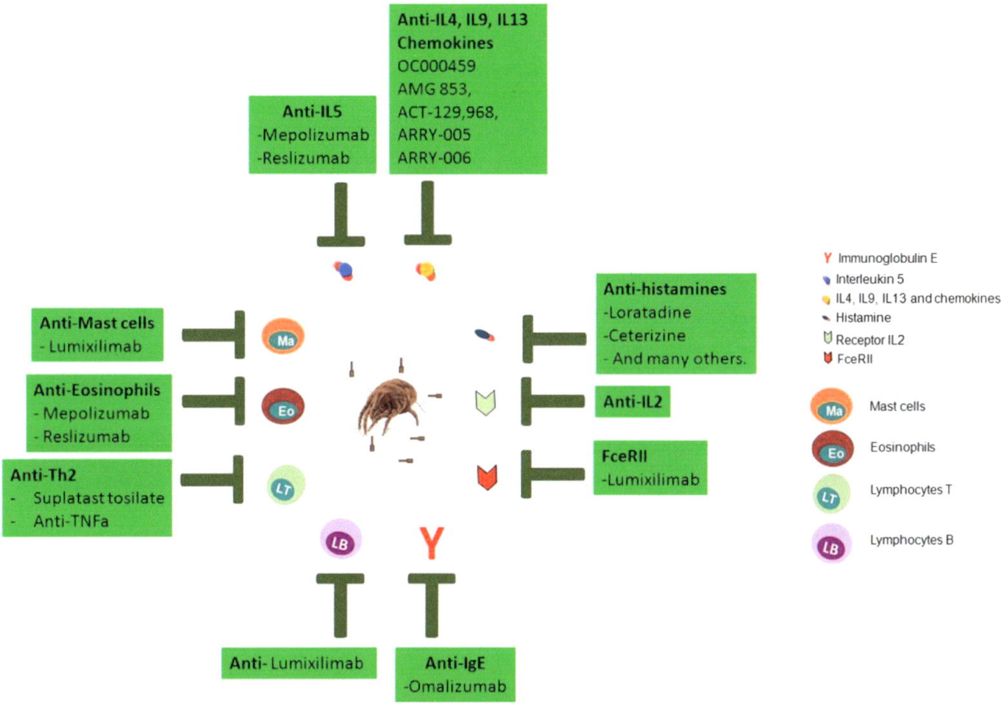

Figure 2: New Drugs in asthma management. Different drugs have been development in recent years and most of them are in clinical trials. Molecules like lumixilimab have effect in different cells because the action is over a receptor present in different cell lines. Other molecules have and indirect effect over other inflammatory mediators like Anti-IL5, that block IL5 and in consequence reduce eosinophil cells production. Omalizumab and Anti-TNFα (Anti-IgE) have a specific action point but have a pleiotropic effect.

ACKNOWLEDGEMENTS

Declared none.

CONFLICT OF INTEREST

The author(s) confirm that this chapter content has no conflict of interest.

REFERENCES

[1] Dennis R, Caraballo L, Garcia E, *et al.* Asthma and other allergic conditions in Colombia: a study in 6 cities. Ann Allergy Asthma Immunol 2004; 93(6): 568-574.

[2] Eder W, Ege MJ, von Mutius E. The asthma epidemic. N Engl J Med 2006; 355(21): 2226-2235.

[3] Büchele G, Genuneit J, Weinmayr G, *et al.* International variations in bronchial responsiveness in children: findings from ISAAC phase two. Pediatr Pulmonol 2010; 45(8): 796-806.

[4] Ballow M, Akdis CA, Casale TB, *et al.* Immune response modifiers in the treatment of asthma: A PRACTALL document of the American Academy of Allergy, Asthma & Immunology and the European Academy of Allergy and Clinical Immunology. J Allergy Clin Immunol 2012; 130(2): 311-324.

[5] Anderson GP. Endotyping asthma: new insights into key pathogenic mechanisms in a complex, heterogeneous disease. Lancet 2008; 372(9643): 1107-1119.

[6] Lötvall J, Akdis CA, Bacharier LB, *et al.* Asthma endotypes: a new approach to classification of disease entities within the asthma syndrome. J Allergy Clin Immunol 2011; 127(2): 355-360.

[7] Springer TA. César Milstein, the father of modern immunology. Nat Immunol 2002; 3(6): 501-503.

[8] Lee SJ, Chinen J, Kavanaugh A. Immunomodulator therapy: monoclonal antibodies, fusion proteins, cytokines, and immunoglobulins. J Allergy Clin Immunol 2010; 125(2 Suppl 2): S314-323.

[9] Sanchez J, Ramirez R, Diez S, *et al.* Omalizumab beyond asthma. Allergol Immunopathol (Madr) 2012; 40(5): 306-315.

[10] Restrepo M, Cardona R, Cardona A. Experience with the use of omalizumab in a patient under 6 years. International Journal on Immunorehabilitation 2011; 13(1): 33.

[11] Lanier B, Bridges T, Kulus M, *et al.* Omalizumab for the treatment of exacerbations in children with inadequately controlled allergic (IgE-mediated) asthma. J Allergy Clin Immunol 2009; 124(6): 1210-1216.

[12] Kulus M, Hébert J, Garcia E, *et al.* Omalizumab in children with inadequately controlled severe allergic (IgE-mediated) asthma. Curr Med Res Opin 2010; 26(6): 1285-1293.

[13] Lin H, Boesel KM, Griffith DT, *et al.* Omalizumab rapidly decreases nasal allergic response and FcepsilonRI on basophils. J Allergy Clin Immunol 2004; 113(2): 297-302.

[14] Rodrigo GJ, Neffen H, Castro-Rodriguez JA. Efficacy and safety of subcutaneous omalizumab *vs.* placebo as add-on therapy to corticosteroids for children and adults with asthma: a systematic review. Chest 2011; 139(1): 28-35.

[15] Prussin C, Griffith DT, Boesel KM, *et al.* Omalizumab treatment downregulates dendritic cell FcepsilonRI expression. J Allergy Clin Immunol 2003; 112(6): 1147-1154.

[16] Djukanović R, Wilson SJ, Kraft M, *et al.* Effects of treatment with anti-immunoglobulin E antibody omalizumab on airway inflammation in allergic asthma. Am J Respir Crit Care Med 2004; 170(6): 583-593.

[17] Slavin RG, Ferioli C, Tannenbaum SJ, *et al.* Asthma symptom re-emergence after omalizumab withdrawal correlates well with increasing IgE and decreasing pharmacokinetic concentrations. J Allergy Clin Immunol 2009; 123(1): 107-113.

[18] Nopp A, Johansson S, Adédoyin J, *et al.* After 6 years with Xolair; a 3-year withdrawal follow-up. Allergy 2010; 65(1): 56-60.
[19] Casale TB, Busse WW, Kline JN, *et al.* Omalizumab pretreatment decreases acute reactions after rush immunotherapy for ragweed-induced seasonal allergic rhinitis. J Allergy Clin Immunol 2006; 117(1): 134-140.
[20] Parks KW, Casale TB. Anti-immunoglobulin E monoclonal antibody administered with immunotherapy. Allergy Asthma Proc 2006; 27(2 Suppl 1): S33-36.
[21] Limb SL, Starke PR, Lee CE, *et al.* Delayed onset and protracted progression of anaphylaxis after omalizumab administration in patients with asthma. J Allergy Clin Immunol 2007; 120(6): 1378-1381.
[22] Cox L, Platts-Mills TA, Finegold I, *et al.* American Academy of Allergy, Asthma & Immunology/American College of Allergy, Asthma and Immunology Joint Task Force Report on omalizumab-associated anaphylaxis. J Allergy Clin Immunol 2007; 120(6): 1373-1377.
[23] Uhm TG, Kim BS, Chung IY. Eosinophil development, regulation of eosinophil-specific genes, and role of eosinophils in the pathogenesis of asthma. Allergy Asthma Immunol Res 2012; 4(2): 68-79.
[24] Wardlaw AJ, Kay AB. The role of the eosinophil in the pathogenesis of asthma. Allergy 1987; 42(5): 321-335.
[25] Leckie MJ, ten Brinke A, Khan J, *et al.* Effects of an interleukin-5 blocking monoclonal antibody on eosinophils, airway hyper-responsiveness, and the late asthmatic response. Lancet 2000; 356(9248): 2144-2148.
[26] Flood-Page P, Swenson C, Faiferman I, *et al.* A study to evaluate safety and efficacy of mepolizumab in patients with moderate persistent asthma. Am J Respir Crit Care Med 2007; 176(11): 1062-1071.
[27] Kips JC, O'Connor BJ, Langley SJ, *et al.* Effect of SCH55700, a humanized anti-human interleukin-5 antibody, in severe persistent asthma: a pilot study. Am J Respir Crit Care Med 2003; 167(12): 1655-1659.
[28] Haldar P, Pavord ID, Shaw DE, *et al.* Cluster analysis and clinical asthma phenotypes. Am J Respir Crit Care Med 2008; 178(3): 218-224.
[29] Pavord ID, Brightling CE, Woltmann G, *et al.* Non-eosinophilic corticosteroid unresponsive asthma. Lancet 1999; 353(9171): 2213-2214.
[30] Flood-Page PT, Menzies-Gow AN, Kay AB, *et al.* Eosinophil's role remains uncertain as anti-interleukin-5 only partially depletes numbers in asthmatic airway. Am J Respir Crit Care Med 2003; 167(2): 199-204.
[31] Wardlaw AJ, Brightling CE, Green R, *et al.* New insights into the relationship between airway inflammation and asthma. Clin Sci (Lond) 2002; 103(2): 201-211.
[32] Nair P, Pizzichini MM, Kjarsgaard M, *et al.* Mepolizumab for prednisone-dependent asthma with sputum eosinophilia. N Engl J Med 2009; 360(10): 985-993.
[33] Haldar P, Brightling CE, Hargadon B, *et al.* Mepolizumab and exacerbations of refractory eosinophilic asthma. N Engl J Med 2009; 360(10): 973-984.
[34] Borish LC, Nelson HS, Lanz MJ, *et al.* Interleukin-4 receptor in moderate atopic asthma. A phase I/II randomized, placebo-controlled trial. Am J Respir Crit Care Med 1999; 160(6): 1816-1823.
[35] Wenzel S, Wilbraham D, Fuller R, *et al.* Effect of an interleukin-4 variant on late phase asthmatic response to allergen challenge in asthmatic patients: results of two phase 2a studies. Lancet 2007; 370(9596): 1422-1431.

[36] Corren J, Busse W, Meltzer EO, *et al.* A randomized, controlled, phase 2 study of AMG 317, an IL-4Ralpha antagonist, in patients with asthma. Am J Respir Crit Care Med 2010; 181(8): 788-796.
[37] Gauvreau GM, Boulet LP, Cockcroft DW, *et al.* Effects of interleukin-13 blockade on allergen-induced airway responses in mild atopic asthma. Am J Respir Crit Care Med 2011; 183(8): 1007-1014.
[38] Corren J, Lemanske RF, Hanania NA, *et al.* Lebrikizumab treatment in adults with asthma. N Engl J Med 2011; 365(12): 1088-1098.
[39] Temann UA, Geba GP, Rankin JA, *et al.* Expression of interleukin 9 in the lungs of transgenic mice causes airway inflammation, mast cell hyperplasia, and bronchial hyperresponsiveness. J Exp Med 1998; 188(7): 1307-1320.
[40] Parker JM, Oh CK, LaForce C, *et al.* Safety profile and clinical activity of multiple subcutaneous doses of MEDI-528, a humanized anti-interleukin-9 monoclonal antibody, in two randomized phase 2a studies in subjects with asthma. BMC Pulm Med 2011; 11: 14.
[41] Davenpeck KL, Berens KL, Dixon RA, *et al.* Inhibition of adhesion of human neutrophils and eosinophils to P-selectin by the sialyl Lewis antagonist TBC1269: preferential activity against neutrophil adhesion *in vitro*. J Allergy Clin Immunol 2000; 105(4): 769-775.
[42] Woodside DG, Vanderslice P. Cell adhesion antagonists: therapeutic potential in asthma and chronic obstructive pulmonary disease. BioDrugs 2008; 22(2): 85-100.
[43] Beeh KM, Beier J, Meyer M, *et al.* Bimosiamose, an inhaled small-molecule pan-selectin antagonist, attenuates late asthmatic reactions following allergen challenge in mild asthmatics: a randomized, double-blind, placebo-controlled clinical cross-over-trial. Pulm Pharmacol Ther 2006; 19(4): 233-241.
[44] Pettipher R. The roles of the prostaglandin D(2) receptors DP(1) and CRTH2 in promoting allergic responses. Br J Pharmacol 2008; 153 (Suppl 1): S191-199.
[45] Singh D, Cadden P, Hunter M, *et al.* Inhibition of the asthmatic allergen challenge response by the CRTH2 antagonist OC000459. Eur Respir J 2012.
[46] Shimizu S, Hattori R, Majima Y, *et al.* Th2 cytokine inhibitor suplatast tosilate inhibits antigen-induced mucus hypersecretion in the nasal epithelium of sensitized rats. Ann Otol Rhinol Laryngol 2009; 118(1): 67-72.
[47] Shahriar M, Mizuguchi H, Maeyama K, *et al.* Suplatast tosilate inhibits histamine signaling by direct and indirect down-regulation of histamine H1 receptor gene expression through suppression of histidine decarboxylase and IL-4 gene transcriptions. J Immunol 2009; 183(3): 2133-2141.
[48] Tanaka A, Minoguchi K, Samson KT, *et al.* Inhibitory effects of suplatast tosilate on the differentiation and function of monocyte-derived dendritic cells from patients with asthma. Clin Exp Allergy 2007; 37(7): 1083-1089.
[49] Ando H, Movérare R, Kondo Y, *et al.* Utility of ovomucoid-specific IgE concentrations in predicting symptomatic egg allergy. J Allergy Clin Immunol 2008; 122(3): 583-588.
[50] Wada M, Nagata S, Kudo T, *et al.* Effect of suplatast tosilate on antileukotriene non-responders with mild-to-moderate persistent asthma. Allergol Int 2009; 58(3): 389-393.
[51] Hoshino M, Fujita Y, Saji J, *et al.* Effect of suplatast tosilate on goblet cell metaplasia in patients with asthma. Allergy 2005; 60(11): 1394-1400.
[52] Sano Y, Suzuki N, Yamada H, *et al.* Effects of suplatast tosilate on allergic eosinophilic airway inflammation in patients with mild asthma. J Allergy Clin Immunol 2003; 111(5): 958-966.

[53] Yoshida M, Aizawa H, Inoue H, *et al.* Effect of suplatast tosilate on airway hyperresponsiveness and inflammation in asthma patients. J Asthma 2002; 39(6): 545-552.

[54] Busse WW, Israel E, Nelson HS, *et al.* Daclizumab improves asthma control in patients with moderate to severe persistent asthma: a randomized, controlled trial. Am J Respir Crit Care Med 2008; 178(10): 1002-1008.

[55] Berry MA, Hargadon B, Shelley M, *et al.* Evidence of a role of tumor necrosis factor alpha in refractory asthma. N Engl J Med 2006; 354(7): 697-708.

[56] Holgate ST, Noonan M, Chanez P, *et al.* Efficacy and safety of etanercept in moderate-to-severe asthma: a randomised, controlled trial. Eur Respir J 2011; 37(6): 1352-1359.

[57] Jacobi A, Antoni C, Manger B, *et al.* Infliximab in the treatment of moderate to severe atopic dermatitis. J Am Acad Dermatol 2005; 52(3 Pt 1): 522-526.

[58] Rosenwasser LJ, Busse WW, Lizambri RG, *et al.* Allergic asthma and an anti-CD23 mAb (IDEC-152): results of a phase I, single-dose, dose-escalating clinical trial. J Allergy Clin Immunol 2003;112(3):563-570.

[59] Bateman ED, Izquierdo JL, Harnest U, *et al.* Efficacy and safety of roflumilast in the treatment of asthma. Ann Allergy Asthma Immunol 2006; 96(5): 679-686.

[60] van Schalkwyk E, Strydom K, Williams Z, *et al.* Roflumilast, an oral, once-daily phosphodiesterase 4 inhibitor, attenuates allergen-induced asthmatic reactions. J Allergy Clin Immunol 2005; 116(2): 292-298.

[61] Bousquet J, Aubier M, Sastre J, *et al.* Comparison of roflumilast, an oral anti-inflammatory, with beclomethasone dipropionate in the treatment of persistent asthma. Allergy 2006; 61(1): 72-78.

[62] Fabbri LM, Calverley PM, Izquierdo-Alonso JL, *et al.* Roflumilast in moderate-to-severe chronic obstructive pulmonary disease treated with longacting bronchodilators: two randomised clinical trials. Lancet 2009; 374(9691): 695-703.

[63] Loh NK, Lucas M, Fernandez S, *et al.* Successful treatment of macrophage activation syndrome complicating adult Still disease with anakinra. Intern Med J 2012; 42(12): 1358-1362.

[64] Lachmann HJ, Kone-Paut I, Kuemmerle-Deschner JB, *et al.* Use of canakinumab in the cryopyrin-associated periodic syndrome. N Engl J Med 2009; 360(23): 2416-2425.

[65] Hoffman HM, Throne ML, Amar NJ, *et al.* Efficacy and safety of rilonacept (interleukin-1 Trap) in patients with cryopyrin-associated periodic syndromes: results from two sequential placebo-controlled studies. Arthritis Rheum 2008; 58(8): 2443-2452.

[66] Stack JH, Beaumont K, Larsen PD, *et al.* IL-converting enzyme/caspase-1 inhibitor VX-765 blocks the hypersensitive response to an inflammatory stimulus in monocytes from familial cold autoinflammatory syndrome patients. J Immunol 2005; 175(4): 2630-2634.

[67] Karjalainen J, Hulkkonen J, Pessi T, *et al.* The IL1A genotype associates with atopy in nonasthmatic adults. J Allergy Clin Immunol 2002; 110(3): 429-434.

[68] Adjers K, Pessi T, Karjalainen J, *et al.* Epistatic effect of IL1A and IL4RA genes on the risk of atopy. J Allergy Clin Immunol 2004; 113(3): 445-447.

[69] Hernández N, Ibero M, Ridao M, *et al.* Safety of specific immunotherapy using a depigmented and polymerised extract of Dermatophagoides pteronyssinus in children under five years of age. Allergol Immunopathol (Madr) 2011; 39(5): 267-270.

[70] Branco Ferreira M, Spínola Santos A, Pereira Santos MC, *et al.* Efficacy and safety of specific immunotherapy with a modified mite extract. Allergol Immunopathol (Madr) 2005; 33(2): 80-85.

[71] Alvarez-Cuesta E, Aragoneses-Gilsanz E, Martín-Garcia C, *et al.* Immunotherapy with depigmented glutaraldehyde-polymerized extracts: changes in quality of life. Clin Exp Allergy 2005; 35(5): 572-578.

[72] Cardona R, Lopez E, Beltrán J, *et al.* Safety of immunotherapy in patients with rhinitis, asthma or atopic dermatitis using an ultra-rush buildup. A retrospective study. Allergol Immunopathol (Madr) 2012. In press.

[73] Terada T. New therapeutic strategies, a chimeric fusion protein inhibits allergic reactivity. Nihon Rinsho 2009; 67(11): 2178-2182.

[74] Edlmayr J, Niespodziana K, Linhart B, *et al.* A combination vaccine for allergy and rhinovirus infections based on rhinovirus-derived surface protein VP1 and a nonallergenic peptide of the major timothy grass pollen allergen Phl p 1. J Immunol 2009; 182(10): 6298-6306.

[75] Gerstmayr M, Ilk N, Jahn-Schmid B, *et al.* Natural self-assembly of allergen-S-layer fusion proteins is no prerequisite for reduced allergenicity and T cell stimulatory capacity. Int Arch Allergy Immunol 2009; 149(3): 231-238.

[76] Okada T, Swoboda I, Bhalla PL, *et al.* Engineering of hypoallergenic mutants of the Brassica pollen allergen, Bra r 1, for immunotherapy. FEBS Lett 1998; 434(3): 255-260.

[77] Swoboda I, De Weerd N, Bhalla PL, *et al.* Mutants of the major ryegrass pollen allergen, Lol p 5, with reduced IgE-binding capacity: candidates for grass pollen-specific immunotherapy. Eur J Immunol 2002; 32(1): 270-280.

[78] Swoboda I, Bugajska-Schretter A, Linhart B, *et al.* A recombinant hypoallergenic parvalbumin mutant for immunotherapy of IgE-mediated fish allergy. J Immunol 2007; 178(10): 6290-6296.

[79] Kussebi F, Karamloo F, Rhyner C, *et al.* A major allergen gene-fusion protein for potential usage in allergen-specific immunotherapy. J Allergy Clin Immunol 2005; 115(2): 323-329.

[80] King TP, Jim SY, Monsalve RI, *et al.* Recombinant allergens with reduced allergenicity but retaining immunogenicity of the natural allergens: hybrids of yellow jacket and paper wasp venom allergen antigen 5s. J Immunol 2001; 166(10): 6057-6065.

[81] Hirahara K, Tatsuta T, Takatori T, *et al.* Preclinical evaluation of an immunotherapeutic peptide comprising 7 T-cell determinants of Cry j 1 and Cry j 2, the major Japanese cedar pollen allergens. J Allergy Clin Immunol 2001; 108(1): 94-100.

[82] Karamloo F, Schmid-Grendelmeier P, Kussebi F, *et al.* Prevention of allergy by a recombinant multi-allergen vaccine with reduced IgE binding and preserved T cell epitopes. Eur J Immunol 2005; 35(11): 3268-3276.

[83] Jutel M, Jaeger L, Suck R, *et al.* Allergen-specific immunotherapy with recombinant grass pollen allergens. J Allergy Clin Immunol 2005; 116(3): 608-613.

[84] Pauli G, Larsen TH, Rak S, *et al.* Efficacy of recombinant birch pollen vaccine for the treatment of birch-allergic rhinoconjunctivitis. J Allergy Clin Immunol 2008; 122(5): 951-960.

[85] Vrtala S, Hirtenlehner K, Susani M, *et al.* Genetic engineering of a hypoallergenic trimer of the major birch pollen allergen Bet v 1. FASEB J 2001; 15(11): 2045-2047.

[86] van Hage-Hamsten M, Kronqvist M, Zetterström O, *et al.* Skin test evaluation of genetically engineered hypoallergenic derivatives of the major birch pollen allergen, Bet v 1: results obtained with a mix of two recombinant Bet v 1 fragments and recombinant Bet v 1 trimer in a Swedish population before the birch pollen season. J Allergy Clin Immunol 1999; 104(5): 969-977.

[87] Van LP, Bardel E, Gregoire S, *et al.* Treatment with the TLR7 agonist R848 induces regulatory T-cell-mediated suppression of established asthma symptoms. Eur J Immunol 2011; 41(7): 1992-1999.

[88] Xirakia C, Koltsida O, Stavropoulos A, *et al.* Toll-like receptor 7-triggered immune response in the lung mediates acute and long-lasting suppression of experimental asthma. Am J Respir Crit Care Med 2010; 181(11): 1207-1216.

[89] Musarra A, Bignardi D, Troise C, *et al.* Long-lasting effect of a monophosphoryl lipid-adjuvanted immunotherapy to parietaria. A controlled field study. Eur Ann Allergy Clin Immunol 2010; 42(3): 115-119.

[90] Rosewich M, Schulze J, Fischer von Weikersthal-Drachenberg KJ, *et al.* Ultra-short course immunotherapy in children and adolescents during a 3-yrs post-marketing surveillance study. Pediatr Allergy Immunol 2010; 21(1 Pt 2): e185-189.

[91] Rosewich M, Schulze J, Eickmeier O, *et al.* Tolerance induction after specific immunotherapy with pollen allergoids adjuvanted by monophosphoryl lipid A in children. Clin Exp Immunol 2010; 160(3): 403-410.

[92] Pfaar O, Barth C, Jaschke C, *et al.* Sublingual allergen-specific immunotherapy adjuvanted with monophosphoryl lipid A: a phase I/IIa study. Int Arch Allergy Immunol 2011; 154(4): 336-344.

[93] Thorburn AN, Foster PS, Gibson PG, *et al.* Components of Streptococcus pneumoniae suppress allergic airways disease and NKT cells by inducing regulatory T cells. J Immunol 2012; 188(9): 4611-4620.

[94] Gupta GK, Agrawal DK. CpG oligodeoxynucleotides as TLR9 agonists: therapeutic application in allergy and asthma. BioDrugs 2010; 24(4): 225-235.

[95] Senti G, Johansen P, Haug S, *et al.* Use of A-type CpG oligodeoxynucleotides as an adjuvant in allergen-specific immunotherapy in humans: a phase I/IIa clinical trial. Clin Exp Allergy 2009; 39(4): 562-570.

[96] Grundström J, Neimert-Andersson T, Kemi C, *et al.* Covalent coupling of vitamin D3 to the major cat allergen Fel d 1 improves the effects of allergen-specific immunotherapy in a mouse model for cat allergy. Int Arch Allergy Immunol 2012; 157(2): 136-146.

[97] Arikan C, Bahceciler NN, Deniz G, *et al.* Bacillus Calmette-Guérin-induced interleukin-12 did not additionally improve clinical and immunologic parameters in asthmatic children treated with sublingual immunotherapy. Clin Exp Allergy 2004; 34(3): 398-405.

[98] Freytag LC, Clements JD. Mucosal adjuvants. Vaccine 2005; 23(15): 1804-1813.

[99] Pizza M, Giuliani MM, Fontana MR, *et al.* Mucosal vaccines: non toxic derivatives of LT and CT as mucosal adjuvants. Vaccine 2001; 19(17-19): 2534-2541.

[100] Van Overtvelt L, Moussu H, Horiot S, *et al.* Lactic acid bacteria as adjuvants for sublingual allergy vaccines. Vaccine 2010; 28(17): 2986-2992.

[101] Van Overtvelt L, Lombardi V, Razafindratsita A, *et al.* IL-10-inducing adjuvants enhance sublingual immunotherapy efficacy in a murine asthma model. Int Arch Allergy Immunol 2008; 145(2): 152-162.

[102] Solano-Parada J, Gonzalez-Gonzalez G, Torró LM, *et al.* Effectiveness of intranasal vaccination against Angiostrongylus costaricensis using a serine/threonine phosphatase 2 A synthetic peptide and recombinant antigens. Vaccine 2010; 28(32): 5185-5196.

[103] Sahoo MK, Sisodia BS, Dixit S, *et al.* Immunization with inflammatory proteome of Brugia malayi adult worm induces a Th1/Th2-immune response and confers protection against the filarial infection. Vaccine 2009; 27(32): 4263-4271.

[104] Pritchard DI, Blount DG, Schmid-Grendelmeier P, *et al.* Parasitic worm therapy for allergy: is this incongruous or avant-garde medicine? Clin Exp Allergy 2012; 42(4): 505-512.

[105] Kim N, Kwon SS, Lee J, *et al.* Protective effect of the DNA vaccine encoding the major house dust mite allergens on allergic inflammation in the murine model of house dust mite allergy. Clin Mol Allergy 2006; 4: 4.

[106] Crameri R, Kündig TM, Akdis CA. Modular antigen-translocation as a novel vaccine strategy for allergen-specific immunotherapy. Curr Opin Allergy Clin Immunol 2009; 9(6): 568-573.

[107] Bousquet J, Scheinmann P, Guinnepain MT, *et al.* Sublingual-swallow immunotherapy (SLIT) in patients with asthma due to house-dust mites: a double-blind, placebo-controlled study. Allergy 1999; 54(3): 249-260.

[108] Kündig TM, Senti G, Schnetzler G, *et al.* Der p 1 peptide on virus-like particles is safe and highly immunogenic in healthy adults. J Allergy Clin Immunol 2006; 117(6): 1470-1476.

[109] Schöll I, Weissenböck A, Förster-Waldl E, *et al.* Allergen-loaded biodegradable poly(D,L-lactic-co-glycolic) acid nanoparticles down-regulate an ongoing Th2 response in the BALB/c mouse model. Clin Exp Allergy 2004; 34(2): 315-321.

[110] Jilek S, Walter E, Merkle HP, *et al.* Modulation of allergic responses in mice by using biodegradable poly(lactide-co-glycolide) microspheres. J Allergy Clin Immunol 2004; 114(4): 943-950.

[111] Saint-Lu N, Tourdot S, Razafindratsita A, *et al.* Targeting the allergen to oral dendritic cells with mucoadhesive chitosan particles enhances tolerance induction. Allergy 2009; 64(7): 1003-1013.

[112] Gómez S, Gamazo C, San Roman B, *et al.* A novel nanoparticulate adjuvant for immunotherapy with Lolium perenne. J Immunol Methods 2009; 348(1-2): 1-8.

[113] Broos S, Lundberg K, Akagi T, *et al.* Immunomodulatory nanoparticles as adjuvants and allergen-delivery system to human dendritic cells: Implications for specific immunotherapy. Vaccine 2010; 28(31): 5075-5085.

[114] Cox L, Calderon MA. Subcutaneous specific immunotherapy for seasonal allergic rhinitis: a review of treatment practices in the US and Europe. Curr Med Res Opin 2010; 26(12): 2723-2733.

[115] Senna G, Ridolo E, Calderon M, *et al.* Evidence of adherence to allergen-specific immunotherapy. Curr Opin Allergy Clin Immunol 2009; 9(6): 544-548.

[116] Martínez-Gómez JM, Johansen P, Erdmann I, *et al.* Intralymphatic injections as a new administration route for allergen-specific immunotherapy. Int Arch Allergy Immunol 2009; 150(1): 59-65.

[117] Senti G, Johansen P, Kündig TM. Intralymphatic immunotherapy. Curr Opin Allergy Clin Immunol 2009; 9(6): 537-543.

[118] Zinkernagel RM. Localization dose and time of antigens determine immune reactivity. Semin Immunol 2000; 12(3): 163-171.

[119] Senti G, Prinz Vavricka BM, Erdmann I, *et al.* Intralymphatic allergen administration renders specific immunotherapy faster and safer: a randomized controlled trial. Proc Natl Acad Sci U S A 2008; 105(46): 17908-17912.

[120] Dickel H, Goulioumis A, Gambichler T, *et al.* Standardized tape stripping: a practical and reproducible protocol to uniformly reduce the stratum corneum. Skin Pharmacol Physiol 2010; 23(5): 259-265.

[121] Nickoloff BJ, Naidu Y. Perturbation of epidermal barrier function correlates with initiation of cytokine cascade in human skin. J Am Acad Dermatol 1994; 30(4): 535-546.

[122] Dickel H, Gambichler T, Kamphowe J, *et al.* Standardized tape stripping prior to patch testing induces upregulation of Hsp90, Hsp70, IL-33, TNF-α and IL-8/CXCL8 mRNA: new insights into the involvement of 'alarmins'. Contact Dermatitis 2010; 63(4): 215-222.

[123] Zhu M, Flynt L, Ghosh S, *et al.* Anti-inflammatory effects of thiazolidinediones in human airway smooth muscle cells. Am J Respir Cell Mol Biol 2011; 45(1): 111-119.

[124] Denning GM, Stoll LL. Peroxisome proliferator-activated receptors: potential therapeutic targets in lung disease? Pediatr Pulmonol 2006; 41(1): 23-34.

[125] Belvisi MG, Hele DJ. Peroxisome proliferator-activated receptors as novel targets in lung disease. Chest 2008; 134(1): 152-157.

[126] Woerly G, Honda K, Loyens M, *et al.* Peroxisome proliferator-activated receptors alpha and gamma down-regulate allergic inflammation and eosinophil activation. J Exp Med 2003; 198(3): 411-421.

[127] Lin CH, Wang MH, Chung HY, *et al.* Effects of acupuncture-like transcutaneous electrical nerve stimulation on children with asthma. J Asthma 2010; 47(10): 1116-1122.

[128] Srivastava K, Zhang T, Yang N, *et al.* Anti-Asthma Simplified Herbal Medicine Intervention-induced long-lasting tolerance to allergen exposure in an asthma model is interferon-γ, but not transforming growth factor-β dependent. Clin Exp Allergy 2010; 40(11): 1678-1688.

[129] Li XM. Traditional Chinese herbal remedies for asthma and food allergy. J Allergy Clin Immunol 2007; 120(1): 25-31.

[130] Palmer DJ, Sullivan T, Gold MS, *et al.* Effect of n-3 long chain polyunsaturated fatty acid supplementation in pregnancy on infants' allergies in first year of life: randomised controlled trial. BMJ 2012; 344: e184.

[131] Krauss-Etschmann S, Hartl D, Rzehak P, *et al.* Decreased cord blood IL-4, IL-13, and CCR4 and increased TGF-beta levels after fish oil supplementation of pregnant women. J Allergy Clin Immunol 2008; 121(2): 464-470. e466.

[132] Furuhjelm C, Warstedt K, Larsson J, *et al.* Fish oil supplementation in pregnancy and lactation may decrease the risk of infant allergy. Acta Paediatr 2009; 98(9): 1461-1467.

Send Orders for Reprints on reprints@benthamscience.net

 Frontiers in Clinical Drug Research-Anti-Allergy Agents, Vol. 1, **2013, 50-117**

CHAPTER 3

Anti-Allergy Agents in Patients Practicing Sports

Mariana Couto[1,2,*], Diana Silva[1], Luís Delgado[1,2] and André Moreira[1,2]

[1]Allergy, Asthma and Sports Unit, Immunoallergology Department, Centro Hospitalar São João, E.P.E. – Porto, Portugal and [2]Immunology Lab, Faculty of Medicine, University of Porto – Porto, Portugal

Abstract: Regular physical activity is recommended for all individuals, but allergic athletes face special challenges managing their diseases while practicing sports. Exercise-induced hypersensitivity disorders are significant problems for both recreational and competitive athletes, occurring with higher prevalence than in the general population. Asthma is the most common chronic condition among athletes.

Athlete's allergic diseases often perplex, frustrate and distress both patients and their physicians. Their treatment frequently poses several issues. In the specific case of asthma, multiple phenotypes exhibiting differences in response to treatment exist, which creates additional difficulties when managing these patients.

Optimal allergic diseases management aims to control both symptoms and inflammation, but when choosing treatment for a specific athletic population compared with the common allergic patient, some additional factors should be taken into account. For the top athlete it is important not only to control symptoms of allergy and prevent its progression, but it becomes equally imperative to reduce the impact upon sports performance, often practiced under extraordinary circumstances. Therefore, the possibility of side effects of the prescribed treatments should also be carefully considered, in a way to allow full participation in physical activity and sports.

Commonly used drugs include antihistamines, corticosteroids or β2-agonists. Oral H1-antihistamines are one of the first-line therapeutic options for allergic rhinitis, however they might affect vigilance and reaction time in athletes. Antileukotrienes efficacy has been questioned in athletes and inhaled corticosteroids are only partially effective. Also, some potential adverse events with the use of inhaled β2-agonists agents have been pointed out, and health care providers should be aware of these concerns. Moreover, as mechanisms and triggers of hypersensitivity disorders can be different in athletes compared to general population, and even vary between athletes practicing different sports, these patients should be managed sometimes in a singular and different way. On the other hand, a careful consideration of available therapies is required in order to

***Address correspondence to Mariana Couto:** Immunology Lab, Faculty of Medicine, University of Porto – Alameda Prof. Hernani Monteiro, 4200-319 Porto, Portugal; Tel: 00351 91 793 22 83; Fax: 00351 225513601; E-mail: marianafercouto@gmail.com

Atta-ur-Rahman (Ed)

comply with World Anti-Doping Agency regulations. Certain medications for athletes with asthma and rhinitis who participate in regulated competitions are not allowed, and as these guidelines often change, sometimes annually, the physician caring for subjects who are active in sports needs regular update.

The aim of this chapter is to increase physicians' awareness of special treatment needs for such a prevalent heath problem among athletes, to demystify this issue and improve doctor's confidence on prescribing anti-allergy agents to sports practicing patients.

Keywords: Anaphylaxis, antihistamines, antileukotrienes, asthma, allergy, beta-2 agonists, corticosteroids, exercise, immunotherapy, rhinitis, sports, urticaria, anti-allergy agents, doping, drugs, athletes.

INTRODUCTION

Regular physical exercise and participation in sports are considered to be important components of a healthy life and are recommended for all individuals. However, allergic athletes face special challenges managing their disorders while practicing sports. Exercise is a frequent trigger of different hypersensitivity events that impair performance. The all-encompassing term exercise-induced (EI) hypersensitivity syndromes include EI-asthma, EI-bronchoconstriction, EI-rhinitis, EI-anaphylaxis and EI-urticaria. These are significant problems for both recreational and competitive athletes, occurring with higher prevalence than in general population [1]. EI-asthma is actually the most common chronic condition among athletes.

Physical exertion is one of many non-pharmacologic and non-immunologic stimuli that can produce episodes of airway obstruction in patients with asthma. In fact, physical activity is the second leading cause of airway constriction [2]. However, unlike other types of triggers, such as upper respiratory tract infections, that function only periodically in the life of patients with the disease, exercise occurs much more frequently, precipitating acute symptoms. EI-asthma is most frequently seen in children and young adults because of their high levels of physical activity, and has been reported to occur in 70-80% of untreated asthmatics [3]. It is even more relevant to patients practicing sports. People with asthma may show less tolerance to exercise due to worsening asthma symptoms during exercise; this can prevent them from playing sports or attempting to keep fit. Evidence has shown that physical training improves cardiopulmonary fitness and shows some positive effects for health-related quality of life [4] and allergic inflammation [5] among people with asthma. Therefore, all efforts must be placed to successfully treat exercise induced symptoms in order to allow them to partake in regular exercise training, without fear of symptom exacerbation.

EI-rhinitis, characterized by itching, sneezing, rhinorrhea and/or postnasal drainage, nasal congestion and occasional anosmia provoked by exercise, is frequently accompanied by eye, ear or throat symptoms [6]. Athletes with rhinitis, particularly congestion, often complain about disturbed sleep, daytime somnolence, fatigue and impaired performance [1]. Treating rhinitis, especially reducing nasal congestion, should improve sleep and thereby improve quality of life and, most likely, athletic performance. Controlling rhinitis also may improve control of asthma. Certain medications for athletes with asthma and rhinitis who participate in regulated competitions are not allowed (Table **1**).

EI-urticaria and EI-anaphylaxis, the later possibly being related to specific food ingestion (a process named food dependent exercise-induced anaphylaxis – FDEIA), are much lesser frequent, but yet with an important impact in performance and quality of life. EI-anaphylaxis is a rare, unpredictable event, and the most serious and potentially life-threatening syndrome associated with exercise [7]; 2–15% of anaphylactic episodes are caused by or associated with exercise [8, 9]. As recurrences might occur under the same conditions, consequently, future exercise-related activities are often curtailed. EI-urticaria also appears in athletes without an associated anaphylactic reaction and is frequently driven by physical and environmental stimuli, like high temperatures (cholinergic urticaria) or even cold environments.

Appropriate management of EI-hypersensitivity disorders relies on correct and prompt diagnosis and proper treatment. The primary aim of the therapy is prophylaxis. Prophylactic management for EI-anaphylaxis is to first avoid the trigger(s), particularly foods in case of FDEIA. Specific food allergens should be avoided for at least 6 h prior to exercise [1]. Acute episodes of asthma can be attenuated by warm up before undertaking strenuous exertion. This works reasonably well for scheduled events, but it is not a practical means of preventing the consequences that follow from the sports undertaken as part of daily life (*e.g.*, athletes). Furthermore, it is not very effective in protecting elite athletes unless the workload approaches that used in competition. The duration of protection is short and seldom exceeds 40 minutes. To provide more effective control, pharmacologic interventions are required.

The aim of this chapter is to provide insight about anti-allergy drugs used in patients practicing sports and how they contribute to appropriate management of EI-hypersensitivity syndromes. Also to increase the awareness of physicians to the special treatment needs for such a prevalent heath problem among athletes, to demystify this issue and improve doctor's confidence on prescribing anti-allergy agents to sports practicing patients.

Table 1: Most frequent medications used to treat asthma and rhinitis [10, 13].

Treatment	WADA Rules	Notes
Controller medication		
Inhaled corticosteroids	Permitted	
Anti-leukotrienes	Permitted	
Nasal corticosteroids	Permitted	
Allergen Immunotherapy*	Permitted	
Reliever medication		
Inhaled beta2-agonists	Prohibited **except** salbutamol, formoterol and salmeterol	Salbutamol maximum 1600μg over 24h and formoterol maximum 36μg over 24h; the presence in urine of salbutamol > 1000 ng/mL or formoterol > 30 ng/mL is presumed not to be an intended therapeutic use of the substance and will be considered as an AAE
Oral beta2-agonists	Prohibited	
Oral corticosteroids	Prohibited	TUE approval is required
Antihistamines	Permitted	Second-generation H1-antihistamines should be preferred to avoid somnolence
Ipratropium bromide	Permitted	Inhaled or nasal formulations are allowed
Decongestants	Nasal application is permitted	Ephedrine, methylephedrine are prohibited when its concentration in urine >10μg/mL. Pseudoephedrine is prohibited when its concentration in urine >150μg/mL.

AAE: Adverse Analytical Finding
TUE: Therapeutic use exemption
WADA: World Anti-Doping Agency.

Drugs which are not allowed by the World Anti-doping Agency to use in athletes [10] are presented in Table **1**. Some of them are, however, relevant to use under certain circumstances (for instance, oral corticosteroids for exacerbations), will be included in this review. Their use requires submitting a Therapeutic Use Exemption to WADA [10].

Xanthines, calcium channel blockers and inhaled furosemide have modest attenuating effects on EI-bronchoconstriction, but side effects generally relegate these classes to the sidelines [11]. Therefore they will not be included in this review. Anti-cholinergics have been considered also third-line treatments and are rarely required or suggested, but as recent data renewed interest for these drugs, with some endurance athletes presenting higher reversibility to inhaled ipratropium bromide than to inhaled beta2-agonists [12] (also unpublished data), some considerations will be included regarding their potential interest.

ANTI-ALLERGY AGENTS

Inhaled Corticosteroids

A joint task force of the European Respiratory Society (ERS) and European Academy of Allergy and Clinical Immunology (EAACI) defined EI-asthma as symptoms and signs of asthma occurring in an asthmatic after exercise, whereas EI-bronchoconstriction was defined as a reduction in forced expiratory volume in one second (FEV1) of 10% after a standardized exercise test [14]. Both EI-asthma and EI-bronchoconstriction are common manifestations of asthma in patients. For the asthmatic athlete, it is important to control EI-asthma without being dependent upon planned pre-medication before scheduled exercise training. Thus, anti-inflammatory treatment controlling asthma becomes important for the daily life accomplishments of asthmatic patients actively participating in sports.

A better understanding of EI-bronchoconstriction will allow the physician to direct the patient towards a type of exercise and medications that can result in a more active lifestyle without the same concern for resulting symptoms. This is especially important for schoolchildren who are usually enrolled in physical education classes, and elite athletes who may desire to participate in competitive sports [15]. EI-asthma is thought to be due to increased ventilation caused by the increase in demand for oxygen as a result of physical exercise [16]. The increased ventilation is accompanied by heat and water loss. The airway surface liquid becomes hyperosmolar, providing a stimulus for water to move from nearby cells. This results in the shrinkage of cells and the consequent release of inflammatory mediators, both newly formed eicosanoids and preformed mediators such as histamine from intracellular granules, that lead to airway smooth muscle contraction [16, 17]. The inflammatory basis of EI-bronchoconstriction was demonstrated by Hallstrand *et al.* [18]. They verified a significant correlation between columnar epithelial cells in induced sputum and severity of EI-bronchoconstriction (r^2=0.174, p=0.043), and between cysteinyl leukotrienes and histamine *vs.* columnar cells in sputum (r^2=0.529, p<0.0001 and (r^2=0.286, p=0.007, respectively), demonstrating the role of mediator's release. Also, the increased ventilatory rate to meet higher muscular oxygen needs results in the inhalation of a large volume of relatively cold air and the loss of heat, besides water, from the respiratory mucosa [17]. Consequently, the airways are cooled, and this mechanic noxious stimulus, together with the osmothic mechanism, could cause epithelial damage, and therefore the influx of inflammatory cells and their mediators' release [17]. Moreover, cooling of the airways also causes reflex parasympathetic nerve stimulation and it has been hypothesized that repeated intensive training could provoke vagal hegemony, predisposing to an increase in the bronchomotor tone [17]. This mechanism will be fully elucidated later. Disruption to the airway epithelium has been implicated in the pathogenesis of EI-asthma, as the airway epithelium of athletes may be injured by strenuous exercise [19, 20]. Also, an increase in the levels of airway vascular permeability has been shown to predict the severity of EI-bronchoconstriction in asthmatics [21], which led to the microvascular theory of EI-bronchoconstriction based on functional abnormalities of endothelial cells in newly generated microvessels in asthmatic airways [22]. Nevertheless, the evidence of similar levels of airway microvascular permeability in competitive swimmers compared with asthmatics, independent of their asthma status, suggests the increased levels of inflammatory cells observed in the airways of athletes may be associated with the airway vascular leakage which, however, does not correlate with lung function or airway hyperesponsiveness [23]. This provides further support to the hypothesis of a "frustrated' inflammatory process in the airways of athletes, suggesting that increased inflammatory airway cells may represent a training adaptation, not necessarily implying detrimental effects on respiratory health [23].

For athletes with asthma, anti-inflammatory treatment with inhaled steroids is most important, both to reduce inflammation and the clinical impact of repeated training and competitions, as well as to possibly improve long-term prognosis [24]. The different mechanisms implicated in EI-asthma and the evidence of increased neutrophil cell counts in induced sputum of swimmers [25] and winter sport athletes (which correlated to the number of training hours per week in both groups) [26], justifies the fact that inhaled corticosteroids are sometimes not totally effective in this population. Nevertheless, presently the most important treatment available and optimal control of EI-asthma is most often obtained with inhaled corticosteroids [16].

Glucocorticoid hormones from the adrenal cortex and their synthetic analogs (steroids) represent the most effective class of drugs in the therapy of inflammatory diseases and are among the most widely used class of drugs for the treatment of atopic diseases. Corticosteroids owe their anti-inflammatory effects to their ability to suppress the expression of a host of inflammatory mediators, including growth factors, cytokines, chemokines, and inflammatory enzymes involved in metabolism of arachidonic acid and nitric oxide [27].

The inhaled formulation is the preferred long-term controller therapy for the management of persistent asthma in children and adults as they act specifically at the application site. The diminished systemic side effects are due to local retention at the application site, high affinity for the glucocorticoid receptor, and rapid metabolism and elimination following absorption. In 1972, beclomethasone dipropionate was the first inhaled corticosteroid to offer superior topical over systemic potency [28]. Ever since, new inhaled corticosteroids, such as budesonide, fluticasone propionate, and mometasone furoate, were designed to provide maximal topical effect in the airways with minimal systemic absorption [29].

The principles for asthma management in athletes are the same as those applicable for general population [30]. This includes a "step-up" approach if worsening of

EI-asthma occur, as in patients with asthma, exercise-induced symptoms can be used as a marker of incomplete asthma control indicating a need for additional controller medications [1]. The first step includes treatment with an as needed-reliever medication (*e.g.,* beta-agonists) and is reserved for untreated athletes with occasional daytime symptoms of short duration related to exercise [30]. Controller medication with inhaled corticosteroids (step 2) is recommended when asthma control is not achieved by reliever therapy alone [31, 32] when the athlete has persistent symptoms, if bronchial hyperresponsiveness and/or inflammation are present, or if bronchodilation therapy is required on a regular basis. Due to tachyphylaxis associated with inhaled beta2-agonists, the use of controller medication will avoid the daily consumption of these drugs, optimizing their rescue or preventive effects when most needed. Regarding EI-bronchoconstriction, the regular use of inhaled corticosteroids is effective [32]. This was shown in children with EI-asthma after 1 week of regular treatment with inhaled budesonide [33]. However, to reduce significantly the fall in maximum mid expiratory flow 25–75% ($MMEF_{25-75}$), longer treatment is needed. Some effect is seen within 4 weeks [34, 35], but the best possible result is not expected to occur until after 8 weeks of regular treatment [35]. A Cochrane Database systematic review of two parallel studies, showed that a duration of at least 4 weeks of inhaled corticosteroids significantly attenuated the percent post-exercise fall index in forced expiratory volume in the first second (FEV1) [35]. Inhaled corticosteroids improve EI-asthma more rapidly than bronchial hyperresponsiveness measured by methacholine bronchial provocation [33].

Although there is no evidence supporting different treatment for EI-bronchoconstriction in asthmatic athletes and nonathletes [36], when choosing treatment for this specific population compared with the ordinary asthma patient, some additional factors should be taken into account. For the top athlete it is important not only to control symptoms of asthma and prevent progression, but it becomes equally imperative to reduce its impact upon sports performance, often under extraordinary circumstances, such as very low temperatures, exposure to high chlorine levels, sustained increased ventilation. The possibility of side effects associated with the prescribed treatment should also be carefully considered [33].

Although the incidence of adverse effects is greatly diminished compared to chronically administered oral corticosteroids therapy, these molecules still have some side-effects. Oral candidiasis and dysphonia are the most commonly encountered adverse effects of inhaled glucocorticoid therapy. However, others should be taken into account when concerning sports, such as adrenal suppression and reduction in bone mineral density. Of course, side effects are dependent on the dose delivered, the pharmacokinetic profile (*i.e.,* degree of first-pass hepatic metabolism), the method of delivery, and individual differences in steroid sensitivity among patients [29]. Although uncommon, adrenal suppression is of particular concern. The degree of suppression of the hypothalamo–pituitary–adrenal axis is largely dependent on the dose and frequency of administration, the duration of treatment, and the time of day of administration. In healthy males inhaling fluticasone proprionate twice daily, 440 μg/d, exercise significantly increased circulating levels of fluticasone, as well as decreased cortisol and adrenocorticotropin; the systemic effects of this topical treatment were demonstrated by an increase in peripheral blood leukocytes and neutrophils, as well as interleukin-6 levels [37]. Adrenal suppression has also been showed in children on low-to-moderate doses of inhaled budesonide [38]. As a result of adrenal suppression, hypoglycaemic convulsions were described in some case reports, especially in patients using fluticasone dipropionate [39-41]. Another side effect, although rare, is reduction in bone mineral density. Many of the available data evaluating the risk of developing osteoporosis with inhaled corticosteroids use comes from cross-sectional studies that often provide contradictory information [42-47]. However, this issue should be considered by clinicians especially when treating asthmatic women practicing endurance sports; this is particularly true in the case of female marathon runners, who have been noted to be at particular risk for osteoporosis [33]. Despite the controversial results, growth retardation in children and adolescents induced by inhaled corticosteroids [29, 48-50], should be also taken into account. More recently, ciclesonide has shown significant efficacy for the treatment of asthma [51, 52] and therefore has attracted the interest of sport practicing patients [24, 34]. Attenuation in exercise-induced decrease of FEV1 can be seen as early as after 1 week of therapy, at doses greater than 40 μg [34]. Ciclesonide is a nonhalogenated parent compound that is converted to its active form in the bronchial epithelium by epithelial esterases to form the biologically potent desisobutyryl-ciclesonide. This conversion facilitates a high concentration of active metabolite at the mucosal surface [53]. *In vitro* comparisons demonstrate that desisobutyryl-ciclesonide exhibits a 100-fold greater glucocorticoid receptor binding than the parent compound ciclesonide [54]. When it passes to blood stream it will be protein bound and inactivated rapidly. Systemic levels of biologically active steroid components are lower in patients administered ciclesonide compared with those administered with fluticasone or budesonide [55]. *In vitro* animal and human studies comparing ciclesonide with alternative inhaled corticosteroids provide evidence that equivalent or lower doses of ciclesonide result in similar clinical responses. These studies also indicate that it induces fewer systemic steroid effects (osteopenia, adrenal suppression, and oral candidiasis) [51, 54, 55]. In combination, these features suggest that ciclesonide might be an attractive therapeutic option for the treatment of athletes, particularly to the potential less suppression of the adrenals, because athletes are dependent upon an optimal stress response from the adrenals [24]. The possibility of side-effects, even if uncommon, substantiates the importance of using inhaled corticosteroids at the lowest possible dose and in appropriate patients.

If control is not achieved, the next step will comprise the increase on corticosteroids dosage (Table **2**) and/or the addition of a long-acting beta2-agonist to inhaled corticosteroids. Inhaled corticosteroids are not among the WADA 2012 list of banned substances (Table **1**) [10].

Inhaled Beta2-Agonists

Adrenergic receptor agonists have been the agent of choice for acute asthma symptoms since the first reported use of "adrenal substance" for acute asthma [56]. The subsequent introduction of aerosol epinephrine provided patients with rapid relief of asthma symptoms, but concerns soon arose about cardiotoxicity and the emergence of tolerance [57]. The development of agents selective for beta2-adrenoceptors, by increasing the bulk of the side chain, provided drugs with greater selectivity for airway smooth muscle and better safety profiles, which produce marked bronchodilation without concomitant tachycardia [58]. These agents act by mimicking the actions of adrenaline (epinephrine). Beneficial effects of the beta2-adrenergic agonists are thought to result primarily from relaxation of bronchial smooth muscle, but they also present several non-bronchodilator actions: increment of air flow, reduction in vascular permeability, increment of mucociliary clearance (ion and water secretion and ciliary beat frequency); protection of respiratory epithelium against bacteria; suppression of microvascular permeability; inhibition of cholinergic neurotransmission; inhibition of inflammatory mediators release; inhibition of functions of different cells, including eosinophils, macrophages, dendritic cells, T-lymphocytes and bronchial epithelial cells; and priming of the glucocorticoid receptor [58]. However, although these effects are useful, they should not be considered to be anti-inflammatory actions that can replace those of inhaled corticosteroids [58].

This class of drugs, especially when administered by inhalation, have shown to be the most effective in protecting against EI-bronchoconstriction [36]. This is the only route of administration allowed by 2012 WADA guidelines (Table **1**) [10]. The major advantage of delivering beta-adrenergic agonists directly into the lungs *via* inhalation is that higher concentrations can be delivered more effectively to the airways and systemic side effects are lessened. On the contrary, although placebo-controlled studies have indicated that, when employed as a sole bronchodilator, oral formulations of beta2-adrenergic agents might improve pulmonary function and ameliorate asthma symptoms [59], it was convincingly demonstrated by the 1970s that they offered a very poor protective effect against EI-bronchoconstriction [36, 60-63]. Studies on the rate of absorption of epinephrine injected by other parenteral routes (intravenous, intramuscular), and in different locations, have shown significant differences in time to peak concentrations, favoring intramuscular injection in the lateral thigh (Sorkness 2008). Moreover, these routes of administration are limited by dose-dependent side effects of tremor, tachycardia, and palpitations [58].

Inhaled beta2-agonists comprises 2 types of agents: the short acting (*e.g.*, salbutamol, terbutaline, isoprenaline, fenoterol) and long acting (*e.g.*, salmeterol, formoterol, indacaterol, arformoterol, carmoterol). Additionally, the time of onset of action is variable among different beta2-agonists, which has implications for treatment (Table **2**).

When only occasional and intermittent symptoms are present (step 1), *as-needed* reliever medication is suitable. Short acting beta2-agonists, such as salbutamol (albuterol) or terbutaline, are effective in this scenario, reversing EI-asthma/EI-bronchoconstriction (it should be noted, however, that for 2012 WADA guidelines, only salbutamol is permitted among inhaled short-acting beta2-agonists [10]). Short-acting inhaled beta2-agonists have an almost immediate action on EI-bronchoconstriction, with a maximum effect 20 minutes after inhalation [33]. The recommended dose of inhaled salbutamol (albuterol) is 0.2–0.4 mg, which corresponds to an inhaled dose of 0.5–1 mg of terbutaline. The effect may still be observed 3 hours after inhalation, but disappears after 4 hours [64] (Table **2**). Therefore, they are also used before exercise, for prevention. It has been shown that short-acting beta2-agonists significantly reduce the percentage fall in FEV1 after exercise in subjects with EI-asthma [65]. Short acting beta2-agonists are more commonly used, but long acting beta-agonists are also effective as prevention strategy, as they protect for up to 12 hours after a single inhalation. Anderson *et al.* [66] compared the short-acting inhaled beta2-agonist salbutamol with the long-acting salmeterol and found salmeterol to be active against EI-bronchoconstriction from 30 minutes to 6.5 hours after inhalation whereas salbutamol was as effective as salmeterol 30 minutes after, but not so from 2.5 to 6.5 hours after inhalation [66]. Another study demonstrated an effect of inhaled salmeterol in children with EI-bronchoconstriction lasting up to 10–12 hours after inhalation [67]. However, only formoterol acts as fast as short acting beta2-agonists. It has a similar long-lasting protective effect as salmeterol on EI-bronchoconstriction and the added benefit of having an onset of protective effect as rapid as salbutamol or terbutaline [68]. Therefore, formoterol or a short acting beta2-agonist should be chosen to reverse EI-asthma/EI-bronchoconstriction.

Nevertheless, it is important to note that there may be potential adverse events with the inhaled use of these agents, and health care providers should be aware of these concerns [11]. Inhaled beta2-agonists may mask worsening airway inflammation. Also, EI-bronchoconstriction is frequently not completely abolished, as exemplified by the study of Carlsen *et al.* with a maximum reduction in FEV1 after exercise of 18–19% after inhaling salmeterol compared with 30% after placebo [67]. In addition, tolerance (tachyphylaxis) occurs with inhaled beta2-agonists regular use, reducing their protective effect [11, 33]. Tolerance is caused by the downregulation of the beta2-receptor gene expression that gives rise to a decreased receptor density and a decreased binding affinity of the receptors to beta2-agonists [36]. A regular use of beta2-agonists leads to increased EI-bronchoconstriction and a suboptimal bronchodilator response to these agents. Although there is little evidence to suggest that this is a problem of clinical importance, current knowledge supports the use of short acting beta2-agonists only as rescue medication, also in elite athletes, as it might be associated with failure to respond to emergency treatment for asthma exacerbations [32]. On the other hand, some concerns regarding cardiovascular side effects in patients who take long-acting inhaled beta2-agonists on a regular basis have been pointed out [69, 70]; a systematic review suggested an increased risk of severe cardiovascular side effects [70]. There is still some controversy [71, 72] regarding this issue, and large, well-designed, controlled, prospective studies evaluating these risks are still lacking. While this question remains unresolved, cardiovascular side effects should be taken into consideration when treating athletes and other patients with inhaled beta2-agonists [13]. Recently, it has been showed that short-term supratherapeutic salmeterol exposure increased oxidative metabolic pathways on skeletal muscle cells, whereas prolonged treatment inhibits cell growth and exerts either a cytostatic or a proapoptotic effect in a time- and dose-dependent way [73]. Furthermore, an increased risk of serious adverse events with regular salmeterol has recently been evidenced, together with an increase in risk of asthma-related mortality in patients not using inhaled corticosteroids [74]. In addition, it has been proposed that airway inflammation could potentiate down-regulation of bronchoprotection in response to beta2-agonists [75]; in this study, asthmatics with EI-bronchoconstriction presenting low airway inflammation (defined by low levels of exhaled nitric oxide) did not lose bronchoprotection in response to regular use of long-acting beta2-agonists. Therefore, long acting beta2-agonists should never be used regularly without an inhaled steroid, and so they should be reserved for a further step-up [30]. In the 2012 WADA guidelines, unrestricted use of inhaled salbutamol, salmeterol, or formoterol is permitted as long as specified doses are not exceeded. Such a change, however, might lead to an increased use of long-acting beta2-agonists, without inhaled corticosteroids. Such a decision has been claimed to introduce safety issues stemming from the unsupervised use of beta2-agonists [76].

Even with the potential for tachyphylaxis or partial loss of efficacy, regular use of long acting beta2-agonists (formoterol or salmeterol) in a combined strategy does have a role in the long-term treatment of asthma. Given the possibility of side-effects associated with the use of inhaled corticosteroids, although uncommon, if adequate asthma control cannot be achieved with low to moderate doses of inhaled corticosteroids therapy alone, an additional long-term controller should be initiated as recommended in national and international asthma guidelines [30]. Within the last few years, there has been a growing appreciation that the function of the glucocorticoid receptor can be modulated by beta2-adrenergic receptor agonists [27]. Recent findings indicate that corticosteroids and beta2-agonists synergistically inhibit airway smooth muscle remodeling, which may contribute to the increased effectiveness of combined treatment with corticosteroids and beta2-agonists in asthma [77]. Also, beta2-agonists can stimulate the glucocorticoid receptor and promote its translocation to the nucleus, resulting in an increased corticosteroid-mediated gene transcription; corticosteroids may also increase the transcription of the beta2-agonists gene in the lung and the nasal mucosa [32, 78]. In fact, patients receiving formoterol or salmeterol, in addition to budesonide or fluticasone, achieved asthma control 10 days sooner, as defined by increased lung function, decreased symptoms (even with exercise), decreased exacerbations and improved quality of life [11]. Reynolds *et al.* reported that the combination of salmeterol and fluticasone was superior to fluticasone alone for the prevention of EI-asthma [79]. In keeping with this observation, Pauwels *et al.* have shown that the combination of formoterol and budesonide is more effective than budesonide alone with regard to symptoms and asthma control [80]. To prescribe a combination of both drugs in the same device may be of interest as a strategy to avoid the possibility of beta2-agonists use only. If a combination inhaler containing formoterol and budesonide is selected, it may be used for both rescue and maintenance [30]. This approach has been shown to reduce exacerbations and improve asthma control in adults and adolescents at relatively low doses of treatment [81-83]; this simplified strategy using budesonide/formoterol for maintenance and reliever therapy is feasible, safe and at least as effective as salmeterol/fluticasone plus salbutamol [84].

The 2012 WADA guidelines establish that all beta-2 agonists (both optical isomers were relevant) are prohibited except salbutamol (maximum 1600 micrograms over 24 hours), formoterol (maximum 36 micrograms over 24 hours) and salmeterol when taken by inhalation in accordance with the manufacturers' recommended therapeutic regime. The presence in urine of salbutamol in excess of 1000 ng/mL or formoterol in excess of 30 ng/mL is presumed not to be an intended therapeutic use of the substance and will be considered as an Adverse Analytical Finding unless the athlete proves, through a controlled pharmacokinetic study, that the abnormal result was the consequence of the use of the therapeutic inhaled dose up to the maximum indicated [10].

Anti-Cholinergics

This class also comprises short acting (*e.g.*, ipratropium bromide) and long acting (*e.g.*, tiotropium) agents. The most used inhaled anti-cholinergic for asthma is ipratropium bromide. Tiotropium is only approved by the Food and Drug Administration for the treatment of chronic obstructive pulmonary disease (COPD) and not for the treatment of asthma (Table **2**). Ipratropium blocks muscarinic acetylcholine receptors and therefore inhibits degradation of cyclic guanosine monophosphate (cGMP), resulting in an intracellular increase in its concentration [85]; this contrasts with the action of beta-adrenergic receptor stimulants, which raise levels of cyclic adenosine monophosphate. Most likely due to actions on intracellular calcium, cGMP results in decreased contractility of smooth muscle in the lung, inhibiting bronchoconstriction and mucus secretion. Ipratropium bromide is a nonselective muscarinic antagonist, binding to muscarinic M2 and M3 receptors with equal affinity. In adults, the maximally bronchodilation effect occurs with a dose of 500 μg.

In most of the older studies, anticholinergics consistently showed no protection against EI-bronchoconstriction [86-89]. A Cochrane systematic review in 2003 concluded that inhaled anti-cholinergics provided significant protection against EI-bronchoconstriction, but the effectiveness was lower than short-acting beta2-agonists and mast cell stabilizers [90]. Those evidences, together with the limitation of ipratropium use by the need for frequent dosing (every 6 hours), resulted in a side-line position of this class of drugs. Recent studies showing that Norwegian competitive endurance athletes responded particularly well to ipratropium bromide with higher reversal of symptoms than seen with inhaled beta2 agonists [12] leads to the proposal that this drug be tried before exercise and competition.

The role of parasympathetic nerves in the etiopathogenesis of asthma was long time ago demonstrated by Molfino *et al.* [91]; in this study, increased airway tone at baseline in patients with asthma could be completely blocked by the inhaled anti-cholinergic agent ipratropium bromide, demonstrating that it is vagally mediated [91].

In the specific case of athletes, the mechanisms proposed to explain the higher occurrence of asthma include the hypothesis of a generalized "dysautonomy" associated with training. The inhalation of cold air and cooling of the airways causes reflex parasympathetic nerve stimulation which leads to bronchoconstriction through stimulation of the vagal nerve, initially causing reflex vasoconstriction of bronchial venules to conserve heat, followed at the end of the exercise by secondary reactive hyperemia (airway rewarming) with vascular bronchial congestion, edema, and further airway narrowing [17]. It has been hypothesized that repeated intensive training could provoke vagal hegemony, which induces not only the well-known resting bradycardia of athletes, but could also predispose to an increase in bronchomotor tone, and consequently susceptibility to bronchospasm [92]. This hypothesis has been supported by an increasing body of evidence. A few years ago, a correlation was observed between vagal activity and maximal oxygen uptake (VO_{2max}) [93]. Later, the pupillary light reflex of endurance runners revealed an increased parasympathetic activity and a reduced sympathetic activity [94]. More recently, Pichon *et al.* demonstrated that subjects with an increased bronchial hyperesponsiveness had a higher vagal tone [95], which was corroborated by Park *et al.* findings of a relationship between methacholine bronchial responsiveness and diminished sweat secretion, tearing and salivary flow rate in healthy athletes [96].

The variability among patients in response to anti-cholinergic treatment of exercise-induced bronchospasm led Knöpfli *et al.* [97] to study the response to ipratropium and correlate it with another measure of vagal activity (using R–R interval variability on electrocardiogram) in children. A significant protective effect of ipratropium was found, with a post-exercise FEV1 being closely correlated (r = 0.9, p<0.002) with vagal activity. Thus, differences among patients in responsiveness to anti-cholinergic treatment can be related to differences in vagal activity. Scrutinizing in advance those athletes who present higher parasympathetic activity could possibly help to predict those who will respond favorably to this class of drugs.

Ipratropium bromide is also available in some countries for intranasal application but it blocks almost exclusively rhinorrhea. It is effective in allergic and nonallergic patients with rhinorrhea and may be beneficial before exercise in rhinitic athletes [98], particularly in vasomotor and cold rhinitis [99]. Local side-effects are minor and there is almost no systemic anti-cholinergic activity.

The overall rate of adverse effects of ipratropium, when administered by inhalation is low [90]. Side effects resembling those of other anti-cholinergics are minimal. However, dry mouth and sedation have been reported. Also, effects such as skin flushing, tachycardia, acute angle-closure glaucoma, nausea, palpitations and headache have been observed. Current use of inhaled anti-cholinergic drugs increases the risk of acute urinary retention, especially if administered *via* a nebulizer [100].

Inhaled ipratropium bromide is not part of prohibited WADA 2012 substances [10].

Anti-Leukotrienes

The cysteinyl leukotrienes, LTC4, LTD4, and LTE4, as well as LTB4, have long been implicated in the pathogenesis of asthma. The cysteinyl leukotrienes are potent bronchoconstrictors (100 to 1000 times more potent than histamine), with additional effects on blood vessels, mucociliary clearance, and eosinophilic inflammation. The cysteinyl leukotrienes are newly generated mediators produced in eosinophils, mast cells, and other cells commonly associated with asthma. As the understanding of the biochemical pathways for the leukotrienes evolved, so did efforts to pharmacologically inhibit or antagonize this pathway, both at the enzyme and receptor level [101]. The compounds which antagonize the cysteinyl leukotrienes 1 receptor that are currently available for clinical use in humans include montelukast, pranlukast and zafirlukast. Of these, montelukast appears to have the highest binding affinity to the cysteinyl leukotrienes 1 receptor in biologic receptor binding models [102]. Zileuton is the only leukotriene modifier available that works by inhibiting the production of leukotrienes (through inhibition of the 5-Lipoxygenase enzyme), and it is available only in the United States. These types of drugs have a broader range of activity as they inhibit the production of all the leukotrienes, including LTB4 [101].

Clinical and physiologic studies of drugs which interfere with the leukotrienes pathway (both cysteinyl leukotrienes 1 receptor antagonists and synthesis inhibitors) confirm their activity as modest bronchodilators and their ability to improve FEV_1, symptoms and exacerbations in adults and children over time [101, 103-108]. However, comparison studies consistently demonstrate that inhaled corticosteroids are superior to anti-leukotrienes drugs [109-111]. Studies also suggest anti-leukotriene drugs can be effective when added to ongoing therapy with inhaled corticosteroids, although the improvements are less than those seen with long-acting beta2-agonists, as retrieved by a Cochrane review [112].

Zafirlukast, the first leukotriene antagonist to be approved in the United States for asthma, showed protection against EI-bronchoconstriction in both adults [113] and children [114] when given eight hours before an exercise test. Pranlukast, mostly used in Japan, showed a similar protective effect after 14 days of treatment [115]. Other inhibitors of the activity of leukotrienes such as zileuton, have also shown beneficial effects in patients with EI-bronchoconstriction [116]. In 2007, a new indication for montelukast sodium, which was approved in the United States since 1998 for the treatment of persistent asthma, was added by Food and Drug Administration: to prevent EI-bronchoconstriction in patients aged above 15 years. In most countries, this is the only leukotriene antagonist that has received approval by drug regulatory agencies for prevention of EI-bronchoconstriction.

In all studies of leukotriene modifiers, it has become apparent that some but not all patients with asthma respond to this class of drugs [109, 117]. This is true also for the prevention of EI-bronchoconstriction in athletes [11], although it should be noted that in athletes only few studies have been performed to assess the effect of montelukast. The first studies reported that anti-leukotrienes consistently reduced by 30 to 60% EI-bronchoconstriction [116, 118-120]. Furthermore, the amount of inhibition is comparable to that produced by pretreatment with cromolyn [121]. In children, inhibition ranged was from 30 to 40% and therefore somewhat less than that seen in adults [114, 122, 123]. However, later studies highlighted the discrepancy of results in this matter. A 12-week study in adults, demonstrated sustained protection against EI-bronchoconstriction when montelukast was taken 16–18 hours prior to exercise [120]; these effects were significantly greater than outcomes with salmeterol administered in the same time frame prior to exercise in 8-week studies [124, 125]. This result is similar to data reported in a later study by Steinshamn *et al.*, in which an improved physical performance was observed with montelukast [126]. Later, another study found no effects of montelukast both on symptoms or objective inflammation parameters of elite ice hockey players [127]. Yet another study found evidence of protection of EI-bronchoconstriction in athletes (91% of protection when exposed to eucapnic voluntary hyperpnoea and 73% when exposed to an exercise test) [128], while another performed in children retrieved 46 to 66% of protection [123].

Also, anti-leukotrienes have consistently proved their beneficial effects in both seasonal and perennial rhinitis [129-132], which led to its approval by the Food and Drug Administration for this indication as well. In athletes with both rhinitis and asthma, this drug could be regarded as an option. Another important focus of research regarding anti-leukotrienes is their potential for treatment of chronic urticaria. Leukotriene receptor antagonists are currently the best-studied group of drugs after the antihistamines, in the therapy of chronic urticaria [101]. However, the leukotriene receptor antagonists are not alternative agents to antihistamines. The excellent safety, absence of required monitoring in the case of montelukast and zafirlukast, and wide availability make leukotriene receptor antagonists the preferred supplementary agents to try with antihistamines. However, although they appear to be useful as both monotherapy and add-on therapy, they are not likely to displace antihistamines from their role as first-line therapy [133]. There is anecdotal evidence of effectiveness of antileukotrienes in primary cold urticaria, delayed pressure urticaria and dermographism, but no evidence exists for other physical urticarias, including EI-anaphylaxis or EI-urticaria [133].

These drugs are dosed orally from one to four times daily (Table **2**), and some data suggest that compliance/adherence is better than with inhaled asthma medications. Zafirlukast is given as a 20mg dose orally twice daily, but can be safely increased to 40 mg daily, as some reports suggest greater efficacy at higher doses, while no indication exist that higher doses of montelukast may be more effective. In the case of zileuton, one study suggested that when clinical stability is achieved, the dose can be reduced to twice daily [117].

In general, anti-leukotrienes are well tolerated [101]. However, as all leukotriene modifiers are metabolized by the hepatic P450 enzyme system, the possibility for significant interactions with other drugs metabolized by this system clearly exists. Although only few such interactions have been reported, it is important to note that Zileuton is metabolized *via* the specific cytochrome P450 system, which metabolizes theophylline. Though theophylline is not common to use for EI-asthma, doctors should bear in mind that recommendations for concurrent use suggest decreasing the theophylline dose by 50% and then checking a theophylline level. Montelukast does not have any known drug interactions [101]. Some increase of transaminases have also been reported, although in very small scale and only for zileuton [104]. Despite the general strong safety profile obtained from a decade of use and the rarity of reported adverse events with montelukast, prescribers should always be aware that recently reports of rare occurrences of neuropsychiatric events have been reported in patients taking montelukast, zafirlukast, and zileuton. These include behavior- and mood-related changes (agitation including aggressive behavior, bad/vivid dreams, depression, feeling anxious, hallucinations, irritability, restlessness, suicidal thoughts and actions, tremor, or trouble sleeping) [15]. Of perhaps greatest concern is the possible association of anti-leukotrienes therapy with Churg-Strauss syndrome, a rare eosinophilic vasculitis. Shortly after marketing, reports of Churg-Strauss syndrome began to appear in some patients taking montelukast and other leukotriene-modifying medications. Although the FDA issued a warning about this syndrome appearing in patients taking leukotriene-modifying medications, the possibility that this condition might be the direct result of treatment with these agents remains unproven [15]. No epidemic of Churg-Strauss syndrome has developed since millions of doses of medications were prescribed over a decade of use. However, this issue has not been resolved and in a recent review of 62 cases, it was concluded that available evidence suggests an association between leukotriene antagonists and Churg-Strauss Syndrome that may be causal [134].

In the particular case of patients practicing sports, it is also of importance to note that no tolerance develops with anti-leukotrienes [123], on the contrary to what often is seen with regular treatment with inhaled beta2-agonists. Currently, no restrictions to anti-leukotrienes use are considered in the WADA Prohibited List [10].

Mast Cell Stabilizers (Chromones)

Cromolyn sodium and nedocromil sodium, members of the chromone group of chemical compounds, were discovered and developed in 1965 and 1979, respectively [135]. These compounds are chemically and pharmacologically distinct from other drugs used in the treatment of allergic disease in patients practicing sports. They act directly on the mucosal surface involved in the allergic disease, by blocking the activation of the calcium channel that follows cross-linking of membrane-bound IgE by antigen; without intracellular calcium, the histamine vesicles cannot fuse to the cell membrane, and the release of histamine and other inflammatory mediators is prevented. This mechanism is distinctly different from that of the corticosteroids: chromones are effective in blocking the acute reaction to allergic challenge, while corticosteroids are not. Both drugs block the late reaction. Single doses of chromones will prevent EI-asthma and other acute challenges; corticosteroids will not [135]. Besides, chromones also act by modulation of nerve reflexes causing symptoms: cromolyn sodium has been shown to inhibit substance P-induced microvascular leakage in the rat trachea [136], while nedocromil sodium inhibits substance P-induced histamine release from human lung mast cells [135]. Moreover, both cromolyn sodium and nedocromil sodium inhibit IgE antibody production [135]. Different formulations are available, to be used in different allergic diseases: inhalers for asthma, nasal sprays to treat allergic rhinitis, eye drops for allergic conjunctivitis and as oral preparations they are used for mastocytosis.

Both cromolyn sodium and nedocromil sodium provide useful protection against an exercise challenge and reduce the degree of bronchoconstriction induced by the inhalation of mannitol; therefore, they are approved in most countries for EI-asthma, although they are not used as frequently today [90, 135, 137-139]. Their popularity was waned in part because of the current availability of more effective, faster, longer acting, and easier to take medications. Because of their excellent safety profile, they were used extensively in children with EI-bronchoconstriction. A systematic review of 20 Randomized Controled Trials (15 studying children and 5 studying adults) with patients aged above 6 years showed that 4 mg of nedocromil inhaled 15 to 60 minutes before exercise significantly reduced the severity and duration of EI-bronchoconstriction compared with placebo [140]. It had a greater effect on patients with severe EI-bronchoconstriction (defined as an exercise-induced fall in lung function >30% from baseline) [140]. They can work alone or in combination when other medications have failed to significantly block the airway response to exercise. Corticosteroid sparing effect was demonstrated by a 50% reduction in inhaled corticosteroid usage use, when nedocromil was added, without loss of effect [135]. Added benefit was also demonstrated in patients inadequately controlled on inhaled corticosteroid treatment [135]. It is important to consider their use especially when other medications have been proven inadequate since mechanisms of action are different [15]. Cromolyn sodium and nedocromil sodium are now generic drugs in all countries and should also be considered when the expense of medication is a concern [15]. Compared to anti-cholinergic agents, mast cell stabilizers are more effective at attenuating bronchoconstriction, providing more individuals with complete protection (73% *vs.* 56% for anti-cholinergics) and clinical protection (defined as 50% improvement over placebo) [90]. When compared to short acting beta2-agonists, mast cell stabilizers are not as effective at preventing deterioration, as evidenced in a systematic review of 24 Randomized Controled Trials, with an average maximum decrease in the FEV1 of 11.9% compared with 4.6% for beta2-agonists. However they had less side effects [90]. Fewer children had complete protection (defined in this study as maximum % decrease in FEV_1 <15% post-exercise) or clinical protection [90]. Combining mast cell stabilizers with a short acting beta2-agonist did not produce significant advantages to pulmonary function over short acting beta-agonists alone. Recently, it has been shown that mast cell activation with release of bronchoconstrictive mediators occurs after hyperpnea in athletes with and without EI-bronchoconstriction, a phenomena that was inhibited by sodium cromoglycate [141]. When compared between each other, both chromones are equally effective in preventing EI-bronchoconstriction in asthmatics [142]. A systematic review including eight Randomized Controlled Trials (5 studying children) with patients aged over 6 years found no significant difference between nedocromil and cromoglycate with regards to decrease in FEV_1, complete protection, clinical protection, or side effects [142].

Kennedy was the first to provide evidence for an anti-inflammatory effect of cromolyn sodium, showing a significant reduction in sputum eosinophils with cromolyn sodium treatment compared with placebo [143]. In the same year, however, Altounyan and Howell, in their report on the first 100 patients treated with inhaled cromolyn sodium, pointed out that the therapeutic effects of cromolyn and corticosteroids are not wholly interchangeable [144]. In fact, when it comes to efficacy of chromones on chronic asthma, a recent Cochrane systematic review found that there is insufficient evidence to be sure about the efficacy of sodium cromoglycate over placebo and that publication bias could have possibly overestimated the beneficial effects of sodium cromoglycate as maintenance therapy in childhood asthma [145]. On the other hand, concerning the efficacy of chromones when compared to inhaled corticosteroids for chronic asthma, comparative trials of the two classes of drugs raise important concerns. First of all, using the two classes of drugs under similar circumstances implies the assumption that all patients with chronic asthma have a common underlying mechanism, which is not the case. Chronic asthma involves more than one type of inflammation, and different mechanisms. Moreover, many of the early trials of inhaled cromolyn sodium in asthma were conducted in asthmatics that were inadequately controlled with inhaled [146, 147] or even oral [135, 148] corticosteroids, or theophylline-dependent asthma patients [149], which probably represent different phenotypes of asthma. Even so, adding cromolyn to existing treatment provided significantly better control of the asthma.

These principles hold good today and are reflected in the use of the two classes of drugs also in vernal keratoconjunctivitis and atopic dermatitis; they are complimentary and not competitive [135]. In a trial of a topical skin lotion of cromolyn sodium in atopic dermatitis [150], the addition of cromolyn resulted in an improvement in the severity of the atopic dermatitis and a significant reduction in the use of topical corticosteroids. Both cromolyn sodium and nedocromil sodium are indicated for the treatment of allergic and nonallergic eosinophilic conjunctivitis, vernal keratoconjunctivitis, and giant papillary conjunctivitis [151, 152]. Both drugs can also be useful in the relief of acute eye symptoms. In the treatment of vernal keratoconjunctivitis, cromolyn and nedocromil eyedrops are used in conjunction with corticosteroid eyedrops and allow a reduced use of the latter [135]. Cromones are available as nasal solution, which has been shown to be better than placebo in controlled trials of patients with seasonal allergic rhinitis and in perennial allergic and non-allergic rhinitis. However, they are less effective than intranasal H1-antihistamines and their effect is short lasting [153]. The use of cromolyn sodium has shown variable results in the prophylactic treatment of patients with EI-anaphylaxis [154-156]. However, it remains unknown if inhaled mast cell stabilizers, administered on a daily basis, maintain sufficient systemic concentration levels necessary to be adequately prophylactic against EI-anaphylaxis.

Efficacy depends upon the efficiency of distribution on the surface affected: bronchial mucosa, nasal mucosa, conjunctivae, or gut mucosa. Therefore in the treatment of EI-asthma efficacy depends on the amount of drug reaching the lungs and the distribution of the drug within the lower airways. As efficacy is related to the amount of drug reaching the airways, the optimal dose of cromolyn sodium with metered-dose inhaler (MDI) will be when used in conjunction with a large (750 mL) spacer [157, 158]. However, since the removal of chloroflurocarbon propellants and the current non-availability of hydrofluoroalkane inhalers for either medication in many countries, chromones are mainly available as dry powder inhalers and nebulizable solution (available in the United States), which further limits their utilization.

The treatment regimen should start with four times a day dosing. Once symptomatic improvement has been achieved, dose frequency can be reduced to 2 to 3 times a day, or dose frequency should be increased if symptom exacerbation occurs. In the case of prevention of EI-asthma, it is recommended that for patients with normal spirometry, the preferred treatment would be either cromolyn sodium 2, 10, or 20 mg, or 4 or 8 mg of nedocromil sodium inhaled immediately before exercise [159].

These drugs are poorly absorbed, not metabolized, excreted unchanged, and have low toxicity. Extensive safety evaluation studies in a range of species by various routes of administration and different durations of dosing at many multiples of the clinical doses have shown a very low order of toxicity for both cromolyn sodium and nedocromil sodium [135]. Both compounds have almost no systemic pharmacologic activity, do not influence the incidence of neoplasia, have no effect on normal host defense mechanisms, and have no teratogenic effects [160, 161]. A summary of human safety considerations showed that nedocromil sodium has an excellent safety profile and is well tolerated and that adverse effects are generally mild [162]. A non-significant difference in side effects was demonstrated with 3% of those receiving mast cell stabilizers compared to 11% of short acting beta-agonist patients experiencing side effects [90]. Hypersensitivity to cromolyn sodium has been reported in individual rare cases [135].

Chromones are not among WADA prohibited substances [10].

Omalizumab

Omalizumab is a humanized monoclonal antibody that binds selectively to the human immunoglobulin E (IgE) in its Cε3 domain, and not through the crystallisable fraction of epsilon receptor 1 (FcεRI) [163]. Lower stimulation of this receptor leads to a decrease in its expression within effectors cells such as mast cells, basophils and dendritic cells. Also, the reduction in free IgE and FcεRI leads to a decrease in allergens processing and their presentation to Th2 lymphocytes, along with a reduction in Th2 cells differentiation and lower expression of cytokines from this profile (IL-4, IL-5, IL-13). In patients with asthma, the most relevant anti-inflammatory effect of omalizumab is the capacity to induce eosinophils apoptosis as well as reducing eosinophilia in sputum and bronchial biopsies [164]. The Food and Drug Administration and the European Medicines Agency approved the use of omalizumab in patients with severe persistent asthma, proven to be allergic and IgE-mediated, with frequent symptoms during the day or waking up during the night and history of many severe ‘exacerbations’ of asthma despite treatment with high doses of inhaled corticosteroids plus a long-acting inhaled beta2-agonist [165]. It was first approved for patients over 12 years of age (these must also have reduced lung function - less than 80% of normal), and lately in patients of over six years. Ever since, a large number of publications have emerged about the use of omalizumab in patients with allergic diseases rather than asthma without response with standard therapy. However, in what concerns to athletes, no report of omalizumab use was presented until now. This is probably related to the strict indications of omalizumab, since athletes typically do not present persistent asthma but rather symptoms triggered by exercise.

Systemic Corticosteroids

Systemic corticosteroids were first shown to be effective in the treatment of acute asthma in 1956 [166]. Ever since, numerous studies have documented their effectiveness in acute asthma. Systemic corticosteroids are most often used as rescue therapy for acute and severe asthma exacerbations and can be given orally, intravenously or intramuscularly. For a given amount of anti-asthmatic efficacy, the development of systemic side effects (*e.g.*, hypothalamo–pituitary–adrenal axis suppression) is greater with oral steroids (approximately four-fold) [27]. Utilization of systemic corticosteroids for treatment of chronic physical urticaria, including delayed pressure urticaria, has a very low quality of evidence [167]. Regarding anaphylaxis, guidelines differ in their recommendations for administration of corticosteroids [168, 169].

Interestingly, a clear consensus regarding the optimal dose and duration of treatment has yet to be reached [29]. Because the duration of treatment is partly related to the severity of the episode, recommendations regarding the duration of treatment are often tailored to the individual case. It often also depends on the individual's response, but should span 4–12 days. Because orally administered corticosteroids are rapidly absorbed and have been found to be as effective as intravenous corticosteroids, oral therapy can be used in most cases [170].

Acute administration of corticosteroids produces central nervous system effects, including changes in mood ranging from euphoria to psychosis, irritability, depression, increased appetite, and suppression of the HPA axis. When these result from brief steroid administration, all symptoms are reversed after discontinuation of medication [27]. Recovery of the hypothalamic–pituitary–

adrenal (HPA) axis is rapid (*i.e.*, requires days) after brief (≤1 week), treatment with high-dose corticosteroids [27].

Table 2: Drugs most frequently used to treat EI-asthma (adapted from Carlsen 2012 [16])

Drug	Type	Notes
Inhaled corticosteroids	**Controller**	Presently the most important treatment available. Ciclesonide may be particularly suited for both children and athletes, due to lack of side-effects. For athletes, the lack of adrenal suppression may be of particular importance for performance
	Budesonide	Daily doses - Low: 200–400µg; Medium: 400–600µg; High: >600µg
	Fluticasone	Daily doses - Low: 88–264µg; Medium: 264–660µg; High: >660µg
	Ciclesonide*	Daily doses - Low: 80-160µg; Medium: 160-320µg; High: >320µg
Anti-leukotrienes	**Controller**	Montelukast protects against EI-asthma without the development of tolerance. Several patients are non-responders. Effect should be controlled through follow-up.
Receptor antagonists	Zafirlukast	Children > 12 years and adults: 20–40mg p.o. twice daily
	Montelukast	Children 2–5 year-old: 4mg p.o. daily; Children 5–10 year-old: 5mg p.o. daily; Children >12year-old and adults: 10mg p.o. daily
	Pranlukast	Children: 3.5 mg/kg bid; Adults: 225mg p.o. twice daily
5-LO inhibitors	Zileuton	Children > 12 year-old and adults: 600mg p.o. four times a day
Cromones	**Controller**	More effective than inhaled anti-cholinergics at attenuating EI-bronchoconstriction, but less than short-acting beta2-agonists
Inhaled beta2-agonists	**Reliever**	Short-acting: Useful for pretreatment before exercise and for reliever treatment of dyspnoea. Regular use may cause tolerance development. Long-acting: Useful with uncontrolled EI-asthma both in schoolchildren and adolescent athletes. Regular use may give tolerance development. Should not be used without concomitant inhaled corticosteroids.
Short-acting	Salbutamol	Time of onset: 2–3 min; Approximate duration of action: 4-6 h
Long-acting	Salmeterol	Time of onset: 30 min; Approximate duration of action: >12 h
	Formoterol	Time of onset: 2–3 min; Approximate duration of action: >12 h
Inhaled anti-cholinergics	**Reliever**	May be particularly useful in athletes due to possible cholinergic involvement in pathogenesis.
	Ipratropium	Can be used as premedication 45 minutes before exercise. Particularly useful in endurance athletes.
	Tiotropium	Not approved for asthma treatment. Not studied for EI-asthma or in athletes. Potentially of importance in athletes.
Omalizumab	**Controller**	Approved for treatment of moderate to severe allergic asthma. Not studied for EI-asthma.

*Approved for adults and adolescent patients with 12 or more years of age.

When systemic corticosteroids use is necessary, doctors should bear in mind that is mandatory to ask for a TUE [10].

Nasal Corticosteroids

Intranasal glucocorticosteroids are the most efficacious medication for rhinitis treatment [153]. The impact of exercise on rhinitis and the effect of rhinitis on exercise has been receiving progressively more attention since the 1984 Olympics; even though nowadays the potential impact of rhinitis on athletic performance is known, it is still under-recognized and under-treated in this population [171, 172].

Rhinitis occurs very frequently in athletes. In several studies published in the last two decades, a prevalence ranging from 13.3 to 48.6% was found [173]. Rhinitis symptoms also vary according to the sports activity practiced, having the highest prevalence in endurance athletes and swimmers [174, 175]. They also depend on environmental conditions as, in most exercise conditions, athletes are strongly and repeatedly exposed to large amounts of aeroallergens, pollutants, including smoke, and different climate conditions [1]. Inhaled air temperature and humidity usually affect this disease [176]. In swimmers, contact with a specific irritant, chlorine derivatives, is also related with increased symptoms [177].

Comprehension of nasal physiology and pathophysiology during exercise enable us to understand why rhinitis is so prevalent in athletes and the role/risk of nasal corticosteroids. Nose is constituted by a mucosa filled with vessels and mucosa glands, which are responsible for filtration, humidification and warming of the inhaled air before it reaches the lungs. This conditioning function is mainly dependent on nasal mucosa blood vessels, which are regulated by autonomic nervous system [173]. Autonomic reflexes usually improve nasal efficiency during training. As nasal sympathetic activity is increased, venous sinusoids constrict, which reduces nasal congestion. Some patients experience improvement with exercise, mediated by the nasal sympathetic tone, while others may have their symptoms worsen. During training, athletes are repeatedly exposed to several risk factors (allergens, cold air and pollutants) by which their contact with this nasal mucosa are responsible for the increasing symptoms of rhinitis in susceptible individuals [173]. Vasomotor rhinitis occurs associated with temperature changes, like in ice sports with the contact with cold air, which is known as “the skiers nose”. This stimuli induces glandular hyper-secretion, nasal discharge and congestion [178]. Constant nasal resistance changes during endurance exercise leads to nasal mucosa dehydration, inducing increase of mucociliary transport system and leads to thickening of secretions; this promotes a rebound increase in nasal secretion as a compensatory mechanism of dehydration, known as “runners nose” [179]. Rhinosinusal problems might also have a traumatic origin in athletes, which is most frequent in recurrent trauma as commonly happens in boxers.

Probably, altered airflow dynamics and ventilation induced by nasal obstruction can potentially have a negative effect in sport activities, mainly in high-intensity [172]. Also, as rhinitis affects sleep, it leads to difficulties in maintaining concentration, which has an understandable impact on sports performance. So, even though a direct association has not yet been proved, an indirect one is easily extrapolated [172]. The nasal corticosteroids are used to prevent these effects due to their close contact with mucosa inflammation.

Management of rhinitis encompasses a multifactor approach, directed to the type of rhinitis: allergic or non-allergic. This approach includes patient education, environmental control and pharmacotherapy, especially nasal corticosteroids [153]. Appropriate management is similar to the treatment of rhinitis in general population [153, 180], but adapted accordingly to WADA guidelines [181]. WADA recommends treatment to be monitored by the treating physician and advices topical intranasal corticosteroids as the main option [182]. If necessary, association with other treatments can be made namely with antihistamines or topical nasal decongestants. Surgery may be also beneficial and is indicated for athletes who have failed medical therapy. Allergy testing is also recommended, especially if an atopic component is suspected, as this information has implications on allergen avoidance measures and other treatment options, namely immunotherapy. In ARIA (Allergic Rhinitis and its Impact on Asthma) guidelines [153], allergic rhinitis treatment is initiated accordingly to: 1) frequency of symptoms: if they are intermittent (less than 4 days a week or less than 4 weeks at a time) or persistent (more than 4 days a week or more than 4 weeks at a time), and 2) severity of the symptoms. Rhinitis is classified as mild if the patient does not feel any impact on quality of life or sleep with symptoms. Otherwise, a moderate-to-severe rhinitis is present if related to sleep disturbance and impairment of daily life activity, work, school or sport practice [153, 180]. For persistent moderate-to-severe rhinitis, nasal corticosteroids are used as first line; in the intermittent or mild rhinitis an option can be made between nasal corticosteroids and antihistamines as the first line [153, 180]. Some authors consider that nasal corticosteroids should be used in athletes as a first-line therapy for all allergic rhinitis types as to accommodate some factors specific to this competitive population [172]. For chronic rhinosinusitis, topical corticosteroids are the first line treatment in both mild and moderate/severe disease [183]. When considering a prescription to an athlete, indications can vary according to efficacy and safety, both at rest and during exercise training [172].

Intranasal glucocorticoids, due to their topic and direct administration, achieve high local concentrations and act directly in the receptors of the nasal mucosa [153]. Intranasal glucocorticosteroids are the most efficacious medication available for allergic and non-allergic rhinitis treatment [153, 184]. They decrease all symptoms of allergic rhinitis as well as ocular symptoms [153]. In rhinosinusitis, they also help to achieve disease control, reducing nasal blockage, rhinorrhea or postnasal drip, increasing smell and preventing bothersome facial pain or headache [183]. They have a relatively slow onset of action (12h) and maximum efficacy over days and weeks. Topical steroids should be given regularly [185]. There is a discussion about prescribing these drugs in a continuous or on-demand treatment. In a recent systematic review [186], that extracted data from 59 randomized controlled trials, therapeutic index reflecting efficacy and safety for different intranasal corticosteroids in allergic rhinitis was studied. The parameters for efficacy included patient rated total nasal symptom score and ocular symptoms. All outcomes were significantly improved. Nasal score showed a better effect with mometasone furoate, followed by budesonide. For the ocular score, budesonide studies were superior to the other nasal corticosteroids; in patient's global assessment, budesonide also had the best effect. It is supported by high quality of evidence [180] and meta-analysis [187] that intranasal glucocorticoids are more effective than oral and topical H1-antihistamines [180]. In a cross-sectional survey in 446 athletes, treatment with corticosteroids was associated with significantly improvement of nasal symptoms and quality of life, as well as performance [188]. Numerous studies have now been published comparing the effect of cysteinyl leukotrienes either alone or in combination with antihistamines to the effect of nasal steroids, in particular nasal fluticasone [189-193]. In every study, the nasal corticosteroid is more efficacious in improving rhinitis symptoms than the cysteinyl leukotrienes.

The current intranasal preparations are well tolerated and adverse effects are few in number, mild in severity and not significantly different from placebo. Even with long-term use, nasal corticosteroids are well tolerated and not associated with mucosal atrophy [194]. Also due to their topic action and small systemic absorption, they do not have other side effects related to oral corticosteroid; namely, no evidence exists of suppression of the hypothalamic pituitary-adrenal axis or bone mineral density loss [153, 195]. Growth in children, however, is a concern. In a clinical trial with a 1 year follow-up, no changes were observed in growth rate with the use of intranasal corticosteroids [196]. The most frequent local side effects are crusting, dryness and minor epistaxis [185, 195]. In a recent systematic review [186], side effects for all in market nasal corticosteroids formulations were studied: epistaxis was associated with all, but this risk was higher with fluticasone furoate. Ocular side effects reported include increase of intraocular pressure and posterior subcapsular cataracts, but this was evidenced only on two case reports; the other trials showed no significant differences regarding intraocular pressure [186]. Side effects, namely the local ones, usually tolerated by normal population might have an impact on athletic performance and well being, so athletes should be followed to prevent them [172].

Swimmers are a specific population and have a significant worsening of nasal function after training experience. This was first reported by Alves *et al.* in a trial that measured peak nasal inspiratory flow and symptoms in swimmers and runners. Swimmers had lower flow and more postnasal drip than the runners, independently of their atopic status [177]. This effect might be explained by continuous chlorine inhalation, as shown in an experimental cross-over design in which chlorine exposure significantly increased nasal airways resistance in seasonal allergic rhinitis patients [197]. Even though individuals with nasal allergy were more likely to have EI-rhinitis, a questionnaire survey about EI-rhinitis symptoms applied to 164 participants, 59 allergic individuals receiving immunotherapy as well as 105 non-allergic revealed that at least 27.7% of non-allergic athletes reported symptoms and almost 53% of these presented indoor EI-rhinitis symptoms, predominantly rhinorrhea [198]. A specific history of indoor and outdoor exercise triggers should be taken into account on athletes complaining of nasal symptoms. In this paper, at least 40% of the participants indicated that their symptoms adversely affected their athletic performance [198].

As athletes are constantly changing their training places, they are frequently submitted to different environments (allergens and irritants) exposures [199]. Therefore, environmental control of the relevant allergens should be promoted, for example through aerobiological records of pollens, like the ones seated up for Athens Olympic Games [200]. Irritants reported to cause nasal symptoms, include tobacco smoke, pollution, chlorine and cold air [201]. To prevent high level exposure to these agents some techniques were tried, namely improvements of ventilation systems in swimming pools and ice arenas [173] and implementation of country level measures to reduce global pollution, similar to what happened in Beijing Olympic Games [202]. Exercise by-itself can pose an increase risk in athletes, as it induces modulation of innate and adaptive immune system, which is dependent on host defence, activity level and disease susceptibility [203]. This might explain why in some cases there seems to be an increased susceptibility of elite athletes to infection, namely upper respiratory tract infection [172, 204] and increase infections complications in already prone athletes with rhinitis.

Though highly trained endurance athletes are indeed at an increased risk, they are frequently under treated. In a cross-sectional survey carried in Finland in 2002 including 494 athletes from the Olympic committee, only half were taking anti-allergic medication; those treated with topical corticosteroid had a significant improvement in nasal symptoms and quality of life [188]. In a clinical trial with 326 Olympic and Paralympics athletes from Australia with diagnostic criteria of seasonal rhinoconjuntivitis, 145 were treated with intranasal budesonide and 91 refused to use any treatment. Those in the intervention group had a significant improvement on nasal and eye symptoms and quality of life scores, but also in performance (accessed by a question about the athlete ability to perform optimally at training and competition), after 8 weeks of treatment. Nasal corticosteroids are fundamental for EI-rhinitis improving nasal and eye symptoms and also performance; their use should be monitored and not delayed.

Nasal corticosteroids do not need currently any TUE [10].

H1-Antihistamines

H1-antihistamines are available worldwide and they are one of the most available drugs for the treatment of allergic diseases, namely rhinitis, urticaria, atopic dermatitis or other skin dermatoses [153]. They have an inverse agonist or neutral antagonist activity at the H1-histamine receptor [172]. The recommended treatment in the most updated guidelines for allergic diseases are the new-generation oral H1-antihistamines that do not have anti-cholinergic, sedative, cognitive and psychomotor side-effects [180]. Athletes benefit the most with these choices, namely endurance athletes, since the sedative effect could impair their psychomotor skills [172, 173]. Some authors even propose a cautious approach in prescription of any antihistamines 24-48 hours before any major competition [172]. Histamine has a multiplicity of roles in human health, namely in allergic inflammation and immune modulation.

Histamine is a low molecular-weight amine, synthesized from L-histidine exclusively by an enzyme, histidine decarboxylase (HDC), that is expressed in cells throughout the body, including central nervous system, gastric-mucosa parietal cells, mast cells, and basophils. Histamine exerts its diverse biologic effects through four types of receptors, inducing different functions accordingly to each receptor and type of cell; most of them induce an increase in pruritus and nasal congestion, except the H2 receptor which is related to gastric acid secretion [205]. H1-receptor (HR1) stimulates the immune cells and leads to a pro-inflammatory activity; also, a more recently found receptor H4-receptor (HR4) has a pro-inflammatory potential. On the other hand, H2-receptor (HR2) is a potent suppressor of inflammatory functions. Histamine modulates neuro-transmissors release through presynaptic H3-receptors (HR3) of the central and peripheral nervous system [206]. Thus, histamine has a central role in allergic-inflammatory responses [207]. Mast cells and basophils are the major source of granule-stored histamine. After the cross-linking of surface IgE by allergen or through mechanisms independent of IgE, these cells degranulate and release histamine with other pre-formed mediators. Most histamine allergic symptoms occur through the link with HR1. Hypotension, tachycardia, flushing and headache occur through both the HR1 and HR2 present in the vessels, whereas cutaneous itch and nasal congestion may occur through both the HR1 and HR3 [208]. Histamine contributes also for the progression of allergic-inflammatory response by enhancing the secretion of pro-inflammatory cytokines, adhesion molecules and migration of inflammatory cells [207, 209]. Antigen presenting cells can be regulated by this molecule, which exerts immunomodulatory effects through the regulation of T-lymphocytes and antibody isotypes [207]. Histamine enhances Th1-type responses by triggering HR1, which is expressed mostly in these cells; then increases IFN-γ production and Th1 proliferation. H2R suppresses both Th1 and Th2 function while promoting T reg cells. Chemotactic functions, which are linked to dendritic cells and leukocytes regulation, are dependent on H4R expression. Specific neuronal activation is mostly mediated by H3R, which alters neurotransmissors release with downstream effects on T cell chemokine secretion. Histamine actions have been recently studied in relation to exercise and exercise-induced fatigue in a mouse model [210]. The link between exercise and histamine role is mediated by H1R and nitric oxide production in the vessels that dilates pre-capillary arterioles and increases capillary permeability, providing the supply of O2 and nutrients when freed at muscular level. Prolonged walking induces HDC enzyme, which produces histamine in mice model and in humans, which might mediate post-exercise hyperaemia by H1R and H2R receptors. In this mice model, treatment with HR1 antagonist lead to lesser endurance capacity with prolonged walking in comparison with the controls, and the same happened in mice deficient in HDC enzyme or in HR1 [210]. It is being now hypothesized that histamine might be involved in the protection against exercise induced fatigue or exhaustion, but this hypothesis has not been studied yet in humans.

H1 antihistamines act as inverse agonists that combine and stabilize the inactive form HR1, maintaining it in an inactive state [205]. Antihistamines can be divided accordingly to their chemical class in alkylamines, piperazine, piperidines, ethanolamines, ethylenediamines and phenotiazines (Table **3**). However, the most used classification is functional as first generation, which are sedating, and second generation which are relatively non-sedating [206]. Besides down-regulation of allergic inflammation, mainly through their action in HR1, they potentially cause adverse effects through their action in the muscarinic, α-adrenergic, serotonin receptors and cardiac-ion channels. These drugs prevent and suppress the response to histamine or allergen in the nasal and conjunctival mucosa, but also allergen-induced wheal appearance and skin flares [206], and that should be bear in mind when it comes to perform skin prick tests to analyse possible sensitizations in athletes. Pre-treatment with oral H1 antihistamines reduces the early response to an allergen challenge in the conjunctiva, nose, lower airway and skin. Oral and topical antihistamines are available topical are frequently adequate for nasal mucosa and conjunctivae symptoms treatment. Duration of action of H1 antihistamines depends on the type, but most second-generation lasts 24h, which facilitates the once-daily-dosing. Specific populations, such as elderly or patients with hepatic and renal dysfunction, might need a reduced dose/dose frequency. After discontinuing treatment and dependent of the agent used, residual suppression on the skin test might be maintained, that varies for 24-48h to one week.

H1-antihistamines are effective and indicated in allergic rhinitis and conjunctivitis, urticaria, atopic dermatitis and other dermatoses related to skin itch, and also can be used in anaphylaxis. Oral H1 antihistamines are the first line treatment for mild to moderate rhinitis, as reported in ARIA guidelines [153, 180]. However, it should be noted that first-generation compounds may impair athletic performance due to their sedative effect that reduces athletes psychomotor skills, and their anti-cholinergic actions, namely mucosal drying and reduced sweating [173]. The first clinical choice for patients, and especially in athletes, should be the second-generation, non-sedating antihistamines that have significant less anti-cholinergic effects. Intranasal H1-antihistamine, like azelastine and levocabastine, are locally effective, reducing itching, sneezing, runny nose and nasal congestion [153]. Their use is recommended in adults with seasonal allergic rhinitis [180]. Due to their rapid and topical effect they can be used on demand by athletes to treat acute unexplained symptoms in the sport field [173]. Ocular medication with antihistamine, for example olopatadine, is quite fast and effective in reducing eye symptoms [185]. Although initial studies suggested that antihistamines in combination with cysteinyl leukotrienes may be more efficacious in allergic rhinitis than single-agent therapy alone, additional studies have not supported added benefit from the combination [101, 130].

Several skin-rashes can be associated with exercise. The commonest non-IgE-mediated rashes that appear with exercise are related to physiological flushing, like cholinergic urticaria. This is one of the physical urticaria variants and is triggered by different mechanisms (sweat, temperature, changes in blood flow, emotional and skin with propensity to hypohydrosis) [211]. Clinically, small wheals, of 2-4mm, surrounded by large areas of erythema are observable, and seldom associated with systemic symptoms. Treatment is adapted to their pathophysiologic mechanism, but the first option is antihistamines [211]. Often, rapid cooling can subside an attack and a refractory period may occur after that. Delayed pressure urticaria is another physical urticaria, but is more associated with angioedema. This is particularly distressful in athletes, as they are often submitted to sustained pressure stimulus, like soles after running, prolonged grips of sports equipment or buttocks after long distance cycling or rowing. Localized deep pressure painful swelling can appear and maintain for several hours after a sustained pressure stimulus [24]. Solar urticaria occurs after sun exposure and can be a problem in patients practicing outdoor sports. Management is based on sunscreen use and antihistamine before sun exposure [212]. A tan can lessen the reaction to sunlight. Swimmers suffer specifically from skin diseases related with water contact, namely pool water dermatitis, goggle dermatitis and also diseases mediated by skin contact dermatitis like the swim cap, nose clip, ear plug or diving mask components, like the isopropylparaphenylenediamine, dethylthiourea and other rubber compounds [213]. Aquagenic urticaria is an uncommon disorder elicited only by water contact, independently of the temperature. It is particularly difficult to treat, as it does not respond to antihistamines [24]. Cold contact urticaria is particularly challenging, despite having good response to antihistamines. It occurs after exposure to cold objects/air/fluid/wind and is a very bothersome condition for swimmers, but also for other sports related to cold exposure [213]. In some cases, it induces severe systemic symptoms like anaphylaxis. Other sports-related rashes can arise through contact with allergens, like some types of clothing, gymnastic or weight lifting chalk, judo carpet, billiard cue and adhesives for athletic tape [214]. Second-generation antihistamines are the first line treatment for most of these subtypes of urticaria and also for skin itch symptoms [167, 215].

Antihistamines are very effective in treating these diseases. They can be used also in topic formulation in the nose, conjunctiva or even skin, which enables them to reduce the systemic side effects and also to increase the local efficacy. Pharmacological research and the emergence of second-generation increased their potential use, since side effects were reduced.

In allergic rhinoconjunctivitis antihistamines are effective against symptoms mediated by histamine, namely rhinorrhoea, sneezing, nasal itching and eye symptoms, but less effective on nasal congestion [153]. There is solid clinical evidence, namely through randomized placebo-controlled trials, for the use of several second-generation H1 antihistamines [216-219] (ceterizine, desloratadine, fexofenadine, loratadine and levocetirizine), as well as for use of intranasal H1-antihistamines like azelastine [206]. Rhinitis treatment improved also quality of life in these patients [218, 220]. The most important advantage in topical treatment is their faster onset of action and can be used "as needed" to treat unexpected symptoms in the sport field [173]. In case of eye symptoms, topical ocular antihistamine can be used, like olopatadine, ketotifen [221], which also combine mast cell stabilizing activity [173].

In acute and chronic urticaria, histamine act as a main mediator of pruritus, so H1-antihistamines provide symptomatic relief of itching, reduce the number, size and duration of individual hives and significantly improve quality of life [167]. In a systematic review of the literature, with a meta-analysis, that included 4 studies, the use of these drugs in acquired cold urticaria decreased the pruritus (OR 10.44; 95% CI 4.39 to 24.84) [222]. On delayed pressure urticaria, desloratadine in a clinical trial with 36 patients showed a significant improvement of urticaria symptoms, in dermographometer challenge test and also in the number of episodes [223]. Efficacy in treatment can be improved in patients with chronic spontaneous urticaria which do not respond to standard doses of antihistamines, by increasing the dosage as high as 4 fold [224], and also in those with acquired cold urticaria [225]. Quality of life is also increased with second generation antihistamine use. This has been most studied with desloratadine in randomized placebo-controlled multicentre trials; the use reduced discomfort, anxiety, social impairment and also health status, including physical functioning. These benefits were maintained with continuous daily therapy [226, 227]. Some physicians recommend an association with second generation antihistamines with first-generation at night, but this type of treatment can still be associated with a "hangover" effect of sedation/cognitive impairment in the morning and is not recommended by the guidelines [167, 206].

For atopic dermatitis and contact dermatitis the use of antihistamines is used to relieve itching symptoms, but they do not treat the disease and often topic corticosteroids are needed. Still due to their safety and less side effects second-generation are the first recommended [205].

In athletes, namely in high competitive levels, the older antihistamines compromise psychomotor skills crucial for an athlete, namely reaction time and visual discrimination [228, 229], so choosing a non-sedating antihistamine is mandatory. Balancing between disease control and antihistamines side-effects in the sports performance is needed.

First-generation antihistamines, chlorpheniramine, diphenydrame and hydroxizine, are lipophilic and with low molecular weight, so they can cross easily the blood-brain-barrier causing fatigue, somnolence, dizziness, impairment of cognitive function and psychomotor performance. On the other hand, the second generation antihistamines are specific for H1R, are lipophobic, and have an affinity to P-glycoprotein efflux pump that prevents them from occupying receptors in the central nervous system. Their propensity to occupy central nervous system receptors can be none or up to 30% in ceterizine, and dose related CNS effects can occur at higher doses [205, 206, 229]. Cardiac toxic effects are related to antimuscarinic effects and blockade of cardiac ion currents with first generation antihistamines, these side effects are rare and usually dose dependent, namely the sinus tachycardia and prolonged QT interval. Also mediated by muscarinic, alpha-adrenergic and serotonin receptors the first generation antihistamines were also related to mydriasis, dry eyes and mouth, constipation and tachycardia, all symptoms that can be bothersome in athletes [205, 206, 229]. Due to these side effects and the inherent risk of first generation antihistamines use, a position paper of EAACI propose a re-examination of the availability of these drugs as over-the-counter, freely disposable to any patient, unaware of their side effects.

H1-antihistamines, both topical and oral formulations, can be used freely in athletes, and no therapeutic use exemption is needed, being specially indicated for rhinitis treatment accordingly to WADA 2012 guidelines [181].

Table 3: H1-antihistamines: chemical and functional classification, adapted from Simons *et al.* [206]

Chemical class	**Functional class**	
	First generation	**Second generation**
Alkylamines	Brompheniramine, chlorpheniramine, dimethindene[b,c], pheniramine[c], triprolidine[a]	Acrivastine[a]
Piperazines	Buclizine, cyclizine, hydroxyzine[a], meclizine, oxatomide[b]	Cetirizine[a], levocetirizine[a]
Piperidines	Azatadine, cyproheptadine, diphenylpyraline, ketotifen[c]	Astemizole[b], bilastine[b], desloratadine[a], ebastine[b], fexofenadine[a], levocabastine[c], loratadine[a], mizolastine[b], olopatadine[c], rupatadine[b], terfenadine[a,b]
Ethanolamines	Carbinoxamine, clemastine, dimenhydrinate, diphenhydramine, doxylamine, phenyltoloxamine[b]	-
Ethylenediamines	Antazoline, pyrilamine, tripelennamine	-
Phenothiazines	Methdilazine, promethazine	
Other	Doxepin[d]	Azelastine[c], emedastine[c], epinastine[c]

[a]Acrivastine is related to triprolidine, cetirizine is a metabolite of hydroxyzine; levocetirizine is an enantiomer of cetirizine; desloratadine is a metabolite of loratadine; and fexofenadine is a metabolite of terfenadine.
[b]In the USA, these H1-antihistamines are either not yet approved, have never been approved, or have had approval withdrawn (*e.g.*, astemizole, terfenadine).
[c]Topical H1-antihistamines: emedastine, epinastine, ketotifen, levocabastine, and olopatadine are applied to the conjunctivae; azelastine, dimethindene, and levocabastine are applied to the nasal mucosa. In some countries, azelastine, dimethindene, and ketotifen are also available in oral formulations.
[d]Doxepin has H1- and H2-antihistamine activities, and is also classified as a tricyclic antidepressant.

Decongestants

Nasal congestion symptoms can be treated with nasal corticosteroids, but their efficacy is not immediate and antihistamines are generally ineffective on this symptom. Nasal congestion is mediated by congestion of the venous sinusoids lining the nasal mucosa. Nasal decongestants, such as α-adrenergic agents, namely pseudoephedrine and phenylephrine, are useful for an immediate improvement of the congestion symptoms. Nasal decongestants can be classified into two major groups: 1) sympathomimetic amines (cocaine, amphethamine, adrenaline, ephedrine) and 2) imidazolines (oxymetazoline and xylometazoline) [230]. These drugs have an agonistic action at α-1 and α-2 adrenergic receptor of endothelial cells of the nasal vessels and induce blood flow reduction, thereby improving nasal congestion associated with mucosal swelling [231]. Of the imidazolines, oxymetazoline, a selective α-1 and partial α-2 agonist, and xylometazoline, an α-2 agonist, are the most popular and clinically used derivatives. The imidazoline derivatives oxymetazoline, xylometazoline and naphazoline are available only as intranasal agents, but cathecolamines, pseudoephedrine and phenylephrine, exist as nasal or oral formulations [230]. These drugs are frequently available alone or in combination with other anti-allergic treatments on medical market and over the counter and are often used in athlete's population. As there are WADA specific anti-doping regulations of their use, athletes should be aware in order to not fall in a non-intentional doping rules violation.

Both oral and topical decongestants are effective in the treatment of allergic rhinitis [232]. In a randomized placebo controlled challenge with grass pollen in a chamber, on 39 grass pollen sensitized patients, a significant improvement was seen with oral pseudoephedrine use [233]. Clinically, they are also widely used in vasomotor rhinitis and chronic rhinosinusitis [234], and in common cold related nasal congestion in adult and children populations [235, 236], frequently associated with antihistamines. In a small clinical trial study in six trained male cyclists, pseudoephedrine use before practice lead to an increase of their cycling time-trial performance by 5%. The mechanism mediating this effect is still unknown, but it is speculated to be due to an increase in central nervous system stimulation [237]. Treatment with this oral decongestant should be reserved for acute exacerbations of sinusitis. Their duration treatment is recommended for up to 8 weeks in an as needed basis for symptom control.

Nasal decongestants are quite effective in nasal congestion and somewhat effective in reducing rhinorrhea, but do not have any effect on sneezing, pruritus or ocular symptoms. Topical formulations have a significantly rapid onset and fewer side effects; overuse might be related to rebound congestion after the withdrawals. In a comparison study of one week with antihistamine *vs.*

diphenydramine use, the latter lead to a superior clinical improvement in moderate to severe allergic rhinitis [238]. Also imidazolines derivatives, namely oxymetazoline were effective in nasal airflow improvement [239]. Increased nasal airflow is related to an improvement of general well-being and therefore perception of decreased impact on nasal symptoms. Although a topical decongestant has a more rapid onset of action, its effect was short-lived compared with the oral drug [232]. Combination of oral/topical H1 antihistamines and topical decongestant is frequent. This combination has a role especially in allergic rhinitis, as the treatment aims at nasal decongestion, where antihistamines are not as effective as nasal decongestants. Also anti-inflammatory drugs can be combined specially in chronic rhinosinusitis treatment [153]. Although no specific randomized controlled trials exist about the efficacy of decongestant in rhinosinusitis and vasomotor rhinitis, a survey including a random sample of Otolaryngologists in United States reported that half of them used oral decongestants and 38% topical decongestants for the treatment of chronic rhinosinusitis [240]. Strong evidence exists of topical decongestants use for treatment of common cold, demonstrating a slight but significant decrease of 6% in patient reported symptoms [241]. In a more recent Cochrane review, combinations of oral antihistamine-decongestant-analgesic formulations in common cold treatment presented general benefits [235, 236]. Athletes can benefit from topical treatment due to their rapid efficacy in solving nasal symptoms; prolonged use of these agents could also be related with a risk of *rhinitis medicamentosa* [173].

Side effects of common topical decongestant include local irritation, nasal dryness and occasionally mucosal ulceration [231]. The most common side effect of topical decongestants is related to their prolonged use (more than 10 days) as intranasal vasoconstrictors can lead to tachyphylaxis and rebound edema of the nasal mucosa, a condition known as *rhinitis medicamentosa*, and this limits the practical utility of these agents to short-term intermittent therapy [153, 232]. Oral decongestants are associated with systemic side effects including nervousness, insomnia, irritability, headache, tachycardia, and hypertension [153]. They interact adversely with monoamine oxidase inhibitors, tricycle antidepressants, indomethacin, beta-blockers and other central nervous system stimulants [242].

Table 4: Pharmacotherapy for the treatment of allergic rhinitis in patients practicing sports, adapted from Mandhne *et al.* [231]

Class	Mechanism of action	Generic name	Major side effects
Antihistamines	HR1 antagonism		
Intranasal		Azelastine HCl Olopatadine HCl	Bitter taste, epistaxis, headache, somnolence
Oral		Diphenhydramine HCl Chlorpheniramine maleate Hydroxyzine HCl Loratadine Desloratidine Cetirizine HCl Fexofenadine HCl	First generation antihistamines cause somnolence, cognitive dysfunction, anti-cholinergic effects. Second generation antihistamines have low potential for these side effects.
Corticosteroids	Glucocorticoid receptor agonism, anti-inflammatory action through multiple effects		
Intranasal		Triamcinolone acetonide Flunisolide Mometasone furoate Budesonide Fluticasone propionate Fluticasone furoate	Transient nasal irritation (burning/stinging), epistaxis, pharyngitis, taste, smell, voice changes.
Oral		Prednisolone Prednisone Dexamethasone Hydrocortisone Betamethasone	Inhibition of growth in children, disturbances of metabolism, glaucoma and cataract formation, immunosuppression, HPA axis suppression, skin thinning/bruising, osteoporosis, behavioral abnormalities
Leukotriene inhibitors (oral)	LT receptor antagonism	Montelukast	Ongoing investigation, none proved so far (see FDA website)
Decongestants	α-Adrenergic receptor agonism		
Intranasal		Oxymetazoline HCl Xylometazoline HCl	Nasal burning, stinging, dryness or mucosal ulcerations and even septal perforations may occur. Rebound congestion (rhinitis medicamentosa) on prolonged use.
Oral		Pseudoephedrine HCl Phenylephrine HCl	Nervousness, insomnia, irritability, headache, tachycardia, hypertension, increased intraocular pressure, and aggravation of urinary obstruction
Mast cell stabilizers (Intranasal)	Mast cell stabilization	Cromolyn sodium	Nasal burning, stinging, or sneezing in ~10% patients
Anti-cholinergics (Intranasal)	Muscarinic receptor antagonism	Ipratropium bromide	Dry mouth/throat, dizziness, ocular irritation, blurred vision, conjunctivitis, hoarseness, cough, and taste perversion in <2% of users

The use of oral decongestants is not recommended during pregnancy, in patients with glaucoma because they increase intraocular pressure, and might increase urinary retention in susceptible patients [153, 231]. In athletes, oral decongestants increased athletic performance and by that may be considered as doping; also, they induce cardiovascular side-effects, mediated by the increase on heart rate and blood pressure [173].

Accordingly to WADA 2012 guidelines, oral decongestants, namely pseudoephedrine, are restricted. In-competition they are prohibited at a urinary concentration above the threshold of 150 ng/mL. The threshold level has been established based on the intake of therapeutic, defined as a maximum daily dose of 240 mg. The risk of doping violation can still occur with higher doses and long type liberation drug pill, so it is recommended that athletes stop using them at least 24h before the in-competition period [177].

Specific Immunotherapy

The management of IgE-mediated hypersensitivity disorders encompasses allergen avoidance, pharmacological treatment and allergen-specific immunotherapy [243]. Allergen-based vaccines, usually referred as Specific Immunotherapy (SIT), using both subcutaneous (SCIT) or sublingual administration (SLIT) at different dosing schedules, have been reported to be effective in reducing allergic symptoms, modifying the natural course of allergic disorders, and inducing long-term clinical tolerance that lasts years after treatment discontinuation [180, 244, 245].

Allergen immunotherapy has been used for at least 100 years. It is a biological response modifier, which induces a specific desensitization to the allergen. It alters the immune response to allergens, inducing immune tolerance through different mechanisms that include modulation of T-and B-cell responses, related antibody isotypes, and both cells and mediators taking part in the allergic inflammation (reviewed by Akdis *et al.* [246]).

SIT is currently advised for symptomatic patients, with proven IgE-mediated allergy (demonstrable by positive skin prick tests and/or high specific IgE to a particular allergen), whose symptoms are not controlled with proper pharmacological therapy and with unavoidable exposure to clinical relevant allergens. Athletes are frequently included in this group, namely in the case of pollen-allergic athletes who train and compete in outdoor environment, and with symptoms that affect their performance [247]. In this selected patients, evidence-based recommendations, supported by systematic reviews and meta-analysis of immunotherapy trials, point toward the use of SIT in allergic rhinitis, allergic conjunctivitis and allergic ("extrinsic") asthma [248-251]. The use of allergy vaccine has not been restricted by organizations that monitor competing athletes [11].

Concerning SCIT, a meta-analysis of randomized, double-masked placebo controlled trials, has shown a consistent small to large effect of SCIT compared to placebo on the symptoms of allergic rhinitis, ocular symptoms, and quality of life in patients with Seasonal Allergic Rhinoconjuntivitis [248]. SCIT is now recommended in adults and children with seasonal allergic rhinitis (pollen-induced), with or without allergic conjunctivitis, and persistent allergic rhinitis caused by house dust mites [180].

However, patients treated with injection immunotherapy are at risk, small but yet increased, of adverse reactions, both local (mostly itching and edema) and systemic (urticaria, rhinitis, asthma exacerbation, and anaphylaxis). In the systematic review of 51 trials of SCIT for patients with Seasonal Allergic Rhinoconjuntivitis [248] the majority of adverse symptoms were readily reversible with appropriate treatment; all subjects fully recovered and none dropped out due to the reactions. Thus, SCIT was considered a safe and valid treatment option [248], as long as administered in settings in which patients can be monitored and, if necessary, promptly and effectively treated for systemic allergic reactions by trained staff (*e.g.,* prompt use of adrenaline with rapidly progressing, severe or anaphylaxis symptoms). For this safety issues, the use of SCIT has been restricted to specialized centers, requiring appropriate resources for its delivery; alternative routes and allergen extracts for SIT, with a better safety profile, have been sought [252-254].

Over the last decades, several trials have focused on the sublingual route - SLIT - and a systematic review [249] including 60 randomized, double-blind, placebo-controlled trials (49 pooled for meta-analyses), with 2333 patients in the active treatment (2256 placebo), on its efficacy and safety was recently published. All patients had allergic rhinitis, with or without allergic conjunctivitis and with or without allergic asthma. SLIT treated patients had significant reductions in symptom scores and medication requirements, compared with placebo. Local adverse events (oral, throat) were more common in the SLIT treated group (the majority were mild to moderate and did not require any treatment). There were no apparent differences of systemic adverse events (rhinitis and/or conjunctivitis, asthma or wheeze) between SLIT and placebo treated participants, with the exception of gastrointestinal symptoms, more common in SLIT group (14% compared to 1.7% in placebo-treated), but none considered serious and largely seen in pediatric trials. There were no reports of serious adverse systemic events, anaphylaxis or adrenaline use. The authors concluded that SLIT is a viable alternative to allergen injection immunotherapy, with a significantly lower risk profile. They found support for the use of SLIT in children and additional support for its use in allergic rhinitis due to seasonal and perennial allergens. In this meta-analysis, a greater effect appeared with perennial allergens (predominantly house dust mites) when compared to seasonal allergens, and data also suggested that treatments for longer than 12 months provided more consistent clinical improvements. Moreover, it seemed that either sublingual drops or tablets were similarly effective [249]. A recent publication from one of the studies of SLIT, using grass allergen tablets for seasonal rhinitis, showed long-term benefit for at least two years following the 3 years of treatment [245], supporting the induction of both clinical and immunological tolerance with SLIT. Although this systematic review excluded trials dealing only with asthma, additional benefits of SLIT may be seen in patients with associated asthma. An open randomized controlled trial in patients with mild persistent asthma and rhinitis due to grass pollen [255] showed that long term SLIT (continuous, up to 5 years) was equally effective as inhaled budesonide in treating asthma symptoms but provided an additional benefit in treating rhinitis symptoms and airways hyperresponsiveness.

SLIT is recommended to be initiated in secondary care and the first dose taken under medical supervision, whereas maintenance treatment is recommended to be self-administered in the patient's home [249]. With this approach, additional concerns with compliance to treatment arise [256], although some studies suggest the patient's adhesion to SLIT is not lower than to injection immunotherapy [257].

Both SCIT and SLIT have also been reported to be effective in the treatment of patients affected by allergic conjunctivitis. The meta-analysis of randomized, double-masked placebo controlled trials of SCIT in seasonal allergic rhinoconjuntivitis [248] have also shown significant reductions in conjunctival symptoms. Moreover, the effects of SLIT (either as drops or sublingual tablets) on symptoms of ocular allergy have been recently established in another systematic review [250], where the authors concluded that it is moderately effective in reducing total and individual ocular symptom scores in patients with allergy conjunctivitis, with or without rhinitis.

Whereas the clinical effectiveness of allergen immunotherapy in allergic rhinitis and conjunctivitis is well accepted, its use in patients with asthma is more controversial. Although beneficial effects upon clinically relevant outcomes have been demonstrated in randomized controlled trials of SCIT in allergic asthma [251], caused by house dust mites, grass pollen, animal dander and moulds (Cladosporium), there remains, for injection immunotherapy, a small but clinical significant risk of severe systemic reactions (1 per million injections) and, very rarely, fatal anaphylaxis (1 per 2.5 million injections). A recent meta-analysis of 88 randomized, controlled trials, published between 1971 and 2004, concluded that there was a significant reduction in asthma symptoms and asthma medication following SCIT. Moreover, allergen immunotherapy significantly reduced allergen specific bronchial hyperresponsiveness, with some reduction in non-specific bronchial hyperresponsiveness as well [251]. From a practical point of view, this systematic review, while confirming the efficacy of SCIT in asthma, recommends that patients should be informed about the risk of significant adverse effects and that other types of allergen immunotherapy, such as SLIT, are available, to allow an informed choice and patient preference. For the SCIT option, patients must be observed and monitored long enough to control any major systemic reactions (usually 30 to 45 minutes), with access at all time to expert advice [248, 251].

In athletes, several expert panels recommend the additional precaution of avoiding physical exercise just before and after receiving the injection immunotherapy [11, 33, 98, 258, 259]. SIT is currently not among the WADA prohibited substances [10]

Adrenaline

Adrenaline is considered, according to evidence based-medicine, the first-line treatment for anaphylaxis [260-265]. Intramuscularly auto-injected into the lateral thigh, it improves airflow and vascular integrity [1]. Its α-adrenergic action allows the increase of peripheral vascular resistance and the reversion of peripheral vasodilation, therefore improving angioedema and urticaria [261, 264-268]. Its β-adrenergic properties induce an increase in heart rate and myocardial contractility and suppress the release of inflammatory mediators from mast cells and basophils [261, 263-268]. The intramuscular route is preferred for both the patient (and families) and professionals because intramuscular adrenaline is rapidly bioavailable, with peak concentrations occurring within 10 min of administration, and has a much better safety profile and longer-lasting action than intravenous adrenaline [260, 263, 264, 267-269]. For the intramuscular route, 1:1000 adrenaline (1 mg/ml) should be used at a dose of 0.01 ml/kg body weight (maximum single dose 0.5 mg). The use of inhaled epinephrine is not an established option [264]; it is not effective as a result of its inadequate systemic bioavailability at doses available from an inhaler or nebulizer.

When a diagnosis of EI-anaphylaxis is established, doctors should teach athletes on how to recognize their first symptoms and signs of EI-anaphylaxis and immediately discontinue exercise. They should learn to assume the Trendelenburg position to facilitate perfusion of vital organs in the face of hypotension, and learn to auto-inject adrenaline. It is recommended for teams or for sporting facilities to have at least one auto-injectable adrenaline device available in their emergency kit.

Systemic adrenaline is part of the Prohibited Substances list for use in sports. Its use requires a Therapeutic Use Exemption (TUE) [10].

Effect of Asthma Drugs Upon Performance in Healthy Athletes and the Relationship to Doping

The question of doping is central to elite athletes. The WADA emits each year a list of prohibited substances in sports, which can be accessed from the website [10]. It is the responsibility of athletes to know the rules and to abide by them. However, as these guidelines often change, sometimes annually, even with minor changes, the physician caring for subjects who are active in sports should also be updated.

The issue of doping is particularly delicate to asthmatic athletes. These subjects are dependent on an optimal and successful management of their asthma to be able to perform effectively in sports. On the other hand, they should not be given advantages over their healthy peers because of the possibility that drugs used in the treatment of asthma might improve physical performance [33]. In this context, it has been long discussed whether asthma drugs have a "doping" effect in non-asthmatic competitive athletes.

In what concerns to beta2-agonists, randomized placebo-controlled trials in non-asthmatic competitive athletes failed to prove performance-enhancing effects of the inhaled beta2-agonists formoterol, salbutamol (albuterol), salmeterol and terbutaline in doses commonly used to prevent EI-bronchoconstriction [33, 270, 271]. In contrast to inhaled beta2-agonists, systemic beta2-agonists may have a positive effect on physical performance in healthy subjects, being able to improve the muscle strength and the endurance performance, although the evidence is weak [270, 271]. From this perspective, it appears to be no justification to prohibit inhaled beta2-agonists from the point of view of the ergogenic effects, and the constant guideline's changes surrounding beta2-agonists use by athletes have been the focus of recent and intense controversy [76, 272]. The use of systemic corticosteroids in any form constitutes doping as they have an anti-inflammatory effect, which would help athlete to restore their joints and muscles after a competition although this, however, does not apply to the inhaled formulation. Regarding inhaled corticosteroids, although they might not contribute significantly to systemic doping, a close similarity between synthetic and natural steroids exists, which could possibly create a problem when performing a doping test [273].

No systemic administration of both these drugs (corticosteroids and beta2-agonists) is permitted in relationship to sports. Besides, those using inhaled beta2-agonists should be instructed only to use the drug in therapeutic doses, as WADA 2012 guidelines clearly state that the presence in urine of salbutamol (albuterol) above 1000 ng/mL or formoterol above 30 ng/mL is presumed not to be an intended therapeutic use of the substance and will be considered as an Adverse Analytical Finding [10].

At present there are no restrictions for the use of inhaled steroids, inhaled ipratropium bromide, leukotriene antagonists and the inhaled beta2-agonists salbutamol, salmeterol and formoterol. However, inhaled terbutaline is restricted in competitive sports and objective measurements of bronchial hyperesponsiveness, EI-bronchoconstriction or bronchodilator reversibility must be documented for approval for its use.

FINAL COMMENTS

EI-hypersensitivity syndromes include EI-asthma, EI-bronchoconstriction, EI-rhinitis, EI-anaphylaxis and EI-urticaria, which are all significant problems for both recreational and competitive athletes. Appropriate management of exercise induced symptoms is mandatory in order to allow them to partake in regular exercise training, without fear of symptom exacerbation.

The best strategy for prevention of EI-bronchoconstriction is optimal control of underlying asthma. Therefore, inhaled corticosteroids are the first-line treatment when asthma control is not achieved by reliever therapy alone, when the athlete has persistent symptoms, if bronchial hyperresponsiveness and/or inflammation are present, or if bronchodilation therapy is required on a regular basis. If even, a patient remains symptomatic during exercise, medication usage should be review, understanding of dosage instructions and administration technique before any changes are made in the treatment regimen. Avoiding known allergens, selecting warm, humid environments for the activities, and proper warm-up and cool-down exercises are also important preventing measures. Inhaled short-acting beta-agonists are most effective in preventing EI-bronchoconstriction, followed by inhaled mast cell stabilizers and anti-cholinergic agents (with evidence arising from multiple randomized control trials). Less evidence supports the use of leukotriene antagonists (recommended on a trial basis with follow-up to evaluate the treatment response). Bronchodilators are frequently needed both as pretreatment before competitions and to relieve symptoms. It is important to assess objective measures like lung function and bronchial hyperesponsiveness when treating competitive athletes, due to the discrepancy between symptoms and clinical objective measures.

EI-rhinitis leads to disturbed sleep, daytime somnolence, fatigue and impaired performance. WADA recommends treatment to be monitored by the treating physician and advices topical intranasal corticosteroids as the main option. Intranasal glucocorticosteroids are the most efficacious medication available for allergic and non-allergic rhinitis treatment, decreasing nasal as well as ocular symptoms. In rhinosinusitis they help to achieve disease control, reducing nasal blockage, rhinorrhea or postnasal drip, increasing smell and preventing bothersome facial pain or headache. If necessary, association with other treatments can be made namely with antihistamines or topical nasal decongestants. In patients practicing sports, namely in high competitive levels, the older antihistamines compromise psychomotor skills crucial for an athlete, namely reaction time and visual discrimination, so choosing non-sedating antihistamine is mandatory. Balancing between disease control and antihistamines side-effects in the sports performance is needed. Controlling rhinitis also may improve control of asthma. Both SCIT and SLIT have shown their efficacy on allergic rhinitis based on multiple systematic reviews and meta-analysis of randomized controlled trials. This efficacy is also seen on allergic conjunctivitis and asthma, although in the specific case of athletes caution should be made regarding extreme exercise before and after administration.

EI-anaphylaxis is a rare, unpredictable event, and the most serious and potentially life-threatening syndrome associated with exercise. Intramuscular adrenaline is the first-line treatment. The use of cromolyn sodium has shown variable results in the prophylactic treatment of patients with EI-anaphylaxis, but it remains unknown if inhaled mast cell stabilizers, administered on a daily basis, maintain sufficient systemic concentration levels necessary to be adequately prophylactic against EI-anaphylaxis. H1-antihistamines are adjunctive treatment therapy for acute anaphylaxis and are an important component of regimens for the prevention of anaphylaxis, although in EI-anaphylaxis prophylaxis regimens are not always effective.

EI-urticaria is much less frequent, but yet with an important impact in performance and quality of life. H1-antihistamines provide symptomatic relief of itching, reduce the number, size and duration of individual hives and significantly improve quality of life and are considered first choice treatment and prophylactic agents.

At all times, physicians who have patients active in sports should be aware of WADA guidelines on prohibited substances and be prepared to give the necessary documentation for the sports authorities. For many years there have been strict regulations for the use of asthma drugs in sports. Initially, there were concerns that these drugs might improve performance, but now it is generally accepted that inhaled steroids and inhaled beta2-agonists do not improve performance, and the regulations have been slacken for most drugs, but not all (such as terbutaline). The constant changes in this field, the emergence of new treatment targets of known anti-allergic therapies and new treatment tools for allergic diseases requires the allergy sports-specialized physician who follows the athlete through their competitive path to be updated.

ACKNOWLEDGEMENTS

Declared none.

CONFLICT OF INTEREST

The authors confirm that this chapter content has no conflict of interest.

REFERENCES

[1] Schwartz LB, Delgado L, Craig T, Bonini S, Carlsen KH, Casale TB, *et al.* Exercise-induced hypersensitivity syndromes in recreational and competitive athletes: a PRACTALL

consensus report (what the general practitioner should know about sports and allergy). Allergy. 2008 Aug;63(8):953-61.

[2] McFadden Jr ER. Approach to the Patient with Exercise-Induced Airway Narrowing. In: Adkinson Jr NF, Bochner BS, Busse WW, Holgate ST, Lemanske Jr. RF, Simons FER, editors. Adkinson: Middleton's Allergy: Principles and Practice. 7th ed. Philadelphia: Mosby; 2008.

[3] Lee TH, Anderson SD. Heterogeneity of mechanisms in exercise induced asthma. Thorax. 1985;40:481-7.

[4] Chandratilleke MG, Carson KV, Picot J, Brinn MP, Esterman AJ, Smith BJ. Physical training for asthma. Cochrane Database Syst Rev. 2012;5:CD001116.

[5] Moreira A, Delgado L, Haahtela T, Fonseca J, Moreira P, Lopes C, *et al.* Physical training does not increase allergic inflammation in asthmatic children. Eur Respir J. 2008 Dec;32(6):1570-5.

[6] Silva D, Moreira A, Delgado L. Allergic Rhinitis and Sports. In: Kowalski ML, editor. Allergic Rhinitis: InTech; 2012.

[7] Del Giacco SR. Exercise induced anaphylaxis: an update. Breathe. 2012;8(4):299-306.

[8] Hompes S, Kohli A, Nemat K, Scherer K, Lange L, Rueff F, *et al.* Provoking allergens and treatment of anaphylaxis in children and adolescents--data from the anaphylaxis registry of German-speaking countries. Pediatr Allergy Immunol. 2011 Sep;22(6):568-74.

[9] Moro Moro M, Tejedor Alonso MA, Esteban Hernandez J, Mugica Garcia MV, Rosado Ingelmo A, Vila Albelda C. Incidence of anaphylaxis and subtypes of anaphylaxis in a general hospital emergency department. J Investig Allergol Clin Immunol. 2011;21(2):142-9.

[10] World Anti-Doping Agency homepage. The World Anti-Doping Agency homepage. Montreal2012 [13 Mar 2012]; Available from: http://www.wada-ama.org/.

[11] Weiler J, Bonini S, Coifman R, Craig T, Delgado L, Capão-Filipe M, *et al.* American Academy of Allergy, Asthma & Immunology Work Group report: exercise-induced asthma. J Allergy Clin Immunol. 2007;119(6):1349-58.

[12] Carlsen K-H. The breathless adolescent asthmatic athlete. Eur Resp J. 2011;38:713-20.

[13] Couto M, Moreira A, Delgado L. Diagnosis and treatment of asthma in athletes. Breathe. 2012;8:286-96.

[14] Carlsen K-H, Anderson S, Bjermer L, Bonini S, Brusasco V, Canonica W, *et al.* Exercise-induced asthma, respiratory and allergic disorders in elite athletes: epidemiology, mechanisms and diagnosis: part I of the report from the Joint Task Force of the European Respiratory Society (ERS) and the European Academy of Allergy and Clinical Immunology (EAACI) in cooperation with GA2LEN. Allergy. 2008;63(4):387-403.

[15] Kemp JP. Exercise-induced bronchoconstriction: The effects of montelukast, a leukotriene receptor antagonist. Ther Clin Risk Manag. 2009;5:923-33.

[16] Carlsen K-H, Carlsen KL. Physical exercise, training and sports in asthmatic children and adolescents. European Respiratory Society Monographs. 2012;56:49-58.

[17] Couto M, Silva D, Delgado L, Moreira A. Exercise and airway injury in athletes. Acta Med Port. 2012 (in press).

[18] Hallstrand TS, Moody MW, Wurfel MM, *et al.* Inflammatory basis of exercise-induced bronchoconstriction. Am J Respir Crit Care Med. 2005;172:679-86.

[19] Carbonnelle S, Francaux M, Doyle I, Dumont X, Burbure C, Morel G, *et al.* Changes in serum pneumoproteins caused by short-term exposures to nitrogen trichloride in indoor chlorinated swimming pools. Biomarkers. 2002;7:464-78.

[20] Bougault V, Loubaki L, Joubert P, Turmel J, Couture C, Laviolette M, *et al.* Airway remodeling and inflammation in competitive swimmers training in indoor chlorinated swimming pools. J Allergy Clin Immunol. 2012 Feb;129(2):351-8, 8 e1.
[21] Kanazawa H, Asai K, Hirata K, Yoshikawa J. Vascular involvement in exercise-induced airway narrowing in patients with bronchial asthma. Chest,. 2002;122(1):166-70.
[22] Kanazawa H. VEGF, angiopoietin-1 and -2 in bronchial asthma: new molecular targets in airway angiogenesis and microvascular remodeling. Recent Pat Inflamm Allergy Drug Discov. 2007;1(1):1-8.
[23] Moreira A, Palmares C, Lopes C, Delgado L. Airway vascular damage in elite swimmers. Respir Med. 2011 Nov;105(11):1761-5.
[24] Del Giacco SR, Carlsen KH, Du Toit G. Allergy and sports in children. Pediatr Allergy Immunol. 2012 Feb;23(1):11-20.
[25] Moreira A, Delgado L, Palmares C, Lopes C, Jacinto T, Rytila P, *et al.* Competitive swimmers with allergic asthma show a mixed type of airway inflammation. Eur Resp J. 2008;31(5):1139-41.
[26] Bougault V, Turmel J, St-Laurent J, Bertrand M, Boulet L. Asthma, airway inflammation and epithelial damage in swimmers and cold-air athletes. Eur Respir J. 2009;33(4):740-6.
[27] Schleimer RP. Pharmacology of Glucocorticoids in Allergic Disease. In: Adkinson Jr NF, Bochner BS, Busse WW, Holgate ST, Lemanske Jr. RF, Simons FER, editors. Adkinson: Middleton's Allergy: Principles and Practice. 7th ed. Philadelphia: Mosby; 2008.
[28] Clark TJH. Effect of beclomethasone dipropionate delivered by aerosol in patients with asthma. Lancet. 1972;1:1361-4.
[29] Spahn JD, Covar R, Szefler SJ. Glucocorticoids: Clinical Pharmacology. In: Adkinson Jr NF, Bochner BS, Busse WW, Holgate ST, Lemanske Jr. RF, Simons FER, editors. Adkinson: Middleton's Allergy: Principles and Practice. 7th ed. Philadelphia: Mosby; 2008.
[30] Global Strategy for Asthma Management and Prevention. Global Initiative for Asthma (GINA). 2011; Available from: http://www.ginasthma.org/.
[31] Grzelewski T, Stelmach I. Exercise-induced bronchoconstriction in asthmatic children: a comparative systematic review of the available treatment options. Drugs. 2009;69:1533-53.
[32] Ali Z, Norsk P, Ulrik CS. Mechanisms and Management of Exercise-Induced Asthma in Elite Athletes. J Asthma. 2012 [Epub ahead of print].
[33] Carlsen KH, Anderson SD, Bjermer L, Bonini S, Brusasco V, Canonica W, *et al.* Treatment of exercise-induced asthma, respiratory and allergic disorders in sports and the relationship to doping: Part II of the report from the Joint Task Force of European Respiratory Society (ERS) and European Academy of Allergy and Clinical Immunology (EAACI) in cooperation with GA(2)LEN. Allergy. 2008 May;63(5):492-505.
[34] Subbarao P, Duong M, Adelroth E, Otis J, Obminski G, Inman M, *et al.* Effect of ciclesonide dose and duration of therapy on exercise-induced bronchoconstriction in patients with asthma. J Allergy Clin Immunol. 2006 May;117(5):1008-13.
[35] Koh MS, Tee A, Lasserson TJ, Irving LB. Inhaled corticosteroids compared to placebo for prevention of exercise induced bronchoconstriction. Cochrane Database Syst Rev. 2007(3):CD002739.
[36] Larsson K, Carlsen K-H, Bonini S. Antiasthmatic drugs: treatment of athletes and exercise-induced bronchoconstriction. European Respiratory Society Monograph: Diagnosis, prevention and treatment of exercise-related asthma, respiratory and allergic disorders in sports. 2005:73-88.

[37] Schwindt CD, Zaldivar F, Eliakim A, Shin HW, Leu SY, Cooper DM. Inhaled fluticasone and the hormonal and inflammatory response to brief exercise. Med Sci Sports Exerc. 2010 Oct;42(10):1802-8.

[38] Priftis KN, Papadimitriou A, Gatsopoulou E, Yiallouros PK, Fretzayas A, Nicolaidou P. The effect of inhaled budesonide on adrenal and growth suppression in asthmatic children. Eur Respir J. 2006 Feb;27(2):316-20.

[39] Drake AJ, Howells RJ, Shield JP, Prendiville A, Ward PS, Crowne EC. Symptomatic adrenal insufficiency presenting with hypoglycaemia in children with asthma receiving high dose inhaled fluticasone propionate. BMJ. 2002 May 4;324(7345):1081-2.

[40] Todd GR, Acerini CL, Buck JJ, Murphy NP, Ross-Russell R, Warner JT, *et al.* Acute adrenal crisis in asthmatics treated with high-dose fluticasone propionate. Eur Respir J. 2002 Jun;19(6):1207-9.

[41] Todd GR, Acerini CL, Ross-Russell R, Zahra S, Warner JT, McCance D. Survey of adrenal crisis associated with inhaled corticosteroids in the United Kingdom. Arch Dis Child. 2002 Dec;87(6):457-61.

[42] Konig P, Hillman L, Cervantes C, Levine C, Maloney C, Douglass B, *et al.* Bone metabolism in children with asthma treated with inhaled beclomethasone dipropionate. J Pediatr. 1993 Feb;122(2):219-26.

[43] Hanania NA, Chapman KR, Sturtridge WC, Szalai JP, Kesten S. Dose-related decrease in bone density among asthmatic patients treated with inhaled corticosteroids. J Allergy Clin Immunol. 1995 Nov;96(5 Pt 1):571-9.

[44] Toogood JH, Baskerville JC, Markov AE, Hodsman AB, Fraher LJ, Jennings B, *et al.* Bone mineral density and the risk of fracture in patients receiving long-term inhaled steroid therapy for asthma. J Allergy Clin Immunol. 1995 Aug;96(2):157-66.

[45] Luengo M, del Rio L, Pons F, Picado C. Bone mineral density in asthmatic patients treated with inhaled corticosteroids: a case-control study. Eur Respir J. 1997 Sep;10(9):2110-3.

[46] Pauwels RA, Yernault JC, Demedts MG, Geusens P. Safety and efficacy of fluticasone and beclomethasone in moderate to severe asthma. Belgian Multicenter Study Group. Am J Respir Crit Care Med. 1998 Mar;157(3 Pt 1):827-32.

[47] Long-term effects of budesonide or nedocromil in children with asthma. The Childhood Asthma Management Program Research Group. N Engl J Med. 2000 Oct 12;343(15):1054-63.

[48] Bisgaard H, Hermansen MN, Loland L, Halkjaer LB, Buchvald F. Intermittent inhaled corticosteroids in infants with episodic wheezing. N Engl J Med. 2006 May 11;354(19):1998-2005.

[49] Guilbert TW, Morgan WJ, Zeiger RS, Mauger DT, Boehmer SJ, Szefler SJ, *et al.* Long-term inhaled corticosteroids in preschool children at high risk for asthma. N Engl J Med. 2006 May 11;354(19):1985-97.

[50] Murray CS, Woodcock A, Langley SJ, Morris J, Custovic A. Secondary prevention of asthma by the use of Inhaled Fluticasone propionate in Wheezy INfants (IFWIN): double-blind, randomised, controlled study. Lancet. 2006 Aug 26;368(9537):754-62.

[51] Pearlman DS, Berger WE, Kerwin E, Laforce C, Kundu S, Banerji D. Once-daily ciclesonide improves lung function and is well tolerated by patients with mild-to-moderate persistent asthma. J Allergy Clin Immunol. 2005 Dec;116(6):1206-12.

[52] Gelfand EW, Georgitis JW, Noonan M, Ruff ME. Once-daily ciclesonide in children: efficacy and safety in asthma. J Pediatr. 2006 Mar;148(3):377-83.

[53] Mutch E, Nave R, Zech K, Williams FM. Esterases involved in the hydrolysis of ciclesonide in human tissues. Eur Respir J. 2003;22(suppl):S267-S8.

[54] Chopra D, Bhandari B, Wardhan N. Ciclesonide--a novel corticosteroid for the management of asthma. Curr Clin Pharmacol. 2012 May;7(2):73-7.

[55] Stoeck M, Riedel R, Hochhaus G, Hafner D, Masso JM, Schmidt B, *et al. In vitro* and *in vivo* anti-inflammatory activity of the new glucocorticoid ciclesonide. J Pharmacol Exp Ther. 2004 Apr;309(1):249-58.

[56] Solis-Cohen S. The use of adrenal substance in the treatment of asthma. J Asthma. 1900;27(6):401-6.

[57] Benson RL, Perlman F. Clinical effects of epinephrine by inhalation. J Allergy Clin. 1948;19:129-40.

[58] Sorkness CA. Beta-Adrenergic Agonists. In: Adkinson Jr NF, Bochner BS, Busse WW, Holgate ST, Lemanske Jr. RF, Simons FER, editors. Adkinson: Middleton's Allergy: Principles and Practice. Philadelphia: Mosby; 2008.

[59] Rachelefsky GS, Katz RM, Siegel SC. Albuterol syrup in the treatment of the young child. Ann Allergy 1981;47:143-6.

[60] Anderson SD, Rozea PJ, Dolton R, Lindsay DA. Inhaled and oral bronchodilator therapy in exercise induced asthma. Aust N Z J Med. 1975;5:544-50.

[61] Anderson S, Seale J, Rozea P, Bandler L, Theobald G, Lindsay D. Inhaled and oral salbutamol in exercise-induced asthma. Am Rev Respir Dis. 1976;114:493-500.

[62] Anderson S, Spiroglou M, Lindsay D. An evaluation of oral hexoprenaline sulphate (Ipradol) in exercise-induced asthma. Med J Aust. 1977;2:825-7.

[63] Konig P, Eggleston P, Serby C. Comparison of oral and inhaled metaproterenol for prevention of exercise-induced asthma. Clin Allergy 1981;11:597-604.

[64] Shapiro GG, Kemp JP, DeJong R, Chapko M, Bierman CW, Altman LC, *et al.* Effects of albuterol and procaterol on exercise-induced asthma. Ann Allergy. 1990 Oct;65(4):273-6.

[65] Anderson S, Lambert S, Brannan J, Wood R, Koskela H, Morton A, *et al.* Laboratory protocol for exercise asthma to evaluate salbutamol given by two devices. Med Sci Sports Exerc. 2001;33:893-900.

[66] Anderson SD, Rodwell LT, Du Toit J, Young IH. Duration of protection by inhaled salmeterol in exercise-induced asthma. Chest. 1991 Nov;100(5):1254-60.

[67] Carlsen K-H, Røksund O, Olsholt K, Nja F, Leegaard J, Bratten G. Overnight protection by inhaled salmeterol on exercise-induced asthma in children. Eur Respir J. 1995;8:1852-5.

[68] Boner AL, Spezia E, Piovesan P, Chiocca E, Maiocchi G. Inhaled formoterol in the prevention of exercise-induced bronchoconstriction in asthmatic children. Am J Respir Crit Care Med. 1994 Apr;149(4 Pt 1):935-9.

[69] Au D, Udris E, Curtis J, McDonell M, Fihn S. Association between chronic heart failure and inhaled beta-2-adrenoceptor agonists. Am Heart J. 2004;148:915-20.

[70] Salpeter S. Cardiovascular safety of beta(2)-adrenoceptor agonist use in patients with obstructive airway disease: a systematic review. Drugs Aging. 2004;21:405-14.

[71] Chinchilli V. General principles for systematic reviews and meta-analyses and a critique of a recent systematic review of long-acting beta-agonists. J Allergy Clin Immunol 2007;119:303-6.

[72] Bermingham M, O'Callaghan E, Dawkins I, Miwa S, Samsudin S, McDonald K, *et al.* Are beta2-agonists responsible for increased mortality in heart failure? Eur J Heart Fail. 2011 Aug;13(8):885-91.

[73] Duranti G, La Rosa P, Dimauro I, Wannenes F, Bonini S, Sabatini S, *et al.* Effects of salmeterol on skeletal muscle cells: metabolic and proapoptotic features. Med Sci Sports Exerc. 2011 Dec;43(12):2259-73.

[74] Cates C, Cates M. Regular treatment with salmeterol for chronic asthma: serious adverse events. Cochrane Database of Systematic Reviews. 2008(3).

[75] Bonini M, Permaul P, Kazani S, Sorkness C, Israel E. Airway Inflammation, As Detected By Exhaled Nitric Oxide, Predicts Loss Of Bronchoprotection Against Exercise-induced Bronchospasm (EIB) From Long-acting β-2 Agonists (LABAs). Am J Respir Crit Care Med. 2010;181:A3722.

[76] Couto M, Horta L, Delgado L, Capão-Filipe M, Moreira A. Impact of Changes in Anti-Doping Regulations (WADA Guidelines) on Asthma Care in Athletes. Clin J Sport Med. 2012;Aug 31. [Epub ahead of print].

[77] Dekkers BG, Pehlic A, Mariani R, Bos IS, Meurs H, Zaagsma J. Glucocorticosteroids and beta2-adrenoceptor agonists synergize to inhibit airway smooth muscle remodelling. J Pharmacol Exp Ther. 2012 Jun 8.

[78] Black J, Oliver B, Roth M. Molecular mechanisms of combination therapy with inhaled corticosteroids and long-acting beta-agonists. Chest 2009;136(4):1095-100.

[79] Reynolds N, Lyseng-Williamson K, Wiseman L. Inhaled salmeterol/fluticasone propionate: a review of its use in asthma. Drugs. 2005;65:1715-34.

[80] Pauwels R, Löfdahl C, Postma D, Tattersfield A, O'Byrne P, Barnes P, *et al.* Effect of inhaled formoterol and budesonide on exacerbations of asthma. Formoterol and Corticosteroids Establishing Therapy (FACET) International Study Group. N Engl J Med. 1997;337(20):1405-11.

[81] Scicchitano R, Aalbers R, Ukena D, Manjra A, Fouquert L, Centanni S, *et al.* Efficacy and safety of budesonide/formoterol single inhaler therapy *vs.* a higher dose of budesonide in moderate to severe asthma. Curr Med Res Opin. 2004 Sep;20(9):1403-18.

[82] O'Byrne PM, Bisgaard H, Godard PP, Pistolesi M, Palmqvist M, Zhu Y, *et al.* Budesonide/formoterol combination therapy as both maintenance and reliever medication in asthma. Am J Respir Crit Care Med. 2005 Jan 15;171(2):129-36.

[83] Rabe KF, Pizzichini E, Stallberg B, Romero S, Balanzat AM, Atienza T, *et al.* Budesonide/formoterol in a single inhaler for maintenance and relief in mild-to-moderate asthma: a randomized, double-blind trial. Chest. 2006 Feb;129(2):246-56.

[84] Vogelmeier C, D'Urzo A, Pauwels R, Merino JM, Jaspal M, Boutet S, *et al.* Budesonide/formoterol maintenance and reliever therapy: an effective asthma treatment option? Eur Respir J. 2005 Nov;26(5):819-28.

[85] Baigelman W, Chodosh S. Bronchodilator action of the anticholinergic drug, ipratropium bromide (Sch 1000), as an aerosol in chronic bronchitis and asthma. Chest. 1977 Mar;71(3):324-8.

[86] Poppius H, Salorinne Y, Viljanen AA. Inhalation of a new anticholinergic drug, SCH 1000, in asthma and chronic bronchitis: effect on airway resistance, thoracic gas volume, blood gases and exercise-induced asthma. Bull Physiopathol Respir (Nancy). 1972 May-Jun;8(3):643-53.

[87] Hartley JP, Davies BH. Cholinergic blockade in the prevention of exercise-induced asthma. Thorax. 1980 Sep;35(9):680-5.

[88] Johnson BE, Suratt PM, Gal TJ, Wilhoit SC. Effect of inhaled glycopyrrolate and atropine in asthma. Precipitated by exercise and cold air inhalation. Chest. 1984 Mar;85(3):325-8.

[89] Poppius H, Sovijarvi AR, Tammilehto L. Lack of protective effect of high-dose ipratropium on bronchoconstriction following exercise with cold air breathing in patients with mild asthma. Eur J Respir Dis. 1986 May;68(5):319-25.

[90] Spooner CH, Spooner GR, Rowe BH. Mast-cell stabilising agents to prevent exercise-induced bronchoconstriction. Cochrane Database Syst Rev. 2003(4):CD002307.

[91] Molfino NA, Slutsky AS, Julia-Serda G, Hoffstein V, Szalai JP, Chapman KR, *et al.* Assessment of airway tone in asthma. Comparison between double lung transplant patients and healthy subjects. Am Rev Respir Dis. 1993 Nov;148(5):1238-43.

[92] Moreira A, Delgado L, Carlsen KH. Exercise-induced asthma: why is it so frequent in Olympic athletes? Expert Rev Respir Med. 2011 Feb;5(1):1-3.

[93] Knöpfli B, Bar-Or O. Vagal activity and airway response to ipratropium bromide before and after exercise in ambient and cold conditions in healthy cross-country runners. Clin J Sport Med. 1999;9(3):170-6.

[94] Capão-Filipe J, Falcão-Reis F, Castro-Correia J, Barros H. Assessment of autonomic function in high level athletes by pupillometry. Auton Neurosci. 2003;104(1):66-72.

[95] Pichon A, Bisschop C, Diaz V, Denjean A. Parasympathetic Airway Response and Heart Rate Variability Before and at the End of Methacholine Challenge. Chest. 2005;127:23-9.

[96] Park C, Stafford C, Lockette W. Exercise-induced asthma may be associated with diminished sweat sectretion rates in humans. Chest. 2008;134(3):552-8.

[97] Knöpfli B, Bar-Or O, Araújo C. Effect of ipratropium bromide on EIB in children depends on vagal activity. Med Sci Sports Exerc. 2005;37(3):354-9.

[98] Bonini S, Bonini M, Bousquet J, Brusasco V, Canonica GW, Carlsen KH, *et al.* Rhinitis and asthma in athletes: an ARIA document in collaboration with GA2LEN. Allergy. 2006 Jun;61(6):681-92.

[99] Bonadonna P, Senna G, Zanon P, Cocco G, Dorizzi R, Gani F, *et al.* Cold-induced rhinitis in skiers--clinical aspects and treatment with ipratropium bromide nasal spray: a randomized controlled trial. Am J Rhinol. 2001 Sep-Oct;15(5):297-301.

[100] Afonso AS, Verhamme KM, Stricker BH, Sturkenboom MC, Brusselle GG. Inhaled anticholinergic drugs and risk of acute urinary retention. BJU Int. 2011 Apr;107(8):1265-72.

[101] Wenzel SE. Antileukotriene Therapy in Asthma. In: Adkinson Jr NF, Bochner BS, Busse W, Holgate ST, Lemanske Jr RF, Simons FER, editors. Middleton's Allergy: Principles and Practice. 7th ed. Philadelphia: Mosby; 2008.

[102] Lynch KR, O'Neill GP, Liu Q, Im DS, Sawyer N, Metters KM, *et al.* Characterization of the human cysteinyl leukotriene CysLT1 receptor. Nature. 1999 Jun 24;399(6738):789-93.

[103] Spector SL, Smith LJ, Glass M. Effects of 6 weeks of therapy with oral doses of ICI 204,219, a leukotriene D4 receptor antagonist, in subjects with bronchial asthma. ACCOLATE Asthma Trialists Group. Am J Respir Crit Care Med. 1994 Sep;150(3):618-23.

[104] Liu MC, Dube LM, Lancaster J. Acute and chronic effects of a 5-lipoxygenase inhibitor in asthma: a 6-month randomized multicenter trial. Zileuton Study Group. J Allergy Clin Immunol. 1996 Nov;98(5 Pt 1):859-71.

[105] Suissa S, Dennis R, Ernst P, Sheehy O, Wood-Dauphinee S. Effectiveness of the leukotriene receptor antagonist zafirlukast for mild-to-moderate asthma. A randomized, double-blind, placebo-controlled trial. Ann Intern Med. 1997 Feb 1;126(3):177-83.

[106] Reiss TF, Chervinsky P, Dockhorn RJ, Shingo S, Seidenberg B, Edwards TB. Montelukast, a once-daily leukotriene receptor antagonist, in the treatment of chronic asthma: a

multicenter, randomized, double-blind trial. Montelukast Clinical Research Study Group. Arch Intern Med. 1998 Jun 8;158(11):1213-20.
[107] Simons FE, Villa JR, Lee BW, Teper AM, Lyttle B, Aristizabal G, *et al.* Montelukast added to budesonide in children with persistent asthma: a randomized, double-blind, crossover study. J Pediatr. 2001 May;138(5):694-8.
[108] Phipatanakul W, Greene C, Downes SJ, Cronin B, Eller TJ, Schneider LC, *et al.* Montelukast improves asthma control in asthmatic children maintained on inhaled corticosteroids. Ann Allergy Asthma Immunol. 2003 Jul;91(1):49-54.
[109] Malmstrom K, Rodriguez-Gomez G, Guerra J, Villaran C, Pineiro A, Wei LX, *et al.* Oral montelukast, inhaled beclomethasone, and placebo for chronic asthma. A randomized, controlled trial. Montelukast/Beclomethasone Study Group. Ann Intern Med. 1999 Mar 16;130(6):487-95.
[110] Bleecker ER, Welch MJ, Weinstein SF, Kalberg C, Johnson M, Edwards L, *et al.* Low-dose inhaled fluticasone propionate *vs.* oral zafirlukast in the treatment of persistent asthma. J Allergy Clin Immunol. 2000 Jun;105(6 Pt 1):1123-9.
[111] Busse W, Raphael GD, Galant S, Kalberg C, Goode-Sellers S, Srebro S, *et al.* Low-dose fluticasone propionate compared with montelukast for first-line treatment of persistent asthma: a randomized clinical trial. J Allergy Clin Immunol. 2001 Mar;107(3):461-8.
[112] Ram FS, Cates CJ, Ducharme FM. Long-acting beta2-agonists *vs.* anti-leukotrienes as add-on therapy to inhaled corticosteroids for chronic asthma. Cochrane Database Syst Rev. 2005(1):CD003137.
[113] Dessanges JF, Prefaut C, Taytard A, Matran R, Naya I, Compagnon A, *et al.* The effect of zafirlukast on repetitive exercise-induced bronchoconstriction: the possible role of leukotrienes in exercise-induced refractoriness. J Allergy Clin Immunol. 1999 Dec;104(6):1155-61.
[114] Pearlman DS, Ostrom NK, Bronsky EA, Bonuccelli CM, Hanby LA. The leukotriene D4-receptor antagonist zafirlukast attenuates exercise-induced bronchoconstriction in children. J Pediatr. 1999 Mar;134(3):273-9.
[115] Suguro H, Majima T, Hattori T, Ichimura K, Hashimoto N, Horie T. [Effect of a leukotriene antagonist, pranlukast hydrate, on exercise-induced asthma for 14 days]. Arerugi. 2000 Aug;49(8):646-52.
[116] Meltzer SS, Hasday JD, Cohn J, Bleecker ER. Inhibition of exercise-induced bronchospasm by zileuton: a 5-lipoxygenase inhibitor. Am J Respir Crit Care Med. 1996 Mar;153(3):931-5.
[117] DuBuske LM, Grossman J, Dube LM, Swanson LJ, Lancaster JF. Randomized trial of zileuton in patients with moderate asthma: effect of reduced dosing frequency and amounts on pulmonary function and asthma symptoms. Zileuton Study Group. Am J Manag Care. 1997 Apr;3(4):633-40.
[118] Finnerty JP, Wood-Baker R, Thomson H, Holgate ST. Role of leukotrienes in exercise-induced asthma. Inhibitory effect of ICI 204219, a potent leukotriene D4 receptor antagonist. Am Rev Respir Dis. 1992 Apr;145(4 Pt 1):746-9.
[119] Reiss TF, Hill JB, Harman E, Zhang J, Tanaka WK, Bronsky E, *et al.* Increased urinary excretion of LTE4 after exercise and attenuation of exercise-induced bronchospasm by montelukast, a cysteinyl leukotriene receptor antagonist. Thorax. 1997 Dec;52(12):1030-5.

[120] Leff JA, Busse WW, Pearlman D, Bronsky EA, Kemp J, Hendeles L, *et al.* Montelukast, a leukotriene-receptor antagonist, for the treatment of mild asthma and exercise-induced bronchoconstriction. N Engl J Med. 1998 Jul 16;339(3):147-52.

[121] Robuschi M, Riva E, Fuccella LM, Vida E, Barnabe R, Rossi M, *et al.* Prevention of exercise-induced bronchoconstriction by a new leukotriene antagonist (SK&F 104353). A double-blind study *vs.* disodium cromoglycate and placebo. Am Rev Respir Dis. 1992 Jun;145(6):1285-8.

[122] Kemp JP, Dockhorn RJ, Shapiro GG, Nguyen HH, Reiss TF, Seidenberg BC, *et al.* Montelukast once daily inhibits exercise-induced bronchoconstriction in 6- to 14-year-old children with asthma. J Pediatr. 1998 Sep;133(3):424-8.

[123] de Benedictis F, del Giudice M, Forenza N, Decimo F, de Benedictis D, Capristo A. Lack of tolerance to the protective effect of montelukast in exercise-induced bronchoconstriction in children. Eur Respir J. 2006;28(2):291-5.

[124] Villaran C, O'Neill SJ, Helbling A, van Noord JA, Lee TH, Chuchalin AG, *et al.* Montelukast *vs.* salmeterol in patients with asthma and exercise-induced bronchoconstriction. Montelukast/Salmeterol Exercise Study Group. J Allergy Clin Immunol. 1999 Sep;104(3 Pt 1):547-53.

[125] Edelman JM, Turpin JA, Bronsky EA, Grossman J, Kemp JP, Ghannam AF, *et al.* Oral montelukast compared with inhaled salmeterol to prevent exercise-induced bronchoconstriction. A randomized, double-blind trial. Exercise Study Group. Ann Intern Med. 2000 Jan 18;132(2):97-104.

[126] Steinshamn S, Sandsund M, Sue-Chu M, Bjermer L. Effects of montelukast on physical performance and exercise economy in adult asthmatics with exercise-induced bronchoconstriction. Scand J Med Sci Sports. 2002 Aug;12(4):211-7.

[127] Helenius I, Lumme A, Ounap J, Obase Y, Rytila P, Sarna S, *et al.* No effect of montelukast on asthma-like symptoms in elite ice hockey players. Allergy. 2004 Jan;59(1):39-44.

[128] Rundell KW, Spiering BA, Baumann JM, Evans TM. Effects of montelukast on airway narrowing from eucapnic voluntary hyperventilation and cold air exercise. Br J Sports Med. 2005 Apr;39(4):232-6.

[129] Donnelly AL, Glass M, Minkwitz MC, Casale TB. The leukotriene D4-receptor antagonist, ICI 204,219, relieves symptoms of acute seasonal allergic rhinitis. Am J Respir Crit Care Med. 1995 Jun;151(6):1734-9.

[130] Meltzer EO, Malmstrom K, Lu S, Prenner BM, Wei LX, Weinstein SF, *et al.* Concomitant montelukast and loratadine as treatment for seasonal allergic rhinitis: a randomized, placebo-controlled clinical trial. J Allergy Clin Immunol. 2000 May;105(5):917-22.

[131] van Adelsberg J, Philip G, Pedinoff AJ, Meltzer EO, Ratner PH, Menten J, *et al.* Montelukast improves symptoms of seasonal allergic rhinitis over a 4-week treatment period. Allergy. 2003 Dec;58(12):1268-76.

[132] Busse WW, Casale TB, Dykewicz MS, Meltzer EO, Bird SR, Hustad CM, *et al.* Efficacy of montelukast during the allergy season in patients with chronic asthma and seasonal aeroallergen sensitivity. Ann Allergy Asthma Immunol. 2006 Jan;96(1):60-8.

[133] Di Lorenzo G, D'Alcamo A, Rizzo M, Leto-Barone MS, Bianco CL, Ditta V, *et al.* Leukotriene receptor antagonists in monotherapy or in combination with antihistamines in the treatment of chronic urticaria: a systematic review. J Asthma Allergy. 2008;2:9-16.

[134] Nathani N, Little MA, Kunst H, Wilson D, Thickett DR. Churg-Strauss syndrome and leukotriene antagonist use: a respiratory perspective. Thorax. 2008 Oct;63(10):883-8.

[135] Edwards AM, Holgate ST. The Chromones: Cromolyn Sodium and Nedocromil Sodium. In: Adkinson Jr NF, Bochner BS, Busse W, Holgate ST, Lemanske Jr RF, Simons FER, editors. Middleton's Allergy: Principles and Practice. 7th ed: Mosby; 2008.

[136] Yamawaki I, Tamaoki J, Takeda Y, Nagai A. Inhaled cromoglycate reduces airway neurogenic inflammation *via* tachykinin antagonism. Res Commun Mol Pathol Pharmacol. 1997 Dec;98(3):265-72.

[137] Morton AR, Ogle SL, Fitch KD. Effects of nedocromil sodium, cromolyn sodium, and a placebo in exercise-induced asthma. Ann Allergy. 1992 Feb;68(2):143-8.

[138] Brannan JD, Anderson SD, Freed R, Leuppi JD, Koskela H, Chan HK. Nedocromil sodium inhibits responsiveness to inhaled mannitol in asthmatic subjects. Am J Respir Crit Care Med. 2000 Jun;161(6):2096-9.

[139] Spooner C, Rowe BH, Saunders LD. Nedocromil sodium in the treatment of exercise-induced asthma: a meta-analysis. Eur Respir J. 2000 Jul;16(1):30-7.

[140] Spooner CH, Saunders LD, Rowe BH. Nedocromil sodium for preventing exercise-induced bronchoconstriction. Cochrane Database Syst Rev. 2002(1):CD001183.

[141] Kippelen P, Larsson J, Anderson SD, Brannan JD, Dahlen B, Dahlen SE. Effect of sodium cromoglycate on mast cell mediators during hyperpnea in athletes. Med Sci Sports Exerc. 2010 Oct;42(10):1853-60.

[142] Kelly K, Spooner CH, Rowe BH. Nedocromil sodium *vs.* sodium cromoglycate for preventing exercise-induced bronchoconstriction in asthmatics. Cochrane Database Syst Rev. 2000(4):CD002731.

[143] Kennedy MC. Disodium cromoglycate in the control of asthma. A double-blind trial. Br J Dis Chest. 1969 Apr;63(2):96-106.

[144] Altounyan R, Howell J. Treatment of asthma with disodium cromoglycate (FPL 670, 'Intal'). Respiration. 1969;26:Suppl:131-40.

[145] van der Wouden JC, Uijen JH, Bernsen RM, Tasche MJ, de Jongste JC, Ducharme F. Inhaled sodium cromoglycate for asthma in children. Cochrane Database Syst Rev. 2008(4):CD002173.

[146] Svendsen UG, Jorgensen H. Inhaled nedocromil sodium as additional treatment to high dose inhaled corticosteroids in the management of bronchial asthma. Eur Respir J. 1991 Sep;4(8):992-9.

[147] Wells A, Drennan C, Holst P, Jones D, Rea H, Thornley P. Comparison of nedocromil sodium at two dosage frequencies with placebo in the management of chronic asthma. Respir Med. 1992 Jul;86(4):311-6.

[148] Goldin JG, Bateman ED. Does nedocromil sodium have a steroid sparing effect in adult asthmatic patients requiring maintenance oral corticosteroids? Thorax. 1988 Dec;43(12):982-6.

[149] Callaghan B, Teo NC, Clancy L. Effects of the addition of nedocromil sodium to maintenance bronchodilator therapy in the management of chronic asthma. Chest. 1992 Mar;101(3):787-92.

[150] Stainer R, Matthews S, Arshad SH, McDonald S, Robinson J, Schapira C, *et al.* Efficacy and acceptability of a new topical skin lotion of sodium cromoglicate (Altoderm) in atopic dermatitis in children aged 2-12 years: a double-blind, randomized, placebo-controlled trial. Br J Dermatol. 2005 Feb;152(2):334-41.

[151] Sorkin EM, Ward A. Ocular sodium cromoglycate. An overview of its therapeutic efficacy in allergic eye disease. Drugs. 1986 Feb;31(2):131-48.

[152] Kari O, Saari KM. Diagnostics and new developments in the treatment of ocular allergies. Curr Allergy Asthma Rep. 2012 Jun;12(3):232-9.

[153] Bousquet J, Khaltaev N, Cruz AA, Denburg J, Fokkens WJ, Togias A, *et al.* Allergic Rhinitis and its Impact on Asthma (ARIA) 2008 update (in collaboration with the World Health Organization, GA(2)LEN and AllerGen). Allergy. 2008 Apr;63 Suppl 86:8-160.

[154] Montgomery LC, Deuster PA. Ingestion of an antihistamine does not affect exercise performance. Med Sci Sports Exerc. 1992;24:383-8.

[155] Juji F, Suko M. Effectiveness of disodium cromoglycate in food-dependent, exercise-induced anaphylaxis: a case report. Ann Allergy. 1994 May;72(5):452-4.

[156] Benhamou AH, Vanini G, Lantin JP, Eigenmann PA. Antihistamine and sodium cromoglycate medication for food cold water exercise-induced anaphylaxis. Allergy. 2007 Dec;62(12):1471-2.

[157] Laube BL, Edwards AM, Dalby RN, Creticos PS, Norman PS. The efficacy of slow *vs.* faster inhalation of cromolyn sodium in protecting against allergen challenge in patients with asthma. J Allergy Clin Immunol. 1998 Apr;101(4 Pt 1):475-83.

[158] Aswania O, Chrystyn H. Relative lung bioavailability of generic sodium cromoglycate inhalers used with and without a spacer device. Pulm Pharmacol Ther. 2001;14(2):129-33.

[159] Anderson SD. Single-dose agents in the prevention of exercise-induced asthma: a descriptive review. Treat Respir Med. 2004;3(6):365-79.

[160] Cox JS, Beach JE, Blair AM, Clarke AJ, King J, Lee TB, *et al.* Disodium cromoglycate (Intal). Adv Drug Res. 1970;5:115-96.

[161] Clark B. General pharmacology, pharmacokinetics, and toxicology of nedocromil sodium. J Allergy Clin Immunol. 1993 Jul;92(1 Pt 2):200-2.

[162] Foulds RA. An overview of human safety data with nedocromil sodium. J Allergy Clin Immunol. 1993 Jul;92(1 Pt 2):202-4.

[163] Holgate S, Casale T, Wenzel S, Bousquet J, Deniz Y, Reisner C. The anti-inflammatory effects of omalizumab confirm the central role of IgE in allergic inflammation. J Allergy Clin Immunol. 2005 Mar;115(3):459-65.

[164] Djukanovic R, Wilson SJ, Kraft M, Jarjour NN, Steel M, Chung KF, *et al.* Effects of treatment with anti-immunoglobulin E antibody omalizumab on airway inflammation in allergic asthma. Am J Respir Crit Care Med. 2004 Sep 15;170(6):583-93.

[165] The European Medicines Agency. 2012; Available from: http://www.ema.europa.eu/ema/.

[166] CONTROLLED trial of effects of cortisone acetate in status asthmaticus; report to the Medical Research Council by the subcommittee on clinical trials in asthma. Lancet. 1956 Oct 20;271(6947):803-6.

[167] Zuberbier T, Asero R, Bindslev-Jensen C, Walter Canonica G, Church MK, Gimenez-Arnau AM, *et al.* EAACI/GA(2)LEN/EDF/WAO guideline: management of urticaria. Allergy. 2009 Oct;64(10):1427-43.

[168] Simons FE. Anaphylaxis pathogenesis and treatment. Allergy. 2011 Jul;66 Suppl 95:31-4.

[169] Simons F. Pharmacologic treatment of anaphylaxis: can the evidence base be strengthened? Curr Opin Allergy Clin Immunol. 2010;10(4):384-93.

[170] Becker JM, Arora A, Scarfone RJ, Spector ND, Fontana-Penn ME, Gracely E, *et al.* Oral *vs.* intravenous corticosteroids in children hospitalized with asthma. J Allergy Clin Immunol. 1999 Apr;103(4):586-90.

[171] Katz RM. Rhinitis in the athlete. Journal of Allergy and Clinical Immunology. 1984;73(5 II SUPPL.):708-10.

[172] Dijkstra HP, Robson-Ansley P. The prevalence and current opinion of treatment of allergic rhinitis in elite athletes. Current Opinion in Allergy and Clinical Immunology. [Classical Review]. 2011(11):103–8.

[173] Delgado L, Moreira A, Capão-Filipe M. Rhinitis and its impact on sports. Allergy and Clinical Immunology International. 2006;18(3):98-105.

[174] Thomas S, Wolfarth B, Wittmer C, Nowak D, Radon K. Self-reported asthma and allergies in top athletes compared to the general population - results of the German part of the GA2LEN-Olympic study 2008. Allergy Asthma Clin Immunol. 2010;6(1):31.

[175] Helbling A, Jenoure P, Muller U. [The incidence of hay fever in leading Swiss athletes]. Schweiz Med Wochenschr. 1990 Feb 17;120(7):231-6.

[176] Bonini S, Bonini M, Bousquet J, Brusasco V, Canonica GW, Carlsen KH, *et al.* Rhinitis and asthma in athletes: An ARIA document in collaboration with GA2LEN. Allergy: European Journal of Allergy and Clinical Immunology. 2006;61(6):681-92.

[177] Alves A, Martins C, Delgado L, Fonseca J, Moreira A. Exercise-induced rhinitis in competitive swimmers. Am J Rhinol Allergy. 2010 Sep;24(5):e114-7.

[178] Dahl R, Mygind N. Mechanisms of airflow limitation in the nose and lungs. Clin Exp Allergy. 1998 Jun;28 Suppl 2:17-25.

[179] Valero A, Serrano C, Valera JL, Barbera A, Torrego A, Mullol J, *et al.* Nasal and bronchial response to exercise in patients with asthma and rhinitis: the role of nitric oxide. Allergy. 2005 Sep;60(9):1126-31.

[180] Brozek JL, Bousquet J, Baena-Cagnani CE, Bonini S, Canonica GW, Casale TB, *et al.* Allergic Rhinitis and its Impact on Asthma (ARIA) guidelines: 2010 revision. J Allergy Clin Immunol. 2010 Sep;126(3):466-76.

[181] The World Anti-Doping Agency homepage. 2012 [cited 2012]; Available from: http://www.wada-ama.org/.

[182] WADA. Medical Information to Support the Decisions of TUEC Asthma. 2011.

[183] Fokkens WJ, Lund VJ, Mullol J, Bachert C, Alobid I, Baroody F, *et al.* EPOS 2012: European position paper on rhinosinusitis and nasal polyps 2012. A summary for otorhinolaryngologists. Rhinology. 2012 Mar;50(1):1-12.

[184] Scadding GK, Durham SR, Mirakian R, Jones NS, Leech SC, Farooque S, *et al.* BSACI guidelines for the management of allergic and non-allergic rhinitis. Clin Exp Allergy. 2008 Jan;38(1):19-42.

[185] van Cauwenberge P, Bachert C, Passalacqua G, Bousquet J, Canonica GW, Durham SR, *et al.* Consensus statement on the treatment of allergic rhinitis. European Academy of Allergology and Clinical Immunology. Allergy. 2000 Feb;55(2):116-34.

[186] Schafer T, Schnoor M, Wagenmann M, Klimek L, Bachert C. Therapeutic Index (TIX) for intranasal corticosteroids in the treatment of allergic rhinitis. Rhinology. 2011 Aug;49(3):272-80.

[187] Weiner JM, Abramson MJ, Puy RM. Intranasal corticosteroids *vs.* oral H1 receptor antagonists in allergic rhinitis: systematic review of randomised controlled trials. BMJ. 1998 Dec 12;317(7173):1624-9.

[188] Alaranta A, Alaranta H, Heliövaaras M, Alha P, Palmu P, Helenius I. Allergic rhinitis and pharmacological management in elite athletes. Medicine and Science in Sports and Exercise. 2005;37(5):707-11.

[189] Nathan RA, Yancey SW, Waitkus-Edwards K, Prillaman BA, Stauffer JL, Philpot E, *et al.* Fluticasone propionate nasal spray is superior to montelukast for allergic rhinitis while neither affects overall asthma control. Chest. 2005 Oct;128(4):1910-20.

[190] Pullerits T, Praks L, Ristioja V, Lotvall J. Comparison of a nasal glucocorticoid, antileukotriene, and a combination of antileukotriene and antihistamine in the treatment of seasonal allergic rhinitis. J Allergy Clin Immunol. 2002 Jun;109(6):949-55.

[191] Di Lorenzo G, Pacor ML, Pellitteri ME, Morici G, Di Gregoli A, Lo Bianco C, *et al.* Randomized placebo-controlled trial comparing fluticasone aqueous nasal spray in mono-therapy, fluticasone plus cetirizine, fluticasone plus montelukast and cetirizine plus montelukast for seasonal allergic rhinitis. Clin Exp Allergy. 2004 Feb;34(2):259-67.

[192] Martin BG, Andrews CP, van Bavel JH, Hampel FC, Klein KC, Prillaman BA, *et al.* Comparison of fluticasone propionate aqueous nasal spray and oral montelukast for the treatment of seasonal allergic rhinitis symptoms. Ann Allergy Asthma Immunol. 2006 Jun;96(6):851-7.

[193] Ratner PH, Howland WC, 3rd, Arastu R, Philpot EE, Klein KC, Baidoo CA, *et al.* Fluticasone propionate aqueous nasal spray provided significantly greater improvement in daytime and nighttime nasal symptoms of seasonal allergic rhinitis compared with montelukast. Ann Allergy Asthma Immunol. 2003 May;90(5):536-42.

[194] Laliberte F, Laliberte MF, Lecart S, Bousquet J, Klossec JM, Mounedji N. Clinical and pathologic methods to assess the long-term safety of nasal corticosteroids. French Triamcinolone Acetonide Study Group. Allergy. 2000 Aug;55(8):718-22.

[195] Demoly P. Safety of intranasal corticosteroids in acute rhinosinusitis. Am J Otolaryngol. 2008 Nov-Dec;29(6):403-13.

[196] Skoner DP, Rachelefsky GS, Meltzer EO, Chervinsky P, Morris RM, Seltzer JM, *et al.* Detection of growth suppression in children during treatment with intranasal beclomethasone dipropionate. Pediatrics. 2000 Feb;105(2):E23.

[197] Shusterman D, Balmes J, Avila PC, Murphy MA, Matovinovic E. Chlorine inhalation produces nasal congestion in allergic rhinitics without mast cell degranulation. Eur Respir J. 2003 Apr;21(4):652-7.

[198] Silvers WS, Poole JA. Exercise-induced rhinitis: A common disorder that adversely affects allergic and nonallergic athletes. Annals of Allergy, Asthma and Immunology. 2006;96(2):334-40.

[199] Sacha JJ, Quinn JM. The environment, the airway, and the athlete. Annals of Allergy, Asthma and Immunology. 2011;106(2):81-8.

[200] Gioulekas D, Damialis A, Papakosta D, Syrigou A, Mpaka G, Saxoni F, *et al.* 15-year aeroallergen records. Their usefulness in Athens Olympics, 2004. Allergy. 2003 Sep;58(9):933-8.

[201] Wallace DV, Dykewicz MS, Bernstein DI, Blessing-Moore J, Cox L, Khan DA, *et al.* The diagnosis and management of rhinitis: An updated practice parameter. Journal of Allergy and Clinical Immunology. 2008;122(2, Supplement 1):S1-S84.

[202] Zhang F, Wang W, Lv J, Krafft T, Xu J. Time-series studies on air pollution and daily outpatient visits for allergic rhinitis in Beijing, China. Science of The Total Environment. 2011;409(13):2486-92.

[203] Walsh NP, Gleeson M, Shephard RJ, Woods JA, Bishop NC, Fleshner M, *et al.* Position statement. Part one: Immune function and exercise. Exerc Immunol Rev. 2011;17:6-63.

[204] Moreira AD, L. ; Moreira, P. ; Haahtela, T. Does exercise increase the risk of upper respiratory tract infections? British Medical Bulletin. [Systematic Review]. 2009(90):111-31.

[205] Simons FE. Advances in H1-antihistamines. N Engl J Med. 2004 Nov 18;351(21):2203-17.

[206] Simons E. Histamine and H1-antihistamine. In: Adkinson F, editor. Middleton`s Allergy: Mosby Elsevier; 2009. p. 1517-47.

[207] Akdis CA, Blaser K. Histamine in the immune regulation of allergic inflammation. J Allergy Clin Immunol. 2003 Jul;112(1):15-22.

[208] Jutel M, Blaser K, Akdis CA. Histamine in chronic allergic responses. J Investig Allergol Clin Immunol. 2005;15(1):1-8.

[209] O'Mahony L, Akdis M, Akdis CA. Regulation of the immune response and inflammation by histamine and histamine receptors. J Allergy Clin Immunol. 2011 Dec;128(6):1153-62.

[210] Niijima-Yaoita F, Tsuchiya M, Ohtsu H, Yanai K, Sugawara S, Endo Y, *et al.* Roles of histamine in exercise-induced fatigue: favouring endurance and protecting against exhaustion. Biol Pharm Bull. 2012;35(1):91-7.

[211] Nakamizo S, Egawa G, Miyachi Y, Kabashima K. Cholinergic urticaria: pathogenesis-based categorization and its treatment options. J Eur Acad Dermatol Venereol. 2012 Jan;26(1):114-6.

[212] Botto NC, Warshaw EM. Solar urticaria. J Am Acad Dermatol. 2008 Dec;59(6):909-20; quiz 21-2.

[213] Tlougan BE, Podjasek JO, Adams BB. Aquatic sports dermatoses: part 1. In the water: freshwater dermatoses. Int J Dermatol. 2010 Aug;49(8):874-85.

[214] Kockentiet B, Adams BB. Contact dermatitis in athletes. J Am Acad Dermatol. 2007 Jun;56(6):1048-55.

[215] Ortonne JP. Urticaria and its subtypes: the role of second-generation antihistamines. Eur J Intern Med. 2012 Jan;23(1):26-30.

[216] Compalati E, Baena-Cagnani R, Penagos M, Badellino H, Braido F, Gomez RM, *et al.* Systematic review on the efficacy of fexofenadine in seasonal allergic rhinitis: a meta-analysis of randomized, double-blind, placebo-controlled clinical trials. Int Arch Allergy Immunol. 2011;156(1):1-15.

[217] Bousquet J, Bachert C, Canonica GW, Mullol J, Van Cauwenberge P, Jensen CB, *et al.* Efficacy of desloratadine in persistent allergic rhinitis - a GA(2)LEN study. Int Arch Allergy Immunol. 2010;153(4):395-402.

[218] Segall N, Gawchik S, Georges G, Haeusler JM. Efficacy and safety of levocetirizine in improving symptoms and health-related quality of life in US adults with seasonal allergic rhinitis: a randomized, placebo-controlled study. Ann Allergy Asthma Immunol. 2010 Mar;104(3):259-67.

[219] Korsgren M, Andersson M, Borga O, Larsson L, Alden-Raboisson M, Malmqvist U, *et al.* Clinical efficacy and pharmacokinetic profiles of intranasal and oral cetirizine in a repeated allergen challenge model of allergic rhinitis. Ann Allergy Asthma Immunol. 2007 Apr;98(4):316-21.

[220] Walter Canonica G, Bousquet J, Van Hammee G, Bachert C, Durham SR, Klimek L, *et al.* Levocetirizine improves health-related quality of life and health status in persistent allergic rhinitis. Respir Med. 2006 Oct;100(10):1706-15.

[221] Borazan M, Karalezli A, Akova YA, Akman A, Kiyici H, Erbek SS. Efficacy of olopatadine HCI 0.1%, ketotifen fumarate 0.025%, epinastine HCI 0.05%, emedastine

0.05% and fluorometholone acetate 0.1% ophthalmic solutions for seasonal allergic conjunctivitis: a placebo-controlled environmental trial. Acta Ophthalmol. 2009 Aug;87(5):549-54.

[222] Weinstein ME, Wolff AH, Bielory L. Efficacy and tolerability of second- and third-generation antihistamines in the treatment of acquired cold urticaria: a meta-analysis. Ann Allergy Asthma Immunol. 2010 Jun;104(6):518-22.

[223] Nettis E, Colanardi MC, Soccio AL, Ferrannini A, Vacca A. Desloratadine in combination with montelukast suppresses the dermographometer challenge test papule, and is effective in the treatment of delayed pressure urticaria: a randomized, double-blind, placebo-controlled study. Br J Dermatol. 2006 Dec;155(6):1279-82.

[224] Staevska M, Popov TA, Kralimarkova T, Lazarova C, Kraeva S, Popova D, *et al.* The effectiveness of levocetirizine and desloratadine in up to 4 times conventional doses in difficult-to-treat urticaria. J Allergy Clin Immunol. 2010 Mar;125(3):676-82.

[225] Siebenhaar F, Degener F, Zuberbier T, Martus P, Maurer M. High-dose desloratadine decreases wheal volume and improves cold provocation thresholds compared with standard-dose treatment in patients with acquired cold urticaria: a randomized, placebo-controlled, crossover study. J Allergy Clin Immunol. 2009 Mar;123(3):672-9.

[226] Grob JJ, Auquier P, Dreyfus I, Ortonne JP. How to prescribe antihistamines for chronic idiopathic urticaria: desloratadine daily *vs.* PRN and quality of life. Allergy. 2009 Apr;64(4):605-12.

[227] Grob JJ, Auquier P, Dreyfus I, Ortonne JP. Quality of life in adults with chronic idiopathic urticaria receiving desloratadine: a randomized, double-blind, multicentre, placebo-controlled study. J Eur Acad Dermatol Venereol. 2008 Jan;22(1):87-93.

[228] Katelaris CH, Carrozzi FM, Burke TV. Allergic rhinoconjunctivitis in elite athletes: Optimal management for quality of life and performance. Sports Medicine. 2003;33(6):401-6.

[229] Church MK, Maurer M, Simons FE, Bindslev-Jensen C, van Cauwenberge P, Bousquet J, *et al.* Risk of first-generation H(1)-antihistamines: a GA(2)LEN position paper. Allergy. 2010 Apr;65(4):459-66.

[230] Eskiizmir G, Hircin Z, Ozyurt B, Unlu H. A comparative analysis of the decongestive effect of oxymetazoline and xylometazoline in healthy subjects. Eur J Clin Pharmacol. 2011 Jan;67(1):19-23.

[231] Mandhane SN, Shah JH, Thennati R. Allergic rhinitis: an update on disease, present treatments and future prospects. Int Immunopharmacol. 2011 Nov;11(11):1646-62.

[232] Meltzer EO, Caballero F, Fromer LM, Krouse JH, Scadding G. Treatment of congestion in upper respiratory diseases. Int J Gen Med. 2010;3:69-91.

[233] Horak F, Zieglmayer P, Zieglmayer R, Lemell P, Yao R, Staudinger H, *et al.* A placebo-controlled study of the nasal decongestant effect of phenylephrine and pseudoephedrine in the Vienna Challenge Chamber. Ann Allergy Asthma Immunol. 2009 Feb;102(2):116-20.

[234] Meltzer EO. Allergic Rhinitis: The Impact of Discordant Perspectives of Patient and Physician on Treatment Decisions. Clinical Therapeutics. 2007;29(7):1428-40.

[235] Shaikh N, Wald ER, Pi M. Decongestants, antihistamines and nasal irrigation for acute sinusitis in children. Cochrane Database Syst Rev. 2010(12):CD007909.

[236] De Sutter AI, van Driel ML, Kumar AA, Lesslar O, Skrt A. Oral antihistamine-decongestant-analgesic combinations for the common cold. Cochrane Database Syst Rev. 2012;2:CD004976.

[237] Pritchard-Peschek KR, Jenkins DG, Osborne MA, Slater GJ. Pseudoephedrine ingestion and cycling time-trial performance. Int J Sport Nutr Exerc Metab. 2010 Apr;20(2):132-8.
[238] Raphael GD, Angello JT, Wu MM, Druce HM. Efficacy of diphenhydramine *vs.* desloratadine and placebo in patients with moderate-to-severe seasonal allergic rhinitis. Ann Allergy Asthma Immunol. 2006 Apr;96(4):606-14.
[239] Vaidyanathan S, Williamson P, Lipworth B. Comparative evaluation of nasal blood flow and airflow in the decongestant response to oxymetazoline. Ann Allergy Asthma Immunol. 2012 Feb;108(2):77-80.
[240] Kaszuba SM, Stewart MG. Medical management and diagnosis of chronic rhinosinusitis: A survey of treatment patterns by United States otolaryngologists. Am J Rhinol. 2006 Mar-Apr;20(2):186-90.
[241] Taverner D, Latte GJ. Nasal decongestants for the common cold. Cochrane Database Syst Rev. 2009(2):CD001953.
[242] Corey JP, Houser SM, Ng BA. Nasal congestion: a review of its etiology, evaluation, and treatment. Ear Nose Throat J. 2000 Sep;79(9):690-3, 6, 8 passim.
[243] Bousquet J, Lockey R, Malling HJ. Allergen immunotherapy: therapeutic vaccines for allergic diseases. A WHO position paper. J Allergy Clin Immunol. 1998 Oct;102(4 Pt 1):558-62.
[244] Wallace DV, Dykewicz MS, Bernstein DI, Blessing-Moore J, Cox L, Khan DA, *et al.* The diagnosis and management of rhinitis: an updated practice parameter. J Allergy Clin Immunol. 2008 Aug;122(2 Suppl):S1-84.
[245] Durham SR, Emminger W, Kapp A, de Monchy JG, Rak S, Scadding GK, *et al.* SQ-standardized sublingual grass immunotherapy: confirmation of disease modification 2 years after 3 years of treatment in a randomized trial. J Allergy Clin Immunol. 2012 Mar;129(3):717-25 e5.
[246] Akdis CA, Akdis M. Mechanisms of allergen-specific immunotherapy. J Allergy Clin Immunol. 2011 Jan;127(1):18-27; quiz 8-9.
[247] Delgado L, Moreira A, Capão-Filipe M. Rhinitis and its impact on sports. Allergy and Clinical Immunology International. 2006;18(3):98-105.
[248] Calderon MA, Alves B, Jacobson M, Hurwitz B, Sheikh A, Durham S. Allergen injection immunotherapy for seasonal allergic rhinitis. Cochrane Database Syst Rev. 2007(1):CD001936.
[249] Radulovic S, Wilson D, Calderon M, Durham S. Systematic reviews of sublingual immunotherapy (SLIT). Allergy. 2011 Jun;66(6):740-52.
[250] Calderon MA, Penagos M, Sheikh A, Canonica GW, Durham SR. Sublingual immunotherapy for allergic conjunctivitis: Cochrane systematic review and meta-analysis. Clin Exp Allergy. 2011 Sep;41(9):1263-72.
[251] Abramson MJ, Puy RM, Weiner JM. Injection allergen immunotherapy for asthma. Cochrane Database Syst Rev. 2010(8):CD001186.
[252] Canonica GW, Passalacqua G. Noninjection routes for immunotherapy. J Allergy Clin Immunol. 2003 Mar;111(3):437-48; quiz 49.
[253] Canonica GW, Bousquet J, Casale T, Lockey RF, Baena-Cagnani CE, Pawankar R, *et al.* Sub-lingual immunotherapy: World Allergy Organization Position Paper 2009. Allergy. 2009 Dec;64 Suppl 91:1-59.
[254] Casale TB, Stokes JR. Future forms of immunotherapy. J Allergy Clin Immunol. 2011 Jan;127(1):8-15; quiz 6-7.

[255] Marogna M, Spadolini I, Massolo A, Berra D, Zanon P, Chiodini E, *et al.* Long-term comparison of sublingual immunotherapy *vs.* inhaled budesonide in patients with mild persistent asthma due to grass pollen. Ann Allergy Asthma Immunol. 2009 Jan;102(1):69-75.

[256] Passalacqua G, Musarra A, Pecora S, Amoroso S, Antonicelli L, Cadario G, *et al.* Quantitative assessment of the compliance with once-daily sublingual immunotherapy in children (EASY project: evaluation of a novel SLIT formulation during a year). Pediatr Allergy Immunol. 2007 Feb;18(1):58-62.

[257] Sieber J, De Geest S, Shah-Hosseini K, Mosges R. Medication persistence with long-term, specific grass pollen immunotherapy measured by prescription renewal rates. Curr Med Res Opin. 2011 Apr;27(4):855-61.

[258] van Cauwenberge P, Palange P, Canonica GW. Prevention: educational issues and recommendations for early recognition. European Respiratory Society Monograph: Chapter 9 (Diagnosis, Prevention and Treatment of Exercise-Related Asthma, Respiratory and Allergic Disorders in Sports). 2005;33:89-101.

[259] Ventura MT, Giuliano G, Buquicchio R, Accettura F, Carbonara M. Local and systemic reactions occurring during immunotherapy: an epidemiological evaluation and a prospective safety-monitoring study. Immunopharmacol Immunotoxicol. 2008;30(1):153-61.

[260] Martelli A, Ghiglioni D, Sarratud T, Calcinai E, Veehof S, Terracciano L, *et al.* Anaphylaxis in the emergency department: a paediatric perspective. Curr Opin Allergy Clin Immunol. 2008 Aug;8(4):321-9.

[261] Ring J, Grosber M, Mohrenschlager M, Brockow K. Anaphylaxis: acute treatment and management. Chem Immunol Allergy. 2010;95:201-10.

[262] Simons FE. Pharmacologic treatment of anaphylaxis: can the evidence base be strengthened? Curr Opin Allergy Clin Immunol. 2010 Aug;10(4):384-93.

[263] Simons F, Ardusso L, Bilo M, El-Gamal Y, Ledford D, Ring J, *et al.* World Allergy Organization Guidelines for the Assessment and Management of Anaphylaxis. W A O Journal. 2011;4:13-36.

[264] Kemp S, Lockey R, Simons F. Epinephrine: the drug of choice for anaphylaxis. A statement of the World Allergy Organization. Allergy. 2008;63(8):1061-70.

[265] Sheikh A, Shehata Y, Brown S, Simons F. Adrenaline for the treatment of anaphylaxis: cochrane systematic review. Allergy. 2009;64(2):204-12.

[266] Muraro A, Roberts G, Clark A, Eigenmann PA, Halken S, Lack G, *et al.* The management of anaphylaxis in childhood: position paper of the European academy of allergology and clinical immunology. Allergy. 2007 Aug;62(8):857-71.

[267] Cheng A, Canadian Paediatric Society Acute Care Committee. Emergency treatment of anaphylaxis in infants and children. Paediatr Child Health 2011;16(1):35-40.

[268] Simons K, Simons F. Epinephrine and its use in anaphylaxis: current issues. Curr Opin Allergy Clin Immunol. 2010;10(4):354-61.

[269] Liberman D, Teach S. Management of anaphylaxis in children. Pediatr Emerg Care. 2008;24(12):861-6.

[270] Pluim BM, de Hon O, Staal JB, Limpens J, Kuipers H, Overbeek SE, *et al.* β2-Agonists and physical performance: a systematic review and meta-analysis of randomized controlled trials. Sports Med. 2011;41(1):39-57.

[271] Kindermann W. Do inhaled beta(2)-agonists have an ergogenic potential in non-asthmatic competitive athletes? Sports Med. 2007;37(2):95-102.

[272] McKenzie D, Fitch K. The Asthmatic Athlete: Inhaled Beta-2 Agonists, Sport Performance, and Doping. Clin J Sport Med. 2011;21:46-50.

[273] Backer V, Lund T, Pedersen L. Pharmaceutical treatment of asthma symptoms in elite athletes - doping or therapy? Scand J Med Sci Sports. 2007 Dec;17(6):615-22.

CHAPTER 4

Omalizumab Therapy for Allergic Diseases

Juan Antonio Martinez-Tadeo*, Eva Perez-Rodriguez and Zulay Almeida-Sanchez

Hospital Universitario Ntra. Sra. De Candelaria, Allergy and Immunology Service, Canary Islands, Tenerife, Spain

Abstract: The antibody omalizumab is a humanized anti-IgE monoclonal binding to IgE circulating preventing binding to receptors and thereby inhibiting the cascade of allergic inflammation. Besides achieving a reduction in expression of IgE receptors on the surface of basophils and expression of high affinity receptor for IgE on the surface of dendritic cells. Its use has been approved for patients aged 6 years old with moderate to severe allergic asthma, also has been effective in other diseases such as asthma of occupational origin, seasonal or perennial allergic rhinitis, chronic urticaria difficult to control and helping to better tolerance immunotherapy. The results obtained in different studies on treatment with omalizumab in severe atopic dermatitis are contradictory. While providing a promising effect in the treatment of food and drug allergy more long-term studies are needed.

Keywords: Omalizumab, asthma, IgE, antiIgE, food allergy, drug allergy, atopic dermatitis, chronic urticaria, immunotherapy, mastocytosis.

INTRODUCTION

IgE was originally described in 1967 by two separate investigators, Ishizaka and Johansson [1]. IgE is important in defense against parasitic diseases, especially those caused by helminthes and some protozoa [2, 3]. However, low or absent levels of IgE do not predispose people to severe parasitic infections [4]. IgE is not believed to play an important role in defense against bacterial infections, since it does not activate complement or participate in opsonization [5]. The importance of IgE in atopic disorders, such as asthma, allergic rhinitis, food allergies and atopic dermatitis has since been established. Elevation of total serum IgE is

***Address correspondence to Juan Antonio Martinez-Tadeo:** Allergy and Immunology Service, Hospital Universitario Ntra. Sra. De Candelaria, Spain; Tel: 34-922602118; Fax: 34-922600089; E-mail: jmartineztadeo@gmail.com

typically found in many atopic patients, and in genetically predisposed individuals allergen-especific IgE is produced. IgE plays a central role in allergic diseases, especially mast cell/basophil activation, and in antigen presentation.

Structure of Immunoglobulin E

Immunoglobulin E is one of five isotypes of human immunoglobulins, IgG, IgA, IgM, IgD, and IgE [6]. The half-life of IgE in the serum is only 2 days and is present in far lower amounts than the rest of immunoglonulins. All immunoglobulins are composed of two light chains and two identical heavy chains (Fig. **1**). The N-terminal portion of heavy and light chains, termed the variable region, binds antigens, whereas the C-terminal portion of the heavy chain, termed the constant region, determines antibody class and effector functions. The heavy chain variable region is encoded in a distinct exon from those that encode the constant region. The variable región exon is assembled early in B-cell development from VH, D, and JH segments through V(D)J recombination. The heavy chain V(D)J exon is first expressed with proximal downstream exons that encode the Cμ constant region, leading to expression of μ IgH chains and IgM antibody. Newly generated B cells express surface IgM and migrate to the periphery where they can be induced to express a different IgH class (*e.g.*, IgG, IgE, or IgA)

The heavy chain differentiates the various immunoglobulin isotypes. The heavy chain in IgE is ε (epsilon). **IgE consists of four constant regions,** in contrast to other immunoglobulins that contain only three constant regions. Due to this extra region, the weight of IgE is 190 kDa compared to 150 kDa for IgG. The Cε2 constant domain is unique to IgE, while the Cε3 region binds to the low and high affinity IgE receptor.

Synthesis of IgE

Antibodies are produced by plasma cells. These cells are programmed to make IgM by default. Both soluble factors and cell surface interactions are critical in inducing B cells to switch isotype while retaining the original antigenic specificity [1, 7, 8]. Genomic DNA is spliced and rejoined in class switch recombination.

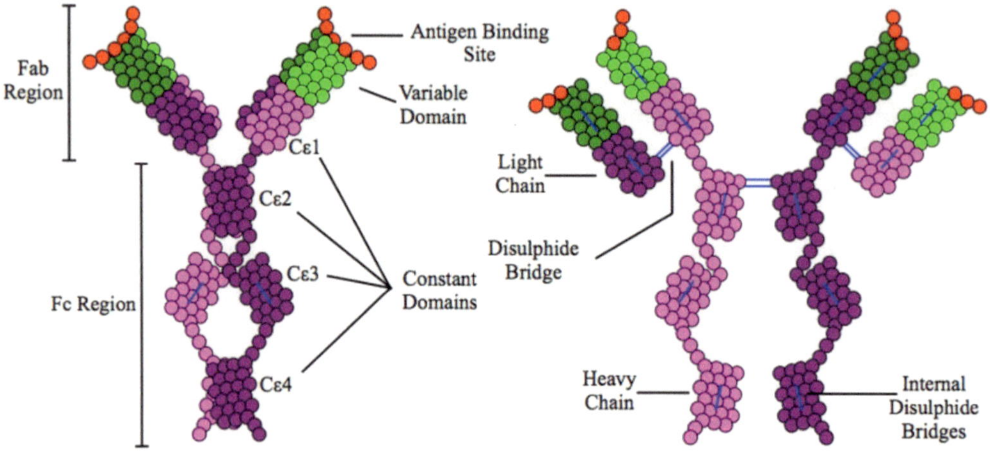

Figure 1: IgE structure.

B cell isotype switching requires two signals:

- The first signal involves the soluble factors interleukin-4 (IL-4) and 13 (IL-13) released by Th2 cells, mast cells, and basophils. Interaction of these cytokines with their respective receptors on B cells activates transcription at the specific ε germline locus *via* signal transducer and activator of transcription (STAT) 6.

- The second signal is the interaction between the B cell CD40 and T cell CD40 ligand (CD154). The second signal results in DNA class switch recombination and IgE expression triggered by nuclear factor κB (NFκB). STAT6 and NFκB synergize to activate B cell activator protein (BSAP), promoting production of IgE. The removal of the unwanted constant regions by splicing and rejoining of the DNA requires AID (activation-induced cytidine deaminase) and UNG (uracil DNA glycosylase). Accessory molecules that amplify IgE production include CD28/CD80-CD86 interactions. In addition there are negative signals that reduce IgE production: ID2 (inhibitor of DNA binding 2) binds to E-box (which contributes on supressing the class switch recombination to IgE); BCL-6 (B cell lymphoma 6) competes with STAT6; and SOCS-1 (suppressor of cytokine signaling 1) regulates STAT-6-dependent eotaxin production (which is a critical mediator for airway inflammation) triggered by IL-4 and TNF-alfa. Interferon gamma can also inhibit IgE production *via* STAT1-mediated activation of SOCS1.

B cell isotype switching to produce antigen-specific IgE occurs primarily in mucosal lymphoid tissues, with the greatest amounts of antigen-specific IgE production in tonsils and adenoids, although some also occurs in peripheral tissues [9]. The newly formed IgE then diffuses through the tissues and into the circulation.

Antigen-specific IgE production occurs locally within the bronchial and nasal mucosa, in addition to the lymphoid tissues, even in patients who are considered nonatopic by skin testing and laboratory tests. This phenomenon of local IgE production may underlie some cases of chronic nonallergic rhinitis and severe asthma [10].

Regulation of Synthesis

The genetic predisposition to develop allergic disease, or atopy, is a complex trait that is not fully understood. Total serum IgE levels and regulation of serum IgE production are strongly influenced by genetic factors. Less is known about other genetic factors important for the development of allergic disease. Genome-wide association studies have identified several loci that may be important for IgE regulation, including loci in the gene encoding the alpha chain of the high affinity receptor for IgE (FCεRIa), STAT6, and in the gene RAD50/IL-13 cluster [11].

IgE Receptors

IgE functions through its high and low affinity receptors on mast cells, basophils and other cells leading to degranulation of mast cells and basophils and antigen presentation [12]. Expression of both receptors is enhanced by IgE binding, so circulating IgE levels are positively correlated with receptor levels on mast cells and basophils. Furthermore, mast cells also express on its surface inhibitory receptors like the IgG receptor FcγRIIb. FcγRIIb crosslinking has been shown to reduce IgE-mediated mast cell activation.

High Affinity Receptor

The high affinity receptor for IgE is FcεRI. IgE binds to the α chain. FcεRI exists in two forms: A tetrameric form (αβγ2) of FcεRI is expressed on mast cells and basophils. In the nonactivated state, these cells are coated with FcεRI receptors bound to various antigen-specific IgE molecules. If that multivalent antigen (allergen) enters the cell's environment, it binds to the IgE, causing the FcεRI receptors to cluster on the cell surface and become cross-linked. Cross-linking leads to activation of the cell and release of preformed mediators from cytoplasmic granules (*e.g.,* histamine), transcription and release of cytokines, and synthesis of leukotrienes and prostaglandins. The strength of the activation signal depends upon the polyvalency of the allergen (ie, number of binding sites for IgE) and the affinity of the IgE for the allergen. The inflammatory mediators released by mast cells and basophils include histamine, tryptases, and tumor necrosis factor α, as well as leukotrienes and prostaglandins (LTC4 and PGD2, respectively). These mediators are responsible for the signs and symptoms of immediate hypersensitivity. In addition, production of the Th2 cytokines IL-4, IL-5, and IL-13 initiates late phase inflammation and promotes more IgE production. These mechanisms underlie the clinical manifestations of allergic diseases, such as allergic rhinitis and conjunctivitis, allergic asthma, food allergy, and anaphylaxis. A trimeric form of FcεRI (αγ2) is expressed on Langerhans cells, dendritic cells, and monocytes. It is important for antigen presentation. In humans, it is theorized that FcεRI on antigen-presenting cells permits the transport of antigens captured by IgE in the tissues into peripheral lymph nodes to initiate immune responses. IgE can upregulate FcεRI expression by a process that depends on stabilization of the surface receptor by IgE. The unoccupied receptor and aggregated receptor are lost from the cell surface by a slow process, which culminates in degradation by a Bafilomycin A-sensitive mechanism, suggesting a role for lysosomal degradation. The unoccupied receptor can recycle to the cell surface under the appropriate conditions.

Low Affinity Receptor

The low affinity IgE receptor, FcεRII (CD23), is present on a variety of cells. The constitutively expressed form, CD23a, is present only on B cells while the inducible form, CD23b, is present on B-cells, T-cells, dendritic cells, monocytes, macrophages, neutrophils, eosinophils, intestinal epithelial cells, and platelets [13].

Functions include regulation of IgE synthesis (binding of IgE to B cell CD23 inhibits IgE synthesis), antigen capture and presentation, and growth and differentiation of B cells. Epithelial cell CD23 transports IgE-allergen complexes from the lumen to the mucosa to interact with mast cells. CD23 can be shed from the cell membrane (sCD23) by endogenous proteases, creating a soluble form that may be important for upregulation of IgE synthesis.

OMALIZUMAB

Elevated total IgE is seen with some allergic disorders, as well as several non allergic diseases. Many patients (although not all) with allergic disorders have elevated levels of total IgE; however, there is no specific cut off value that discriminates patients with allergic disease from those without and there is considerable overlap. Allergen specific IgE is usually detectable several years before a person becomes reactive to that allergen, although only a subset of sensitized people will ever develop symptons. The role of total and allergen-specific IgE levels in pathogenesis and diagnosis differs among the leading allergic disorders. Asthma correlates with increased total IgE levels, regardless of atopic status. Allergic rhinitis is associated with allergen-specific IgE antibodies, although not with total IgE levels. Patients with atopic dermatitis may have very elevated levels of total IgE, although only a minority of patients (mostly children with severe AD) has clinically-apparent allergic reactions to food

Omalizumab is a humanized monoclonal antibody that recognizes and binds to the Fc portion of the IgE molecule [14]. Approximately 5% of omalizumab is composed of murine sequences which were engrafted onto a human IgGκ framework; it is these Fab portions that contain the antigen (IgE)-binding regions of the molecule (Fig. **2**). Nowadays, omalizumab is the only available anti-IgE therapy in use [15].

Mechanism of Action

Omalizumab binds to the CH3 domain of the IgE molecule, which is conserved among all of IgE molecules [1]. This is the same site where IgE binds to FcεRI. The binding of omalizumab to IgE results in the formation of soluble immune complexes that are subsequently cleared by the reticuloendothelial system. Typically, omalizumab forms trimers of two omalizumab molecules per IgE antibody, but can form other complexes. In essence, binding of omalizumab to free IgE blocks the binding of IgE to FcεRI and the subsequent expression of IgE on the surface of allergic effector cells. Because omalizumab binds to the same site that IgE molecules use to attach to FcεRI, it cannot cross-link cell surface expressed IgE. In other words, omalizumab can bind only to soluble IgE, and therefore cannot initiate degranulation of effector cells. The amount of cell-bound IgE declines over the course of omalizumab treatment owing to the reduced amount of free IgE available.

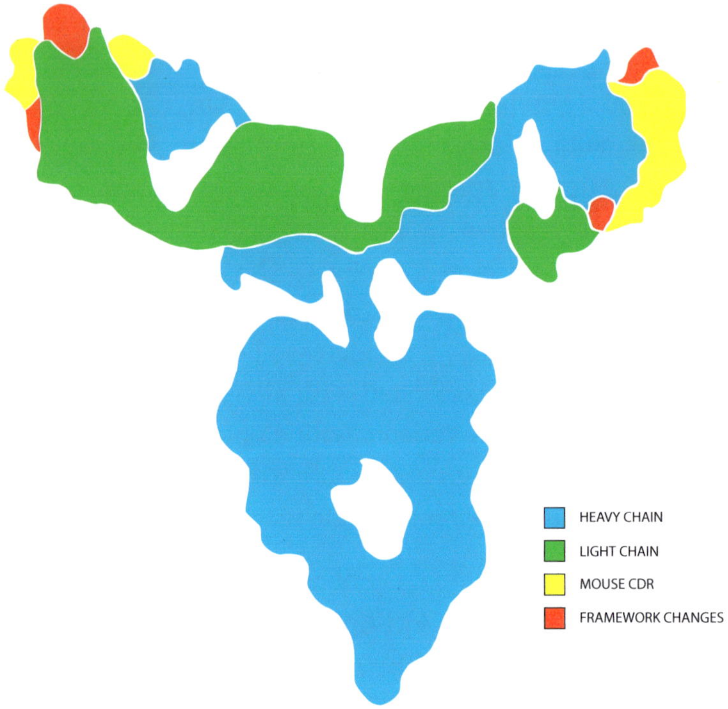

Figure 2: Structure of omalizumab.

The administration of omalizumab results in a rapid and substantial decrease in free IgE in serum and reduces the expression of FcεRI on several cell types. A 99% reduction in free serum IgE levels has been noted within 2 hours of omalizumab administration. Furthermore, within 3 months of therapy, human basophil responsiveness (histamine releasability) was reduced by 90%. The antibody is specific to IgE and does not bind to IgG or IgA. An important property of omalizumab is that it cannot bind to IgE receptors or to IgE already attached to FcεRI, and therefore does not interact with cell-bound IgE or activate mast cells or basophils by interacting with FcεRI. Free IgE must be reduced to extremely low levels to achieve clinical efficacy. This is because there are 10,000 to 1,000,000 FcεRI on mast cells and basophils and nearly all are occupied by IgE. Only 2000 IgE molecules are needed for half-maximal release of histamine from basophils; therefore, a marked reduction in IgE is needed to prevent mast cell and basophil activation. Omalizumab administration results in reductions in allergen-induced nasal challenge responses and expression of FcεRI on basophils within 7 days. Djukanovic *et al.* [16] found that active treatment resulted in a reduction of bronchial biopsy IgE+ cells in the airway mucosa, tissue eosinophil numbers and CD3+, CD4+, and CD8+ T lymphocytes in 55 patients with mild to moderate asthma with sputum eosinophilia of 2% or more. Omalizumab treatment was not associated however, with improvement in airway hyperresponsiveness to methacholine. A reduction in induced sputum eosinophils, bronchial biopsy eosinophil numbers, IgE-bearing cells plus early and late bronchoconstrictor response to inhaled allergen, has been reported, but omalizumab does not attenuate airway responsiveness to methacholine post-allergen challenge [17]. A pattern of improved clinical outcomes, associated with decreased peripheral blood eosinophils and worse clinical outcomes associated with increased peripheral blood eosinophils has been described, in keeping with the efficacy of omalizumab being due, at least in part, with an inhibitory effect on eosinophils. Treatment of allergic subjects with omalizumab also reduces the release of Th2 cytokines from peripheral blood basophils. All these data suggest that treatment with omalizumab reduces eosinophilic airway inflammation and IgE-bearing cells, but does alter airway responsiveness. Possible mechanisms for the reduction in eosinophil numbers, although not established, could be explained by a reduction in high affinity IgE receptor numbers on dendritic cells causing less antigen presentation to T cells, by decreased release of eosinophilic chemotactic factors from mast cells and basophils and by the induction of eosinophil apoptosis. Two subtypes of dendritic cells, DC1 and DC2, appear to be instrumental in the phenotypic development of Th1 and Th2 cells, respectively, and both subtypes showed a significant decreased in FcεRI expression as early as day 7 of treatment with omalizumab. In addition, omalizumab blocks low affinity IgE receptors on epithelial cells and airway smooth muscle, which may decrease the release of eosinophil chemokines such as eotaxin. There is limited information on the effects of omalizumab on airway remodeling. Prevention of degranulation of allergen bound mast cells by omalizumab prevents the release of pro-inflammatory cytokines, including IL-4, IL-13 and IL-5 that are associated with airway remodeling. Omalizumab reduces exhaled breath condensate levels of endothelin-

1, a proinflammatory mediator also implicated in asthmatic airway inflammation and remodelling, suggesting a potential mechanism by which this therapy could reduce structural changes to the airways. In a study of 30 patients with severe persistent asthma, which used computed tomography (CT) to assess airway dimensions, found that treatment with omalizumab (16 weeks) compared to usual care was associated with a reduction in indices of airway wall thickness. Interestingly, the decrease in airway wall thickness was associated with improvements in lung function and decrease in sputum eosinophil count. A longterm randomized controlled trial (EXPLORED study) is underway in patients with moderate to severe allergic asthma to examine the effects of 78 weeks treatment with omalizumab on bronchial biopsy sub-epithelial eosinophils, mast cell and CD4+ T-lymphocytes as well as thickness of the lamina reticularis, as an index of airway remodelling. The findings of this study should provide insights into the effects of long-term treatment with omalizumab on airway inflammation and remodeling. In summary, omalizumab decreases allergic airway inflammation by reducing the expression of high affinity IgE receptors on inflammatory cells and eosinophil numbers within the airways. Research is underway to help establish whether long-term treatment with omalizumab also reduces airway remodelling [18].

Current Guidelines

The US National Asthma Education and Prevention Expert Panel Report 3 (EPR-3) guideline, the international Global Initiative for Asthma (GINA) [19] guideline and the British guideline on the management of asthma [20] have similar recommendations on the management of chronic asthma, with step-wise treatment aimed at controlling symptoms. Steps 4 to 6 of the EPR-3 [21] guideline and Steps 4 and 5 of the GINA and British guidelines are the stage at which asthma is considered severe. Anti-IgE therapy is recommended by the EPR-3 guidelines at steps 5 and 6 and the GINA and British guidelines for patients at step 5.

Dosing and Administration

Omalizumab is administered by subcutaneous injection every two to four weeks in a dose that is determined by body weight and the levels of serum IgE (0.016 mg/kg per IU/mL of IgE per month). It should not be initiated in the setting of an acute exacerbation of asthma, nor should it be self-administered. Therapy requires a dose of 150 to 375 mg injected subcutaneously every two to four weeks. Peak serum concentration is reached in seven to eight days. No more than 150 mg should be administered at a single site, to prevent local reactions. The elimination half-life of the drug is one to four weeks after subcutaneous administration. Total serum IgE levels should be between 30 and 700 international units/mL (IU/mL), although case reports describe benefit in patients with IgE levels below and above this range. For patients with serum IgE levels above 300 IU/mL, there are upper limits of body weight beyond which administration is not recommended. Sensitization to a perennial aeroallergen (*e.g.*, dust mite, animal danders, cockroach, molds) must be demonstrated by positive skin testing or *in vitro* IgE testing. Baseline FEV1, peak flow, or other pulmonary function testing is recommended.

Omalizumab is approved for administration by subcutaneous injection. Initial trials demonstrated that aerosolized omalizumab was ineffective in protecting against allergen challenge and had no effect on circulating IgE. Although in human subjects with atopy, intravenous omalizumab seems to have similar efficacy than subcutaneous, the subcutaneously route of delivery was chosen for practical reasons. A minimum of 12 weeks of treatment is needed to determine the efficacy of anti-IgE therapy. Some patients may respond only after months of treatment, but this appears to be atypical [22]

Indications

In 2003, omalizumab was approved by the FDA for the treatment of adults and adolescents aged 12 years and above with moderate to severe persistent allergic asthma whose symptoms are poorly controlled with inhaled corticosteroids. A Black Boxed adverse effects warning issued in 2007 advising of the risk of the delayed development of anaphylaxis after administration of omalizumab and a further warning issued in 2009 notified of interim safety findings from the EXCELS study of a possible increase in the number of cardiovascular and cerebrovascular adverse events in treated patients. The European Medicines Agency (EMA) licensed omalizumab in 2005 for the treatment of severe allergic asthma in patients aged 12 years or older in whom symptoms are poorly controlled, including a history of multiple exacerbations, despite inhaled high dose corticosteroids and inhaled longacting β2 agonist bronchodilators and in whom the FEV1< 80%. In 2009 the licence was extended to include children aged 6 to 12 years as an add-on treatment for poorly controlled asthma in patients with severe persistent allergic asthma. In addition to the US and Europe, omalizumab is licensed for treating patients with moderate to severe allergic asthma in a large number of other countries worldwide including Australia, Canada and Brazil.

For the purpose of using omalizumab the term allergic is defined as a positive skin test or *in vitro* reactivity to a perennial aeroallergen and in addition the serum total IgE levels should be in the range 30 to 700 IU/ mL in the US. In Europe the serum total IgE ranges are ≥30 to ≤1500 IU/mL in adults and children >12 years and <1300 IU/mL for children over 6 years. The dose (mg) of omalizumab and dose frequency is based on the serum total IgE level (IU/mL) and the patient's body weight (kg). Based on this calculation, omalizumab is given at a dose of 150 to 375 mg by subcutaneous injection every 2 or 4 weeks. The main contraindication is a past history of a severe hypersensitivity reaction to omalizumab. There is limited data on the efficacy of omalizumab in active cigarette smokers with allergic asthma, as this group is usually excluded from clinical trials of omalizumab, although it is likely that the efficacy will be similar to that reported in non-smokers with allergic asthma [23].

Assessment of Therapeutic Response

Several studies have tried to identify clinical or immunological factors that predict a good therapeutic response to omalizumab. Based on a pooled analysis from seven randomized controlled omalizumab trials, Bousquet and colleagues concluded that treatment benefits were not related to baseline total IgE levels. However, in the INvestigatioN of Omalizumab in seVere Asthma TrEatment (INNOVATE) study undertaken in patients with severe allergic asthma and included in the pooled analysis, baseline total IgE was the only predictor of efficacy and levels of specific IgE for individual allergens were of no additional benefit in predicting a positive response. On the contrary, Steiss *et al.* [24] describes a significant decrease of the total IgE concentration after six months of therapy in children and adolescents. In this study, a reduction in frequency of asthma exacerbations and rescue medications were found. The presence of sensitization and exposure to cockroach allergen predicted a very good response to omalizumab in inner-city US children, adolescents, and young adults with persistent allergic asthma. It has been reported that patients receiving longterm oral corticosteroids or frequent courses of oral corticosteroids respond poorly to omalizumab, although there is some limited evidence to support an oral corticosteroid sparing effect of omalizumab. An open-label study of 82 patients with severe allergic asthma, found the addition of omalizumab therapy resulted in lower mean (SD) percent maintenance oral corticosteroid use after 32 weeks of treatment (−45.0%) compared with that in 23 patients who received usual care (18.3%). It is recommended that a decision is made whether to continue long-term treatment based on assessment of response made after 16 weeks of treatment, although a recent study reported that the maximum effect of omalizumab occurred within 4 weeks of starting treatment. In several studies of omalizumab, the physician's overall assessment at 16 weeks following a course of treatment was the best predictor of a continuing beneficial response. Nevertheless the combination of objective measurements of efficacy, such as ACQ, as well as the physicians' and patients' overall assessment are often used to assess response, although these tools have not been validated. Cardiopulmonary exercise testing has been advocated as an additional method to assess and confirm a clinical response to omalizumab in patients with severe asthma although to date the utility of exercise testing as not been investigated in a large number of patients [25, 26].

Duration of Treatment

Once a patient is considered to respond to omalizumab, treatment is then continued often for several years. It remains uncertain when treatment can be discontinued or whether prolonged treatment is required. Certainly a dose reduction at 6 months, in patients who were responders at 16 weeks, is associated with a recurrence of symptoms. A small study of patients with severe cat allergen-induced asthma reported good symptom control and reduced basophil allergen sensitivity three years following completion of six years treatment with omalizumab, suggesting that treatment may not need to be indefinite, although whether this conclusion applies to patients who do not have cat allergen-induced asthma is not known. Long-term dosing should be adjusted for changes in body weight. Reductions in the omalizumab dose below the recommended formula (0.016 mg/kg per IU/mL of IgE per month) are likely to result in a loss of efficacy. Once omalizumab therapy is discontinued, serum free IgE levels and skin test responses gradually return to baseline [27, 28].

OMALIZUMAB DISEASE-SPECIFIC EFFECTS

Asthma

In Europe guidelines omalizumab is authorized for patients since 6 years and older with moderate-severe allergic asthma that is not controlled with corticosteroids inhaled and β_2 agonist bronchodilators. Several studies to date suggest that treatment with omalizumab manages to reduce the dose of inhaled corticosteroids, even in some cases stop it, and long acting B2 agonist, also reducing the number of asthma exacerbations. Consequently, this entails reduction in rescue medication needs, fewer emergency room visits and hospitalizations, and improve quality of life of these patients [18].

Two large systematic reviews published in 2006 and 2011, involving respectively 3143 and 3429 children and adults with moderate to severe asthma poorly controlled with treatment at high doses of inhaled corticosteroids, observed that treatment with omalizumab caused a reduction in asthma exacerbations. and there was a high percentage of patients who could reduce or withdraw treatment with inhaled corticosteroids [29, 30].

Lanier *et al.* published a randomized, double-blind, placebo-controlled trial enrolled children age 6 to <12 years with perennial allergen sensitivity and history of exacerbations and asthma symptoms despite at least medium-dose inhaled corticosteroids. During the first 24 weeks omalizumab reduced the rate of clinically significant asthma exacerbations by 31% *vs.* placebo (when the inhaled corticosteroids dose remained stable) and over a period of 52 weeks, the exacerbation rate was reduced by 43% *vs.* placebo. Over a period of 52 weeks, omalizumab had an acceptable safety profile, with no difference in overall incidence of adverse events compared with placebo [31].

Bardelas *et al.* published in 2012 a double-blind, placebo-controlled study, with patients ≥12 years received omalizumab or placebo every 2 or 4 weeks for 24 weeks. The main variable that was studied was changes in the baseline in Asthma Control Test (ACT) total score. ACT score improved more with omalizumab compared with placebo; however, the difference was not significant. Significant benefits were observed for omalizumab compared with placebo for change in ACT score at in a subgroup of patients with very poorly controlled asthma at baseline [32].

Has also raised the possible benefit of treatment with omalizumab in allergic asthma origin. Van den Berge *et al.* reported a case with severe asthma from non-allergic (high levels of total IgE, specific IgE and skin test negative) than after treatment with omalizumab improved their symptoms with subsequent relapse after treatment withdrawal [33].

Other current studies support the data shown above. Eisner *et al.* conducted an observational cohort study in which patients were followed for two years. Approximately 5000 omalizumab-treated and 2500 non-omalizumab-treated patients aged $\geq$ 12 years with moderate to severe asthma. Over a 2-year period, patients initiating omalizumab therapy experienced clinically relevant improvements in asthma control, which were maintained during 2 years of longitudinal follow-up. Established users of omalizumab asthma control maintained over the 2-year period with a small improvement similar to that omalizumab seen in non-users [34]. Brodlie *et al.* studied 34 children with severe asthma in treatment with prednisolone; the Omalizumab treatment for 16 weeks allowed a significant reduction in daily prednisolone dose and was associated with improvements in Asthma Control and Quality of Life [35]. Wittchen *et al.* conducted a study in patients with severe allergic asthma, using the same sample size (n = 53) for patients treated with Omalizumab as control group of usual-care (naturalistic treatment). They observed beneficial effects similar to those observed in previous controlled trials; to regard the reduction of asthma attacks, persistence of symptoms, asthma monitoring and reduction of concomitant asthma medications [36].

In conclusion, published studies to date support the benefits of treatment with omalizumab in patients with moderate to severe asthma not controlled with other therapies.

Occupational Asthma

Occupational asthma is defined as reversible airway obstruction to airflow associated with bronchial hyperresponsiveness caused by exposure in the workplace; the first treatment option in these patients would be a change in the workplace. After leaving the workplace the indications for anti-IgE therapy are the same as those for asthma not related to occupational exposure. In those patients unable to leave their place of work, the first serious document that IgE plays an important role in the pathophysiology of the disease. There are some case reports of patients with occupational asthma that have not abandoned their jobs and have been treated with omalizumab [37].

In a double blind, randomized, placebo-controlled study whose study population was 18 health care workers who had clinical symptoms of occupational latex allergy for at least 1 year. The patients were treated with omalizumab, remaining unchanged in its labour. At study end, the patients treated with omalizumab exhibited mean relative decreases in skin reaction and improvements in conjunctival challenge test compared with the placebo group [38].

Pérez Pimiento *et al.* report a case of a male baker with professional asthma which starts with omalizumab after stopping specific immunotherapy by systemic reaction. It was found that the patient had high levels of IgE, and skin test positivity and specific IgE to flours. The patient reported clinical improvement, a reduction in the need for systemic corticosteroids, and fewer emergency room visits. Changes in FEV1, PEF, and FeNO, however were irregular [39]. M Olivieri *et al.* also described a similar case of a baker who developed occupational asthma with a poor control their symptoms despite high doses of inhaled corticosteroids. After starting treatment with omalizumab patient has improvement in all symptoms (assessed through the Asthma Control Test), is able to reduce inhaled therapy and FEV1 increased progressively during the treatment reaching normal values after 4 months of treatment. Skin prick test became negative to wheat flour [40].

Allergic Rhinitis and Nasal Polyposis

Published studies on the use of omalizumab in patients with allergic rhinitis suggest promising results. It has been reported to produce improvement in symptoms, reducing the need for rescue medication and consequently improves the quality of life in these patients. However, more studies are still needed to determine its long-term effects [41].

One randomized trial evaluated response to omalizumab among 536 patients with seasonal allergic rhinitis by ragweed pollen. Patients were randomly assigned to the subcutaneous administration of placebo or omalizumab administered prior to ragweed season and repeated during the season every four weeks throughout the pollen season. Symptoms were significantly improved among those receiving high dose (300 mg) *vs.* patients given lesser doses or placebo. A dose-dependent decrease in serum free IgE levels was also observed [42]. In another randomized study included 92 patients with seasonal allergic rhinitis, was that the group had greater improvement was that omalizumab was added to treatment with specific immunotherapy [43]. Omalizumab has also been used in perennial rhinitis, although there are fewer studies about it: in a study of 289 patients with perennial rhinitis were randomized to receive omalizumab or placebo. The improvement in daily clinical practice and the decline in the use of rescue medication were significantly higher in the group receiving omalizumab than the placebo group [44].

Penn R performed a retrospectively study on two groups of patients with atopic asthma and nasal polyposis who underwent endoscopic sinus surgery, including a control group and an anti-IgE treatment group (treatment postoperatively). They observed significant improved in omalizumab group the nasal polyp scores relative to preoperative values, whereas the control group showed no significant improvement. The results arise from the inclusion of anti-IgE therapy in the postpolypectomy management of atopic asthmatic individuals may reduce the severity of nasal polyposis recurrence [45].

Chronic Urticaria

Urticaria is defined by pruritic wheals with or without angioedema, that appear in minutes or hours, usually transient, disappearing within 24 hours. It is considered chronic if duration is more than 6 weeks.

Standard managements of chronic urticaria primarily include H1 antihistamines, although to achieve an optimal control is sometimes necessary to combine with H2 antihistamines and leukotriene modifiers or other adjunctive agents. Is sometimes necessary to use short courses of corticosteroids to control exacerbations. Patients whose symptoms are not controlled over time using with these standard therapies are considered to have refractory symptoms. In this situation, the clinician should consider other therapies such as immunomodulatory agents, antiinflammators or immunosuppressant. In these patients, omalizumab has shown in some studies promoting effects [46, 47]:

- In a randomized study, placebo-controlled, that included 90 patients aged between 12 to 75 years and with persistent moderate-to-severe chronic urticaria symptoms were treated with a single dose of omalizumab (doses of 75, 300, or 600 mg subcutaneously) or placebo and observed for 16 weeks. Omalizumab group showed greater improvement *vs.* the placebo group, although there were no significant differences from placebo at a dose of 75 mg [48].

- In a multicenter, randomized, double-blind, placebo-controlled study who incluyed 49 pacients, all subjects had demonstrable IgE autoantibodies to thyroid peroxidase, although the role of this antibody in the pathogenesis of chronic urticaria has not been demonstrated. Were randomly administered omalizumab (dosed according to weight and serum IgE levels, according to scheme used in asthma) or placebo. Full protection was observed in 70.4% patients omalizumab group compared with only 4.5% patients in the placebo group [49].

The optimal dose and duration of therapy with omalizumab in chronic urticaria has not been determined. Also has been reported on beneficial effects of therapy omalizumab in patients with chronic physical urticaria. Physical urticaria is characterized by onset of itching, hives and / or angioedema after application of appropriate physical stimulus (solar radiation, mechanical friction, cold,...). A study proceeds to treat 7 patients with chronic urticaria with sparse physical response to standard therapies (solar urticaria (n = 2), urticaria factitia/symptomatic dermographism (n = 2), cold urticaria, delayed pressure urticaria and localized heat urticaria); gaining complete control of symptoms in 5 patients with the first dose, one patient improved after increasing the dose and other significant changes were not obtained [50].

Atopic Dermatitis

Atopic dermatitis is a chronic inflammatory skin condition that relates with a genetic defect in the proteins supporting the epidermal barrier. The most patients obtain good control of the disease with adequate cutaneous hydration, topical therapies for inflammation, the elimination of exacerbating factors and antihistamine treatment to reduce itching. However, a small percentage of these patients develop severe symptoms that do not respond to conventional therapies. They could benefit from alternative therapies among which include immunosuppressive agents, phototherapy or biologic therapies [51-53].

Studies of biologics agents for the treatment of atopic dermatitis are limited and the results obtained so far are conflicting. Omalizumab has shown some improvement in clinical trials with small number of patients; in a study of three patients with severe atopic dermatitis and high levels of IgE were treated with omalizumab for twelve weeks, referring improvement after 2 weeks of treatment initiation [54]. However, a randomized study placebo-controlled and double blind of 20 patients found that treatment did not significantly alter several measures of disease activity [55]. In another study with three patients with severe atopic dermatitis (with asthma and / or allergic rhinitis associated) there was no change in skin condition after 4 months of treatment with omalizumab. Failure in this trial could be related to an insufficient dosage of omalizumab, as these patients had extremely high values of serum IgE prior to initiation of treatment [56]. Currently, efficacy of omalizumab in patients with extremely high levels of serum IgE is unknown.

Omalizumab Plus Immunotherapy

Although specific immunotherapy is an important treatment option for patients with allergic diseases, the potential for systemic allergic reactions has limited its use, especially for patients with symptomatic disease. In several studies it has been found that the addition of omalizumab to immunotherapy (either prior to or during treatment) is able to reduce the number of systemic reactions due to administration of immunotherapy, thereby allowing patients to tolerate treatment. However, such therapy is limited by high costs and the requirements for permanent or every-season treatment [57].

Kontou-Fili reports a case of a patient with systemic mastocytosis presenting severe reaction following administration of bee venom immunotherapy. It was decided to administer a dose twice according to the corresponding weight and IgE level, seven days before immunotherapy and slowly got cut this time to an hour before inmunotherapy. Finally getting the patient tolerated the maintenance dose without reactions [58].

Massanari *et al.* performed a study for evaluate omalizumab's effect on the tolerability of specific immunotherapy in patients with symptomatic persistent asthma not adequately controlled with inhaled corticosteroids. It was a multicenter, double-blind study in which patients were allocated randomly to treatment with omalizumab or placebo, after which they received specific immunotherapy to at least 1 of 3 perennial aeroallergens (cat, dog, and house dust mite). Patients receiving omalizumab experienced significantly fewer systemic allergic reactions to immunotherapy than those receiving placebo and had fewer respiratory-related systemic allergic reactions. Furthermore, patients with omalizumab were able to reach the target maintenance immunotherapy dose [59].

Casale TB and al. also observed like effects in a similar study but in patients with allergic rhinitis who were receiving rush immunotherapy regimen against ragweed pollen. Patients received either 9 weeks of omalizumab or placebo, followed by 1-day rush (maximal dose 1.2-4.0 mug Amb a 1) or placebo immunotherapy, then 12 weeks of omalizumab or placebo plus immunotherapy. Patients receiving immunotherapy and omalizumab had fewer adverse events than those receiving immunotherapy alone; post hoc analysis of groups receiving immunotherapy demonstrated that addition of omalizumab resulted in a 5-fold decrease in risk of anaphylaxis caused by rush immunotherapy [60].

Drug Allergy

A case report of a man with type I diabetes mellitus diagnosed to insulin allergy. After performing a desensitization to insulin successfully (nine months later) he presented allergic symptoms after an episode of diabetic ketoacidosis. The symptoms were not controlled despite treatment with antihistamines. The corticosteroids were avoided to prevent any increase in insulin requirement. Omalizumab treatment began and after 20 weeks, the patient was taking only 5 mg every 24 hours of levocetirizine without allergic symptoms. The omalizumab in the treatment of other IgE-mediated conditions, such as severe drug allergy, has a promising future, although more trials are needed [61].

Food Allergy

Currently it is estimated that food allergy affects about 2% of adults and 6% of children, affecting their quality of life significantly. The probability of eating the food inadvertently is high and this can trigger fatal reactions. In the United States the peanut allergy is estimated to affect 1.5 million people and cause 50 to 100 deaths per year.

Studies have explored the use of omalizumab for the treatment of food allergy. A multi-center randomized trial evaluated another humanized monoclonal anti-IgE mouse IgG1 antibody (TNX-901) in 84 patients with a history of immediate hypersensitivity to peanut. Patients were randomly assigned to receive either TNX-901 (150, 300, or 450 mg) or placebo every four weeks for four doses. Later patients underwent a second oral peanut challenge; only the high dose group (450 mg) the sensitivity threshold increased from a level equal to approximately half a peanut to one equal to almost nine peanuts. However, even at the highest dose of TNX-901, approximately 25 percent were not protected [62]. Sampson *et al.* designed a multicenter and randomized trial, double-blind, placebo-controlled, to assess the efficacy of omalizumab (given at a minimum dose of 0.016 mg/kg/IgE) in reducing the risk of peanut-induced allergic reactions. The study was designed to compare changes in peanut tolerability thresholds in subjects with proven peanut allergy who were treated with either omalizumab or placebo although the study was discontinued prematurely because of safety issues related to anaphylactic reactions [63].

Further studies would be needed to determine whether further dose increases might confer protective effect in these patients (some patients have extremely high IgE levels that do not fall within the ranges for current approved dosing), to confirm and optimize the protective effect of anti-IgE against food anaphylaxis, establish a safety profile in young children, and identify markers for selecting food-allergic subjects most likely to benefit from anti-IgE therapy [64].

Omalizumab in Other Diseases

Allergic Bronchopulmonary Aspergillosis

Allergic bronchopulmonary aspergillosis (ABPA) is a disease characterized by reversible obstruction of the airways, transient pulmonary infiltrates, eosinophilia, and fever, caused by hypersensitivity response against *Aspergillius fumigatus* antigens, that are colonizing the bronchial tree. This disease occurs frequently in patients with asthma or cystic fibrosis.

Tillie-Leblond *et al.* performed a open-label studied with 16 patients with ABPA without CF, with a mean age of 56 years, in which treatment with omalizumab during a year resulted in a reduced number of exacerbations and the need for systemic corticosteroids [65].

Zirbes *et al.* presented their experience with three children suffering from cystic fibrosis and ABPA under prolonged treatment with corticosteroids. The start of omalizumab achieved a significant improvement and allowed discontinuation of corticosteroids [66]. Van der Ent CK et cols. describe a case of similar characteristics in which a single dose of omalizumab produces a dramatic and rapid improvement of respiratory symptoms and lung function [67]. However, in another case report of a child with CF and ABPA treated with omalizumab, glucocorticoids were not able to be weaned over a 12-month period while the patient was receiving 300 mg every four weeks of the drug [68]

Published studies are still just as scarce and more tests are needed to see the effectiveness of omalizumab in the treatment of ABPA.

Eosinophilic Esophagitis

The management of eosinophilic esophagitis includes elimination and elemental diets to decrease allergen exposure, acid suppression to treat gastroesophageal reflux disease, esophageal dilation to treat strictures and topical glucocorticoids to decrease esophageal inflammation. Rocha *et al.* reported two cases with multiple food allergies (very restrictive diet) and eosinophilic esophagitis who receiving treatment with omalizumab. Observed an improvement in allergic symptoms but not in endoscopic or histologic features of eosinophilic esophagitis. Omalizumab may improve the quality of life of patients with severe food allergy by improving symptoms, but it does not appear to change endoscopic and histological features. More tests would be needed to test the effects of omalizumab in this pathology [69].

Mastocytosis

Melody C. Carter demonstrated preliminary data showing that omalizumab might have efficacy in the prevention of spontaneous episodes of anaphylaxis in patients with systemic mastocytosis. They reported two cases, both patients with systemic mastocytosis and recurrent anaphylaxis episodes. They started omalizumab treatment with 300 mg every 4 weeks. The drug had been well tolerated and not experienced any episodes of anaphylaxis since starting therapy, also showed decreases of their basal medication [70]. Frank Siebenhaar *et al.* also report a case of a female, 56-year-old, cutaneous mastocytosis and Ménière disease diagnosed. She started treatment with omalizumab (150mg every 14 days for the first 4 shots and she has continued receiving similar shots as maintenance therapy once every 4 weeks). After initial doses and 6 months with therapy, no further wheal formation or pruritus has occurred, and there have been no more attacks of vertigo or nausea, but the unilateral poor hearing and slight tinnitus remain [71].

ADVERSE EFFECTS

Introduction

Concern about security of biologic therapies has existed since they were introduced. In the last years some cases of severe adverse effects during clinical trials with biologics have transcended the media and created social alarm [72].

Most therapies in clinical use have demonstrated efficacy with an acceptable tolerance profile, but they are still relatively new and data about long-term use effects are lacking.

One problem of most biologic is the lack of knowledge about all the consequences of blocking a therapeutic target. If the molecular target has important functions the probably of adverse effects is higher. This could be the case of anti-TNF or interferon therapies for example.

Omalizumab mechanism of action consists in blocking IgE and down- regulating Fc RI ε receptor in mast cells. Physiologic functions of IgE are not completely elucidated. It is supposed to have a role in defense against parasitic infections and could be part of other defense mechanism. Theoretically the blockage of an immune system target may elicit an immune suppression status and predispose to neoplasm and infections.

In addition, usage of monoclonal humanized antibodies could be associated with adverse effects as allergic reaction or serum sickness.

Since the first clinical trials and during the post-commercialization period, thousand of patients have received treatment with omalizumab with a relatively low number of adverse effects reported [73].

In clinical trials, unspecific adverse events as myalgia, pyrexia, pain in extremities, cephalea or abdominal pain presented with similar frequency in both groups of active treatment and placebo. These events were mild and self-limited, and the relation with the study drug was not clear [73].

Local Reaction

The most common omalizumab associated adverse events are mild and associated with the place of injection. Local fever, pain and swelling are relatively frequent and reported by 44-45% of patients in studies, usually with no significant differences between placebo and treatment groups. Reactions are usually mild to moderate (1.5-3 cm) and appear within one hour after administration. They last about 3-14 days and rarely are a cause of discontinuation of the drug [73, 74].

Rash and Urticaria

Skin rash of any type presented in 6.9% of omalizumab treated patient and 5.3% of placebo patient with no significant differences [73]

Urticaria develops in approximately 1% of patient. Relationship between urticaria and predisposition to anaphylaxis has not been evaluated [75].

Anaphylaxis

The underlying mechanism of omalizumab-induced anaphylaxis is not clear yet. It had been related with pre-existing antiallotypic or anti-idiotypic antibody (IgE or IgG) against omalizumab. In other cases these antibodies might be generated *de novo* after exposition.

The polysorbate used as excipient could cause anaphylaxis too. In at least two cases it had been identified as the sensitization antigen [76].

Anaphylactic reactions occur in a low percentage of patients. During the clinical trials an incidence of at least 0.2% was reported [77]. Review of post-commercialization studies and spontaneous reports data could show a lower incidence (0.09%) [73, 78]. Most episodes (78%) occur in the first two hours after the injection but in a 5% of cases anaphylaxis presented in the 1-4 days after the injection. Reactions most frequently occurred during the first three injections (78%) [77], but there are reports in patients who were on treatment for at least a year [76]. No fatalities have been attributed to this cause to the date.

No predictor factor for omalizumab anaphylaxis had been identified. It is supposed that asthma and previous episodes of anaphylaxis could be risk factors. Skin sensitivity to mouse antigens had not been correlated with reactions after omalizumab administration [79].

The joint task force of the American Academy of Allergy Asthma and Immunology and the American College of Allergy Asthma and Immunology for omalizumab-related anaphylaxis made some recommendation to prevent or minimize the impact of these reactions [78]:

1. Obtaining written informed consent and giving complete information to the patients. The risk, benefits and alternatives should be discussed before starting therapy with omalizumab.

2. Education of patients on signs and symptoms of anaphylaxis.

3. Prescribing epinephrine auto injector to be carried for at least 24 hours after the injection.

4. Checking the health status of the patient before administration, including physical examination and lung function test if indicated.

5. Monitoring the patient after the injection. A time of two hours for the three first doses and 30 minutes for the next doses is considered appropriate.

Other recommendation includes reviewing concomitant medications (avoidance of beta-blockers and checking of asthma treatment compliance) and assuring that the dose and preparation of the medication are correct. Physicians trained in managing anaphylaxis must do Omalizumab administration, and medication and equipment to treat a reaction must be available. If a reaction appears, it should be treated according to the usual guidelines and recommendations for anaphylaxis management, and omalizumab administration should be stopped.

Skin prick test (SPT) can be done with the undiluted drug. Intradermal skin testing with a 1: 100 000 solution of omalizumab (1.25 µg/ mL) has been proved to be safe and non-irritant [80] in healthy volunteers and patients with asthma, but usefulness of these test in patients with previous anaphylaxis to omalizumab is yet to be proved. Intradermal testing can be performed with polysorbate and other excipients [76].

Helminth Infections

Helminth parasites are widely distributed with a greater prevalence in warmth and moisture areas in tropical and subtropical regions. The most prevalent species are *Ascaris lumbricoides*, *Trichuris trichura*, hook worm and *Strongiloides stercoralis*. Other relevant infections are schistosomiasis and filariasis.

IgE has been related with defense against helminthes. It is known that infection with these agents induce an Ig E elevation and Th2 response activation, with increment of eosinophils and mast cell in the infected tissues and elevation of IL-5 and IL-13. For some species of helminthes a high level of Ig E and Th2 cytokines is associated with resistance to re-infection. In endemic areas children with resistance to ascaris infection usually have higher levels of specific Ig E against ascaris antigen ABA-1, while chronically infected children have a low Th2 response [78].

Hypothetically anti-IgE therapy could reduce natural protection against helminthes increasing the risk and severity of infections and impairing the efficacy of treatments.

Paradoxically, studies in several animal models of helminthic infection showed a reduction in the parasitic burden [82, 83]; except for one study which showed an increase in survival of L3 stage *Oncocerca volvulus* larvae after treatment with anti-IgE [84].

In humans, a randomized, double-blind, placebo-controlled study in an endemic area was carried out to determine if the use of omalizumab increases the risk of parasitic infection. The study population consisted in 137 Brazilian patients, with allergic asthma and/ or rhinitis who were randomized to receive either omalizumab or placebo during a 52 weeks period. Prior the study patients were screened to rule out the presence of helminthic infection and treated if indicated. The study showed a slightly higher prevalence of infection (OR 1.47) and a potential increased risk of re-infection with common geohelminth parasites in the omalizumab group but no increment in morbidity or resistance to treatment [85].

Clinical trials population represents an exposure of more than 60 000 patients-years in non high risk population. The rate of helminthic infection is about 0.03% in these studies. There have not been post- commercialization reports of parasitic infection in USA in over 50 000 patients treated with omalizumab [81].

Anyway, observational studies are required to confirm the security of omalizumab in areas with high risk of parasitic infection.

For patients living in areas with low prevalence of parasitic infection, no specific caution is required before start omalizumab therapy. Patients who have stayed in endemic areas for a short period of time do not require parasitic screening too.

If the patient has recently emigrated from a high risk area or passes long periods in these areas, parasitic screening can be considered, especially if a history of filariasis, schistosomiasis or strongiloidosis exists. Strongiloidosis can cause a hyperinfection syndrome that is potentially lethal. Immune suppression can precipitate these status, so if *S. stercoralis* infection is suspected, it should be rule out before starting omalizumab [81].

Malignancy

Other theoretically consequence of immune suppression by omalizumab could be the apparition of neoplasm.

In the phase I to III studies an imbalance in the number of malignancies was observed between placebo and active groups. This is reflected in omalizumab labels both in the US and EU [73].

Recently a cluster association study has been performed to assess this association [86]. Data from 67 clinical trials have been analyzed including a total number of 11,459 patients, 7, 789 of them who received omalizumab. The time of exposition was 5,800 patient-years for the omalizumab group. In this study no relation was found between omalizumab exposure and cancer. The incidence rate of cancer were 4.14 (95% CI, 2.26-6.94) and 4.45 (95% CI, 2.22-7.94), respectively for the placebo and omalizumab group.

The duration of exposure and the cumulative dose of omalizumab were not found related with the apparition of malignancy.

All malignancies were solid tumours, which usually requires a longer time of exposition to develop. The incidence and prevalence of cancer between omalizumab treated patients were not different from general population.

The authors conclude that the relation between omalizumab and cancer is unlikely for the patients included in this study. Anyway more studies are required with a longer follow-up period to rule out this association [86].

Interestingly, no cases of myeloid or lymphoid neoplasm have been reported in patients taking omalizumab. A case of myeloid cell elevation with no evidence of malignancy was reported in a patient who suffered from common variable immune deficiency, after 29 months of omalizumab treatment. The cell count came to normality after omalizumab was stopped [87].

Arteriothrombotic Events

In 2009 an interim safety analysis performed by the FDA detected an apparent increase in cardiovascular disorders (ischemic heart disease, arrhythmias, cardiomyopathy and embolic and thrombotic events) in the patients taking omalizumab with respect to the placebo group. This effect was no statistically significant. This data were taken from an unpublished cohort trial (EXCELS) and analysis of the randomized clinical trials. As a result, the UK Medicines and Healthcare Products Regulatory Agency advised prescribers to be vigilant about the possible occurrence of arterial thrombotic events in patients exposed to omalizumab, and to report suspected relevant adverse reactions to the UK spontaneous adverse event reporting system [88].

A new study assessing the safety profile of omalizumab with respect to arterial thrombotic events recorded in the FDA Adverse Event Reporting System (AERS) database have published recently [89]. This work analyses all arterial thrombotic events reported in relation with asthma medication over a period of 6 years. They conclude that omalizumab was the second drug, after inhaled corticosteroid, associated with thrombotic events risk, with an odds ratio of 2.75 (2.39–3.16) and 1.09 (0.95–1.24) with respect to all asthma drugs and all drugs in AERS. This study has a number of limitations, as the lack of data in some cases, difficult to assure of the nature of events and its real relation with the drug, and under-reporting of adverse events.

To the date, FDA has not included specific recommendation for arterial thrombotic events risk in the omalizumab label. More epidemiological studies, as the results of the EXCELS study are needed to confirm or rule out this association.

Serum Sickness

To the date, at least two cases of omalizumab induced serum sickness has been described, one of them with a fatal outcome [90, 91]. The patient's death was caused by myocardial infarction and was supposed to be due to diabetes complication and not to omalizumab therapy [90]. In the other case, mild serum sickness appeared after desensitization was tried in a patient with previous anaphylactoid reaction [91].

Although these events remain unfrequent, they may be in mind of physicians. More data from post-commercialization surveillance are needed.

COST-EFFECTIVENESS

In the last years a high number of new health technologies have arisen. As a consequence, patient's expectations have substantially improved for some chronic and disabling diseases but at the price of a strong increment in healthcare costs. Pharmaco-economy science tries to provide information about the costs and benefits of different treatment options in order to take a decision about using a new technology.

The benefits of a treatment are usually evaluated in quality of life adjusted years (QALY). This is a measure of the number of healthy life years gained with an intervention, and is calculated multiplying the number of life years gained by a factor obtained with the application of a quality of life questionnaire.

The cost is measured in monetary units. There are direct costs as the cost of the intervention and additional treatments and hospitalizations, and indirect costs as the loss of days of work and pain and suffering from the patients.

The results are expressed in ICER (index of cost-effectiveness ratio) that is a measure of the economic cost per QALY if the intervention is performed. This is calculated with the formula ICER= (C1- C2)/ (E1-E2); where C1 and C2 are the costs and E1 and E2 the benefits of two different interventions.

Economic studies can be done from different perspectives; patients, society or payers (insurance company or public health service). They define an scenario, where the cost-effectiveness of the intervention is measured, take data of mortality, morbidity and complications from clinical trials or statistical recordings and use mathematical models to extrapolate them to the real world.

One way-sensitivity analysis consists in re-calculate the ICER adjusting a variable- per example mortality or cost of therapy- in a wide range of values, so we can analyse the consistency of the model and how our conclusions can be modified if the values assigned to variables are different from real world ones.

Willingness-to-pay is a pre-determined monetary value defined as the maximum amount of money that we are disposed to pay to gain one QALY [92].

Omalizumab is a high cost therapy. The price of 150 mg vial rounds € 436.99 in Spain and $561.96 in US. Patients can require one to four vials once of twice per month depending on the weight and IgE levels so the cost of treatment ranges from $7 000 to $54 000 per year.

However, severe non-controlled asthma represents a high cost too. Total direct and indirect annual costs are approximately €18 billion in Europe [93] and US$13 billion in the USA [94].

A study performed in Spain estimates total cost of asthma in €1489 million per year. The same study found that annual cost of illness for Spanish asthmatic patients comes to €1726 per patient from a societal perspective and €1533 from the perspective of the National Health Service. Severe asthma consumed most resources with a medium cost of €2635 per patient. Most of these resources are consumed in medication, hospitalizations and diagnostic tests [95]. The cost increases in patients with severe non-controlled asthma.

Omalizumab cost-effectiveness has been the object of several studies and systematic reviews recently. Most of these studies are financed by the pharmaceutical industry, although some of them are independent.

In 2004, a study by Oba *et al.* found that omalizumab cost was about $523 to obtain an additional successfully controlled day. This is a high cost compared with other asthma medication. For example, the incremental costs per symptom-free day gained were $3.35 to $7.5 with inhaled corticosteroids. The cost to maintain a clinical significant improvement (at least 0.5 points in the Asthma Quality of Life Questionnaire) was $ 140 000 per year. They concluded that it could be cost-effective only in non-smokers patients who are hospitalized 5 or more times or 20 days or longer per year despite maximal asthma therapy. Main limitation of this work is that their results are not presented in cost per QALY, so it is difficult to make comparisons with other studies [96].

Wu *et al.* in 2007 found that omalizumab was not cost-effective at its current price. They report a cost of $821 000 per QALY. In the sensitivity analysis, the omalizumab cost and the improvement in quality of life questionnaires punctuation had the greatest effect on the incremental cost-effectiveness ratios. This study used a societal point of view and takes into account the fact that there are a number of non-responders patients [97].

Other studies found that omalizumab can be cost-effective. A Swedish study used the data from the INNOVATE clinical trial to estimate cost-effectiveness from a societal perspective in severe asthma population. They report an incremental cost-effectiveness ratio of €56,091 [€31,328; €120,552 with 95% CI] which seems a more attractive ICER in these patients [98].

Another study uses data from ETOPA clinical trial and takes Canada as country of reference. It reports an ICER of $31 209 per QALY if 5 years of treatment are given, concluding that omalizumab is cost-effective and compares favourably with other biologics used in treatment of rheumatoid arthritis, hepatitis B or cancer. The limitation of this work is that the analysis was based on a small open-label trial and limited to the participants who were responders to omalizumab [99].

A recent study calculates cost-effectiveness from the perspective of US payer. They report an ICER of $287 200 per QALY for all patients and $172 300 in the responder scenario and concludes that omalizumab cost-effectiveness is similar to other biologics [100].

The National Institute for Health and Clinical Excellence (NICE) of the UK reviewed evidence submitted from the manufacturer in 2009. They recommend consider adding omalizumab in non-smokers patients with severe allergic non controlled asthma despite optimal treatment, who has had at least two asthma attacks within the past year needing admission to hospital, or three or more severe asthma attacks within the past year, one of which has needed admission to hospital and the other two have needed additional treatment in an accident and emergency department [101].

The NICE review and all published analysis agree in recommend evaluating the response to treatment at week 16 and stop it in non responder patients [99-101].

Cost- effectiveness studies for the paediatric indication (6-11 years) are still lacking. A NICE analysis for this population performed in 2011 found that omalizumab is not cost effective in this group of age but most studies are needed [102].

As a conclusion, it seems that omalizumab as add-on therapy could be cost-effective in a selected population of non-smokers patients with severe non-controlled asthma. Cost-effectiveness increases when the response at week 16 is used to guide the decision of continuing therapy. Sensitivity- analysis showed that cost-effectiveness is very sensible to the price of omalizumab, so a decrease in its price should make it a more reliable therapy for a higher number of patients [95, 100]

Anyway more studies are needed, especially for paediatric population and for new indications. It is desirable a greater proportion of studies not depending on the pharmaceutical companies funding.

OTHER APPROACHES TO ANTI-IG E THERAPY

To the date omalizumab is the only anti-Ig E therapy approved to be used in humans and commercially available worldwide.

However, other options of treatment have been investigated. Some of them seem to be promising while others have been abandoned due to lack of efficacy and/ or adverse events.

Theoretically it is possible to intervening in all steps of IgE synthesis; from blocking or activating transcription factors, blocking Th-2 cytokines or its receptors and increasing levels of Th-1 cytokines, to targeting Ig E itself. Strategies at almost all these levels have been assayed [103].

Transcription Factor Targeting Approaches

Cytokines production and Ig E synthesis are regulated by transcription factors. GATA-3 and T-bet are known to be critical in regulating Th-2 and Th-1 responses respectively and some strategies to modulate their activity have been tried [104].

GATA-3 expression is known to be reduced by the activation of peroxisome proliferators-activated receptor (PPAR). PPAR are ligand-activated transcription factors that belong to the nuclear receptor super-family. The PPAR-γ and α agonists have been shown to decrease antigen-induced airway hyper-responsiveness, lung eosinophilia and eosinophil chemotaxis, GATA-3 expression, Th-2 cytokine production, and antigen-specific IgE production in animal models. Activation of PPAR gamma was capable of reducing GATA-3 and T-bet expression and inducing Foxp3 expression in CD4+ T cells. PPAR gamma agonist inhibits the production or release of key Th1 and Th2 cytokines in a PPAR gamma-dependent fashion. Induction of Tregs by PPAR gamma activation may be one of the possible mechanism by PPAR gamma agonist suppresses allergic inflammation. In the anti-IgE way, PPAR ligands negatively regulate the expression of the high-affinity IgE receptor FcεRI [105].

Some of these agents are rosiglitazone and pioglitazone- in use for type 2 diabetes- and statins. Their use in human allergic airway diseases should be studied [104-107].

T-bet transcription factor switches immune response from Th-2 to Th-1 [104]. Expression of T-bet is induced by CpG motif through the toll-like receptor 9. Immunotherapy with conjugated CpG and allergen had been used in clinical trials with good results [107].

Cytokines Inhibitors

1. Suplatast tosilate is a relatively selective inhibitor of the synthesis of IL-4 and IL-5 and inhibits Ig E synthesis. It is administered orally in two daily doses. This drug has been developed in Japan where is currently under clinical trials. It has demonstrated to reduce Ig E levels, serum and sputum eosinophils, bronchial hyper-responsiveness, symptoms scores and exhaled nitric oxide (NO) in several studies [108, 109]. It has been evaluated as monotherapy in mild asthma [110] and as add-on therapy in moderate and severe asthma [107]. A small study with 10 patient showed it could be effective in patients who are not responders to anti-leucotriene therapy [110]. It has been used too for others diseases in which eosinophils

play a role, as eosinophilic pneumonia [111], hypereosinophilic syndrome [112] and Kimura syndrome [113].

2. Altrakincept is a soluble IL-4 receptor. Initial phase I/ II studies with nebulized altrakincept showed an improvement in lung function, asthma symptoms scores and exhaled NO levels [114, 115]. In posterior clinical trials it failed to reach the clinical endpoints and was subsequently abandoned [103].

3. Pitrakinra is a mutated IL-4 protein which blocks the common IL-4 and IL-13 receptor. In published studies inhaled pitrakinra has proved to reduce exacerbations in eosinophilic asthma and late phase asthmatic response after bronchial challenge [116]. Recently, a pharmacogenetic study suggested that it could be possible to identify patients who respond to pitrakinra by the polymorphisms in the *IL-4RA* gene [117].

4. Lebrikizumab is a monoclonal anti-IL-13 Ig G_4 humanized antibody. A randomized, double-blind, placebo controlled clinical trial showed a significant improvement in FEV1 values in the lebrikizumab group at 12 weeks but not at 24 weeks [118]. High pre-treatment levels of periostin were associated with good response to the drug. However, no significant changes in quality of life questionnaires punctuation, symptoms scores or exacerbation rates were assessed. Lebrikizumab therapy was associated with a higher rate of musculoskeletal adverse events compared with placebo.

Th1 Cytokines

Intravenous infusion of recombinant human IL-12 markedly reduced blood and sputum eosinophilia following bronchial challenge but had no effects on late asthmatic responses to inhaled allergens or airways responsiveness to histamine. Significant adverse events as arrithmias and increase in mortality were observed, so this approaching has been abandoned [119, 120]. Currently, DNA plasmids to induce endogenous production of IL-12 in murine models are under investigation [121].

IFN-γ has not been effective in asthma treatment and is also associated with adverse events [122].

Anti CD23

CD23 is the low affinity Ig E receptor or FcεRII. When CD23 on B cells is stimulated by Ig E it enhances antigen presentation and amplifies Ig E synthesis; but the cross linking of membrane-bound CD23 molecules down-regulates Ig E synthesis [103].

Lumiliximab (also known as IDEC-152) is a primatized Ig G_1 anti-CD23 monoclonal antibody consisting of primate variable region and human constant region. In a placebo controlled clinical trial, the administration of a single dose of lumiliximab produced a dose-dependent and sustained reduction of Ig E levels but no effect on FEV1 was observed [123].

In vitro, lumiliximab reduced allergen-induced proliferation of peripheral mononuclear cells and pro-inflammatory cytokines [124].

This agent is also in clinical trials for the treatment of chronic lymphocytic leukaemia. Its role in allergic disease remains to be established.

Fc Fusion Proteins

FcεRI cross-linking stimulates the release of allergic mediators and FcγRIIb can block FcεRI-mediated reactivity by co-aggregating with FcεRI. FcγRIIb is expressed in mast cells and basophils. In 2002 Zhu *et al.* developed a Fcγ- Fcε chimeric fusion protein which was able to bound to the FcεRI and FcγRII receptors. It showed dose- and time-dependent inhibition of antigen-driven IgE-mediated histamine release from fresh human basophils and inhibition of cutaneous passive anaphylaxis in a transgenic mice expressing human FcεRIα [125].

In other work non human primates with dust mites sensitization were used, Fcγ-Fcε fusion protein administration increased the concentration of allergen needed to enhance an early phase asthmatic response. It also was able to reduce the number of circulating basophils and expression of FcεRI on them after 4 weeks of treatment. However, repeated administration induced sensitization to the Fcε and Fcγ domains and anaphylaxis like reactions [126].

Other approach has been using a Fcγ-Der f 2 fusion protein in a murine model of asthma. The levels of specific Ig E in blood and cytokines in blochoalveolar lavage were lower in the treatment group compared with control group. Inflammatory cell infiltration in airways and blood vessels was also lower [127].

Vaccines Targeting Ig E

Omalizumab acts as a passive immunization against Ig E. It has some disadvantages: high cost of therapy, needing of continuous injections to maintain its effects and risk of adverse effects as anaphylaxis or serum sickness. These problems could be avoided with an active immunization strategy. Since 1985 several groups have been working in different methods for the development of anti-Ig E vaccines.

Ig E vaccines can be obtained by coupling or fusing a significantly large portion of rat IgE to a heterogonous carrier protein forming a chimeric IgE molecule or a fusion protein. Administration of this molecule in ovoalbumin (OVA) sensitized rats induced a strong polyclonal response against Ig E but may cross react with other immunoglobulins containing the same epitopes.

Peptide-based vaccines use short and Ig E specific sequences coupled to a carrier protein as keyhole limpet hemocyanin (KLH). They have been tried in several animal models demonstrating ability to reduce serum Ig E levels, histamine release and passive cutaneous anaphylaxis. The problem with this approach is that these vaccines are not very immunogenic and requires the use of strong adjuvant CFA/ IFA (Freund's adjuvant) which is not reliable for human administration.

Ig E- peptide- based virus-like particle vaccines are synthesized by coupling peptides to the carrier protein of hepatitis B surface antigen (Hbs Ag) using the glutharaldehyde method to create a vaccine conjugate. It was able to reduce Ig E production and reverse elevated Ig E in sensitized rats and mice.

Ig E vaccines are still in animal research phase. If they are eventually developed for human use they could be a safe and low cost method to treat allergic diseases. Their main advantage compared with passive immunization would be the induction of a polyclonal response of 100% natural human antibodies against Ig E, so the possibility of adverse events- at least in theory- would be lower [128].

CONCLUSIONS

Omalizumab is a recombinant humanized monoclonal antibody that binds circulating IgE antibody. It is approved in patients with moderate to severe persistent allergic asthma, whose symptoms are poorly controlled with inhaled corticosteroids.

Omalizumab decreases allergic airway inflammation by reducing the expression of high affinity IgE receptors on inflammatory cells and eosinophil numbers within the airways.

Recent long-term clinical trials confirm the benefits of omalizumab in reducing exacerbations and symptoms in adults and in children with moderate to severe allergic asthma. Clinical trials are in progress to determine whether omalizumab has efficacy in the treatment of non-allergic asthma

No clinical or immunological factors consistently predict a good therapeutic response to omalizumab in allergic asthma. In responders, the duration of treatment is unclear.

The main adverse effect of omalizumab is anaphylaxis. Preliminary data from a five year safety study raised concerns about increased cardiovascular events and a final report is awaited

Omalizumab seems to be cost-effective in non smokers patients with severe allergic asthma.

ACKNOWLEDGEMENTS

This is to acknowledge Mr. Diego Moguel for his contribution to figures treatment.

CONFLICT OF INTEREST

The author(s) confirm that this chapter content has no conflict of interest.

REFERENCES

[1] Vercelli D. Immunobiology of IgE. In: Middleton's allergy: Principles and practice, 7th ed, Adkinson NF, Bochner BS, Busse WW, *et al* (Eds), Mosby Elsevier, 2009.

[2] McSharry C, Xia Y, Holland CV, Kennedy MW. Natural immunity to Ascaris lumbricoides associated with immunoglobulin E antibody to ABA-1 allergen and inflammation indicators in children. Infect Immun 1999; 67: 484.

[3] Lynch NR, Hagel IA, Palenque ME, *et al.* Relationship between helminthic infection and IgE response in atopic and nonatopic children in a tropical environment. J Allergy Clin Immunol 1998; 101: 217.

[4] Watanabe N, Katakura K, Kobayashi A, *et al.* Protective immunity and eosinophilia in IgE-deficient SJA/9 mice infected with Nippostrongylus brasiliensis and Trichinella spiralis. Proc Natl Acad Sci U S A 1988; 85: 4460.

[5] Stone KD, Prussin C, Metcalfe DD. IgE, mast cells, basophils, and eosinophils. J Allergy Clin Immunol 2010; 125: S73.

[6] Schroeder HW Jr, Cavacini L. Structure and function of immunoglobulins. J Allergy Clin Immunol 2010; 125: S41.

[7] Vercelli D. Genetic regulation of IgE responses: Achilles and the tortoise. J Allergy Clin Immunol 2005; 116: 60.

[8] Geha RS, Jabara HH, Brodeur SR. The regulation of immunoglobulin E class-switch recombination. Nat Rev Immunol 2003; 3:721.

[9] Smith P, Ownby DR. Clinical significance of IgE. In: Middleton's allergy: Principles and practice, 7th ed, Adkinson NF, Bochner BS, Busse WW, *et al.* (Eds), Mosby Elsevier, 2009

[10] Takhar P, Corrigan CJ, Smurthwaite L, *et al.* Class switch recombination to IgE in the bronchial mucosa of atopic and nonatopic patients with asthma. J Allergy Clin Immunol 2007; 119: 213.

[11] Granada M, Wilk JB, Tuzova M, *et a*l. A genome-wide association study of plasma total IgE concentrations in the Framingham Heart Study. J Allergy Clin Immunol 2012; 129: 840.

[12] Dullaers M, De Bruyne R, Ramadani F, *et al.* The who, where, and when of IgE in allergic airway disease. J Allergy Clin Immunol 2012; 129: 635.

[13] Hibbert RG, Teriete P, Grundy GJ, *et al.* The structure of human CD23 and its interactions with IgE and CD21. J Exp Med 2005; 202: 751.

[14] Presta LG, Lahr SJ, Shields RL, *et al.* Humanization of an antibody directed against IgE. J Immunol 1993; 151: 2623.

[15] Buhl R. Anti-IgE antibodies for the treatment of asthma. Curr Opin Pulm Med 2005; 11: 27.

[16] Djukanović R, Wilson SJ, Kraft M, *et al.* Effects of treatment with anti-immunoglobulin E antibody omalizumab on airway inflammation in allergic asthma. Am J Respir Crit Care Med. 2004;170(6): 583–93.

[17] Van Rensen ELJ, Evertse CE, Van Schadewijk WAAM *et al.* Eosinophils in bronchial mucosa of asthmatics after allergen challenge: effect of anti-IgE treatment. Allergy. 2009; 64(1): 72–80

[18] Thomson NC, Chaudhuri R. Omalizumab: Clinical Use for the Management of Asthma. Clin Med Insights Circ, Respir Pulm Med 2012 6: 27–40

[19] GINA report, global strategy for asthma management and prevention http://www.ginasthma.com, 2010. Accessed February 25, 2012.

[20] British guideline on the management of asthma. British Thoracic Society Scottish Intercollegiate Guidelines Network. Thorax. 2008; 63: iv 1–121.

[21] Expert Panel Report 3 (EPR-3): Guidelines for the Diagnosis and Management of Asthma-Summary Report 2007. J Allergy Clin. Immunol. 2007; 120(5 Suppl 1): S94–138.

[22] Tan R, Corren J. Omalizumab in the treatment of asthma. Expert Rev Respir Med 2011 Dec;5(6): 747-56

[23] Spears M, Cameron E, Chaudhuri R, Thomson NC. Challenges of treating asthma in people who smoke. Expert Rev Clin Immunol. 2010; 6(2): 257–68.

[24] Steiss JO, Strohmer P, Zimmer KP, Lindermann H. Reduction of the total Ig E level by omalizumab in children and adolescents. J Asthma 2008;45 (3): 233-6

[25] Bousquet J, Wenzel S, Holgate S, *et al.* Predicting response to omalizumab, an anti-IgE antibody, in patients with allergic asthma. Chest 2004; 125(4): 1378–86.

[26] Bousquet J, Rabe K, Humbert M, *et al.*.Predicting and evaluating response to omalizumab in patients with severe allergic asthma. Resp Med. 2007;101(7): 1483–92

[27] Slavin RG, Ferioli C, Tannenbaum SJ, *et al.* Asthma symptom re-emergence after omalizumab withdrawal correlates well with increasing IgE and decreasing pharmacokinetic concentrations. J Allergy Clin Immunol. 2009;123(1): 107–13.

[28] Nopp A, Johansson SGO, Adédoyin J, *et al.* After 6 years with Xolair; a 3-year withdrawal follow-up. Allergy. 2010; 65(1): 56–60.

[29] Walker S, Monteil M, Phelan K, Lasserson T, Walters E. Anti-IgE for chronic asthma in adults and children. Cochrane Database of Systematic Reviews. 2006;2: CD003559. doi: 10.1002/14651858.CD003559.pub3.

[30] Rodrigo GJ, Neffen H, Castro-Rodriguez J. Efficacy and safety of subcutaneous omalizumab *vs.* placebo as add-on therapy to corticosteroids for children and adults with asthma. Chest. 2011; 139(1): 28–35.

[31] Lanier B, Bridges T, Kulus M, *et al.*. Omalizumab for the treatment of exacerbations in children with inadequately controlled allergic (IgE-mediated) asthma. J Allergy Clin Immunol. 2009; 124(6): 1210–6.

[32] Bardelas J, Figliomeni M, Kianifard F, Meng X. A 26-Week, Randomized, Double-Blind, Placebo-Controlled, Multicenter Study to Evaluate the Effect of Omalizumab on Asthma Control in Patients with Persistent Allergic Asthma. J Asthma. 2012; 49(2): 144–52.

[33] Van den Berge M, Pauw RG, de Monchy JGR, *et al.*. Beneficial effects of treatment with anti-IgE antibodies (omalizumab) in a patient with severe asthma and negative skin-prick Test Results. Chest. 2011; 139(1): 190–3.

[34] Eisner MD, Zazzali JL, Miller MK, Bradley MS, Schatz M. Longitudinal changes in asthma control with omalizumab: 2-year interim data from the EXCELS Study. J Asthma. 2012 Aug;49(6): 642-8

[35] Brodlie M, McKean MC, Moss S, Spencer DA. The oral corticosteroid-sparing effect of omalizumab in children with severe asthma. Arch Dis Child. 2012 Jul;97(7): 604-9

[36] Wittchen HU, Mühlig S, Klotsche J, *et al.*.Omalizumab *vs.* 'usual care': results from a naturalistic longitudinal study in routine care. Int Arch Allergy Immunol. 2012;159(1): 83-93

[37] Slavin RG. Update on occupational rhinitis and asthma, Allergy Asthma Proc 2010 Nov-Dec; 31 (6): 437-43

[38] Leynadier F, Doudou O, Gaouar H, *et al.* Effect of omalizumab in health care workers with occupational latex allergy. J Allergy Clin Immunol. 2004;113(2): 360.

[39] Pérez Pimiento A, Bueso Fernández A, García Loria J, *et al.* Effect of omalizumab treatment in a baker with occupational asthma. J Investig Allergol Clin Immunol. 2008;18(6): 490.

[40] Olivieri M, Biscardo CA, Turri S, Perbellini L. Omalizumab in persistent severe bakers' asthma. Allergy. 2008; 63(6): 790.

[41] Félix Toledo R,Martínez López R, Negro Álvarez JM, Ramírez Hernández M, Mérida Fernández C. [Anti Ig E (omalizumab) in the treatment of allergic rhinitis]. Alergol Inmunol Clin 2004; 19: 133-139.

[42] Casale TB, Condemi J, LaForce C *et al.* Omalizumab Seasonal Allergic Rhinitis Trail Group: Effect of omalizumab on symptoms of seasonal allergic rhinitis: a randomized controlled trial. JAMA. 2001; 286(23): 2956.

[43] Kopp MV, Brauburger J, Riedinger F *et al.* The effect of anti-IgE treatment on *in vitro* leukotriene release in children with seasonal allergic rhinitis. J Allergy Clin Immunol. 2002; 110(5): 728.

[44] Chervinsky P., Casale T., Townley R., *et al;* Omalizumab, an anti-IgE antibody, in the treatment of adults and adolescents with perennial allergic rhinitis. Ann Allergy Asthma Immunol 2003; 91: 160-167.

[45] Penn R, Mikula S The role of anti-IgE immunoglobulin therapy in nasal polyposis: a pilot study. Am J Rhinol. 2007; 21(4): 428.

[46] Metz M, Maurer M. Omalizumab in chronic urticaria. Curr Opin Allergy Clin Immunol 2012 Aug; 12 (4): 406-11

[47] Boyce JA. Successful treatment of cold-induced urticaria/anaphylaxis with anti-IgE. J Allergy Clin Immunol. 2006;117(6): 1415.

[48] Saini S, Rosen KE, Hsieh HJ *et al.* A randomized, placebo-controlled, dose-ranging study of single-dose omalizumab in patients with H1-antihistamine-refractory chronic idiopathic urticaria. J Allergy Clin Immunol. 2011;128(3): 567.

[49] Maurer M, Altrichter S, Bieber T *et al.* Efficacy and safety of omalizumab in patients with chronic urticaria who exhibit IgE against thyroperoxidase. J Allergy Clin Immunol. 2011; 128(1): 202.

[50] Metz M, Altrichter S, Ardelean E *et al.* Anti-immunoglobulin E treatment of patients with recalcitrant physical urticaria. Int Arch Allergy Immunol. 2011; 154(2): 177.

[51] Ring J, Alomar A, Bieber T *et al.* Guidelines for the treatment of atopic eczema (atopic dermatitis). J Eur Acad Dermatol Venereol 2012; Sep 26 (9): 1176-93

[52] Sheinkopf LE. Rafi AW, Do LT, Katz RM, Klaustermever WB. Efficacy of omalizumab in the treatment of atopic dermatitis; a pilot study. Allergy Asthma Proc 2008 Sep-Oct; 29 (5): 530-7

[53] Kopp MV. Omalizumab: anti Ig E therapy in allergy. Curr Allergy Asthma Report 2011 apr; 11(2); 101-6

[54] Lane J.E., Cheyney J.M., Lane T.N., *et al*: Treatment of recalcitrant atopic dermatitis with omalizumab. J Am Acad Dermatol 2006; 54: 68-72.

[55] Heil PM, Maurer D, Klein B, Hultsch T, Stingl G. Omalizumab therapy in atopic dermatitis: depletion of IgE does not improve the clinical course - a randomized, placebo-controlled and double blind pilot study. J Dtsch Dermatol Ges. 2010;8(12): 990

[56] Krathen R.A., Hsu S. Failure of omalizumab for treatment of severe adult atopic dermatitis. J Am Acad Dermatol 2005; 53: 338-340.

[57] Fitzhugh DJ, Lockey RF. Allergen immunotherapy: a history of the first 100 years. Curr Opin Allergy Clin Immunol 2011 Dec; 11 (6): 554-9

[58] Kontou-Fili K High omalizumab dose controls recurrent reactions to venom immunotherapy in indolent systemic mastocytosis. Allergy 2008; 63 (3): 376-378

[59] Massanari M, Nelson H, Casale T *et al*. Effect of pretreatment with omalizumab on the tolerability of specific immunotherapy in allergic asthma. J Allergy Clin Immunol. 2010;125(2): 383.

[60] Casale TB, Busse WW, Kline JN *et al.* Omalizumab pretreatment decreases acute reactions after rush immunotherapy for ragweed-induced seasonal allergic rhinitis. Allergy Clin Immunol. 2006; 117(1): 134.

[61] Matheu V, Franco A, Perez E, Hernández M, Barrios Y: Omalizumab for drug allergy. J Allergy Clin Immunol. 2007 Dec; 120(6): 1471-2; author reply 1472-3. Epub 2007 Sep 12.

[62] Leung DY, Sampson HA, Yunginger JW *et al.* Avon Longitudinal Study of Parents and Children Study Team. N Engl J Med. 2003; 348(11): 986.

[63] Sampson HA, Leung DY, Burks AW *et al* A phase II, randomized, double-blind, parallel-group, placebo-controlled oral food challenge trial of Xolair (omalizumab) in peanut allergy DA. J Allergy Clin Immunol. 2011; 127(5): 1309.

[64] Sicherer SH, Leung DY, Advances in allergic skin disease, anaphylaxis and hypersensitivity reactions to food, drugs and insects in 2009. J Allergy Clin Immunol 2010; 125 (1): 85-97

[65] Tillie-Leblond I, Germaud P, Leroyer C *et al.* Allergic bronchopulmonary aspergillosis and omalizumab. Allergy. 2011;66(9): 1254

[66] Zirbes JM, Milla CE: Steroid-sparing effect of omalizumab for allergic bronchopulmonary aspergillosis and cystic fibrosis. Pediatr Pulmonol. 2008;43(6): 607

[67] Van der Ent CK, Hoekstra H, Rijkers GT: Successful treatment of allergic bronchopulmonary aspergillosis with recombinant anti-IgE antibody. Thorax. 2007; 62(3): 276

[68] Brinkmann F, Schwerk N, Hansen G, Ballmann M: Steroid dependency despite omalizumab treatment of ABPA in cystic fibrosis. Allergy. 2010; 65(1): 134.

[69] Rocha R, Vitor AB, Trindade E *et al.* Omalizumab in the treatment of eosinophilic esophagitis and food allergy. Eur J Pediatr. 2011 Nov;170(11): 1471-4. Epub 2011 Aug 2.

[70] Carter MC, Robyn JA, Bressler PB, *et al.* Omalizumab for the treatment of unprovoked anaphylaxis in patients with systemic mastocytosis. J Allergy Clin Immunol 2007 Jun; 119(6) : 1550–1

[71] Siebenhaar F, Kühn W, Zuberbier T, Maurer M.Successful treatment of cutaneous mastocytosis and Ménière disease with anti-IgE therapy. J Allergy Clin Immunol. 2007 Jul; 120 (1): 213–5

[72] Goodyear M. Learning from the TGN1412 trial. BMJ. 2006 Mar 25; 332(7543): 677-8.

[73] Corren J, Casale T B, Lanier B, Buhl R, Holgate S.Jiménez P. Safety and tolerability of omalizumab. Clin Exp Allergy 2009; 39: 788-797

[74] Ayres JG, Higgins B, Chilvers ER, Ayre G, Blogg M, Fox H. Efficacy and tolerability of anti-immunoglobulin E therapy with omalizumab in patients with poorly controlled (moderate-to severe) allergic asthma. Allergy 2004; 59:701–8.

[75] United States Food and Drug Administration. 2007 Safety alerts for drug, biologics, medical devices, and dietary supplements. www.fda.gov/medwatch/safety/2007/safety07.htm#Xolair (Accessed on August 2, 2012).

[76] Price KS, Hamilton RG. Anaphylactoid reactions in two patients after omalizumab administration after successful long-term therapy. Allergy Asthma Proc. 2007 May-Jun; 28(3): 313-9.

[77] Limb SL, Starke PR, Lee CE, Chowdhury BA. Delayed onset and protracted progression of anaphylaxis after omalizumab administration in patients with asthma. J Allergy Clin Immunol 2007;120: 1378–81.

[78] Cox L, Platts-Mills T, Finegold I *et al.* American Academy of Allergy, Asthma & Immunology/American College of Allergy, Asthma and Immunology Joint Task Force Report on omalizumab-associated anaphylaxis. J Allergy Clin Immunol 2007; 120 (6): 1373-7.

[79] Varghese M, Lieberman P. The effects of repeat omalizumab administration on skin test positivity and the assessment of the safety of administration in patients with positive skin tests to mouse antigen. Allergy Asthma Proc. 2007 May-Jun;28(3): 320-3.

[80] Lieberman P, Rahmaoui A, Wong D. The safety and interpretability of skin test with omalizumab. Ann Allergy Asthma Immunol 2010; Dec 105: 493-5

[81] Cooper P, Ayre G, Martin C, Rizzo JA, Ponte EV, Cruz A. Geohelminth infections: a review of the role of IgE and assessment of potential risks of anti-IgE treatment. Allergy 2008; 63: 409–417

[82] Amiri P, Haak-Frendscho M, Robbins K, McKerrow JH, Stewart T, Jardieu P. Anti-immunoglobulin E treatment decreases worm burden and egg production in Schistosoma mansoni-infected normal and interferon-c knockout mice. J Exp Med 1994; 180: 43–51.

[83] Korenaga M, Watanabe N, Tada I. Effects of anti-IgE monoclonal antibody on a primary infection of Strongyloides ratti in mice. Parasitol Res 1991;77: 362–363.

[84] Abraham D, Leon O, Schnyder-Candrian S *et al.* Immunoglobulin E and eosinophil-dependent protective immunity to larval Onchocerca volvulus in mice immunized with irradiated larvae. Infect Immun 2004; 72:810–817.

[85] Cruz AA, Lima F, Sarinho E *et al.* Safety of anti immunoglobulin E therapy with omalizumab in allergic patients at risk of geohelminth infection. Clin Exp Allergy 2007; 37: 197–207.

[86] Busse W, Buhl R, Fernández Vidaurre C *et al.* Omalizumab and the risk of malignancy: Results from a pooled analysis. J Allergy Clin Immunol 2012; 129 (4): 983-9

[87] Banh HL, Trevoy J, Pabst H, Beach J, Vethanayagam D. Persistent elevation of peripheral blood myeloid cell counts associated with omalizumab therapy. Am J Health Syst Pharm. 2012 Feb 15; 69(4): 302-6.

[88] Medicines and Healthcare Regulatory Agency. Omalizumab: Potential risk of arterial thrombotic events. Availablefrom: http://www.mhra.gov.uk/home/groups/dsu/documents /publication/con108718.pdf. (Accessed on August 12, 2012).

[89] Ali Ak, Hartzema A. Assessing the association between omalizumab and arteriothrombotic events through spontaneous adverse event reporting. J Asthma Allergy 2012; 5 : 1-9

[90] Pilette C, Coppens N, Houssiau F, Rodenstein D. Severe serum sickness–like syndrome after omalizumab therapy for asthma. J Allergy Clin Immunol 2007; 120(4): 972-3

[91] Dreyfus D, Randolph C. Characterization of an anaphylactoid reaction to omalizumab. Ann Allergy Asthma Immunol 2006; 96: 624–627.

[92] López- Bastida J. [Economic evaluation of health technologies]. In: [An introduction to investigation methodology in the evaluation of health technologies] 1st ed Santa Cruz de Tenerife, Spain: Servicio Canario de la Salud 2010; pp 129-148.

[93] European Respiratory Sociey and the European Lung Foundation. European lung white book. Brussels, Belgium: European Respiratory Society and the European Lung Foundation 2003.

[94] Beasley R. The burden of asthma with specific reference to the United States. J Allergy Clin Immunol 2002; 109 (Supl B): S482-9

[95] Martínez-Moragón E, Serra Batllés J, De Diego A *et al.* Economic cost of treating the patient with asthma in Spain: The AsthmaCost study. Arch Bronconeumol. 2009; 45(10): 481-486

[96] Oba Y, Salzman G. Cost-effectiveness analysis of omalizumab in adults and adolescents with moderate-to-severe allergic asthma. J Allergy Clin Immunol 2004; 114 (2): 265-9

[97] Wu A, Paltiel D, Kuntz K, Weiss S, Fuhlbrigge A. Cost- effectiveness of omalizumab in adults with severe asthma: Results from the Asthma Policy Model. J Allergy Clin Immunol 2007; 120(5): 1146-1152

[98] Dewilde S, Turk F, Tambour M, Sandström T. The economic value of anti-IgE in severe persistent, IgE-mediated (allergic) asthma patients: adaptation of INNOVATE to Sweden. Curr Med Res Opin. 2006 Sep; 22(9): 1765-76

[99] Brown R, Turk F, Dale P, Bousquet J. Cost-effectiveness of omalizumab in patients with severe persistent allergic asthma. Allergy 2007; 62: 149-153

[100] Campbell JD, Spackman DE, Sullivan SD. The costs and consequences of omalizumab in non-controlled asthma from a USA payer perspective. Allergy 2010; 65: 1141–1148

[101] Jones J, Sheperd J, Hartwell D *et al.* Omalizumab for the treatment of severe persistent allergic asthma. Health Technology Assessment 2009; 13 (Suppl. 2): 31- 9.

[102] Walker S, Burch J, McKenna C, *et al.* Omalizumab for the treatment of severe persistent allergic asthma in children aged 6-11 years. Health Technol Assess. 2011 May;15 Suppl 1:13-21.

[103] Stokes J, Casale T. Rationale for new treatments aimed to Ig E immunomodulation. Ann Allergy Asthma Immunol. 2004; 93: 212-7

[104] Escoubet-Lozach L, Glass C, Wasserman S. The role of transcription factors in allergic inflammation. J Allergy Clin Immunol. 2002;110:553–564

[105] Woerly G, Honda K, Loyens M, *et al.* Peroxisome proliferator-activated receptors γ and α down-regulate allergic inflammation and eosinophil activation. J Exp Med. 2003; 198:411–421

[106] Paumelle R, Blanquart C, Briand O *et al.* Acute antiiflammtory properties of statins involve peroxisome-activated receptor alpha *via* inhibition of the protein kinase C signalling pathway. Cir Res 2006; 98: 361-9

[107] Senti G, Johansen P, Haug S *et al.* Use of type-A CpG oligodeoxynucleotides as an adjuvant in allergen-specific immunotherapy in humans: a phase I/ IIa clinical trial. Clin Exp Allergy 2009 Aprl; 39 (4): 562-70.

[108] Tamaoki J, Kondo M, Sakai N *et al.* Effect of suplatast tosilate; a Th2 cytokine inhibitor on steroid dependent asthma: a double-blind randomized study. Tokyo Joshi-Idai Asthma research group. Lancet 2000; Jul 22; 356(9226): 273-8

[109] Shiga M, Horiguchi T, Kondo R *et al.* Long-term monotherapy with suplatast tosilate in patients with mild atopic asthma: A pilot comparison with low-dose inhaled fluticasone. Asian Pac J Allergy Immunol 2011; 29: 134-42

[110] Wada M, Nagata S, Kudo T, Shimizu T, Yamashiro Y. Effect of suplatast tosilate on antileukotriene non-responders with mild-to-moderate persistent asthma. Allergology International 2009; 58: 389-393

[111] Watanabe N, Hirata A, Makino S, Fukuda T. A case of eosinophilic pneumonia successfully treated with suplatast tosilate alone. Int Arch Allergy Immunol 2009; Suppl 1: 94-101.

[112] Yamada Y, Yoshihara S, Arisaka O. Successful treatment of paediatric hypereosinophilic syndrome with suplatast tosilate. Ann Allergy Asthma Immunol 2007 Oct; 99(4):380-1

[113] Ueda T, Arai S, Amoh Y, Katsuoka K. Kimura's disease treated with suplatast tosilate and loratadine. Eur J Dermatol 2011 Nov-Dec; 21(6): 1020-1

[114] Borish L, Nelson H, Lanz M *et al.* Interleukin-4 receptor in moderate atopic asthma: A phase I/ II randomized placebo-controlled trial. Am J Respir Crit Care Med. 1999; 160: 1816-23

[115] Borish L, Nelson L, Corren J *et al.* Efficacy of soluble IL-4 receptor for the treatment of adults with asthma. J Allergy Clin Immunol 2001; 107 (6): 963-970

[116] Wenzel S, Wilbraham D, Fuller R, Getz E B, Longphre M. Effect of an interleukin-4 variant in late phase asthmatic response to allergen challenge in ashmatic patients: Results of two phase IIa studies. Lancet 2007; Oct 20; 370(9596):1422-31

[117] Slagger R, Otulana B, Hawkins G *et al.* IL-4 receptor polymorphisms predict reduction in asthma exacerbations during response to an anti IL-4 receptor α antagonist. J Allergy Clin Immunol 2012; 130 (2): 516-522

[118] Corren J, Lemanske R, Hanania N *et al.* Lebrikizumab treatment in adults with asthma. N Engl J Med 2011; 365 (12): 1088-1098

[119] Bryan SA, O'Connor BJ, Matti S, *et al.* Effects of recombinant human interleukin-12 on eosinophils, airway hyper-responsiveness, and the late asthmatic response. Lancet 2000; 356: 2149–2153

[120] Leonard JP, Sherman ML, Fisher GL, *et al.* Effects of a singledose interleukin-12 exposure on interleukin-12 associated toxicity and interferon- production. Blood 1997; 90: 2541-8

[121] Kumar M, Behera A, Hu J, Lockey RF, Mohapatra SS. IFN-and IL-12 plasmid DNAs as vaccine adjuvant in a murine model of grass allergy. J Allergy Clin Immunol 2001; 108: 402- 8

[122] Boguniewicz M, Martin RJ, Martin D, *et al.* The effects of nebulized recombinant interferon-gamma in asthmatic airways. J Allergy Clin Immunol 1995; Jan; 95(1 Pt 1):133-5

[123] Rossenwasswer L, Busse W, Lizambri R, Olejnic T, Totoritis M. Allergic asthma and an anti CD23 mAb (IDEC 152): Results of a phase I single-dose, dose-scalating clinical trial. J Allergy Clin Immunol 2003; 112 (3): 563-570

[124] Poole J, Meng J, Reff M, Spellman M, Rossenwasser L. Anti-CD23 monoclonal antibody, lumiliximab, inhibited allergen induced responses in antigen presenting cells and T cells from atopic subjects. J Allergy Clin Immunol 2005; 116 (4): 780- 8

[125] Zhu D, Kepley CL, Zhang M, Zhang K, Saxon A. A novel human immunoglobulin Fcγ-Fcε bifunctional fusion protein inhibits FcεRI-mediated degranulation, Nat Med 2002 May; 8 (5); 518-21

[126] Van Scott MR, Merstching E, Negrou E *et al.* Systemic administration of an Fc gamma-Fc epsilon fusion protein in house dust mites sensitive non human primates. Clin Immunol 2008 Sep; 128 (3): 340-8

[127] Lin LH, Zheng P, Yuen JW *et al.* Prevention and treatment of allergic inflammation by an Fcγ- Der f2 fusion protein in a murine model of house dust induced asthma, Immunol Res 2012 Jun; 52 (3); 276-83

[128] Peng Z. Vaccines targeting Ig E in the treatment of asthma and allergy. Human vaccines 2009 May; 5 (5): 302-9

CHAPTER 5

Therapeutics for Allergy Management

Sagar Laxman Kale and Naveen Arora*

Allergy and Immunology Section, CSIR-Institute of Genomics and Integrative Biology, Delhi University Campus, Mall road, Delhi-110007, India

Abstract: Allergy is defined as an inappropriate immune response in atopic individuals to antigens called as allergens capable of mediating type I hypersensitive reactions. Prevalence of allergic diseases is on the rise and has reached epidemic proportions. Extensive research over the past few decades on pathogenesis of allergic diseases and the molecular mechanisms involved has led to many therapeutic approaches. Management of allergic diseases includes allergen avoidance, pharmacotherapy and allergen specific immunotherapy (SIT). Though allergen avoidance has proved to be effective, it is not feasible to control the exposure of allergens. Pharmacotherapy includes a vast range of strategies and therapies for managing allergic diseases of which inhaled corticosteroids (ICSs) form the first line of treatment. Though ICSs are highly effective, in severe asthma cases other class of medications like β_2 agonists, anti-histamines, omalizumab *etc.*, in combination with ICSs are recommended. Allergen specific immunotherapy (SIT) is the only treatment modality that acts on effector cells and prevents progression of mild allergy to severe allergic diseases. Inspite of these therapies for allergic disease many patients have poorly controlled symptoms. A better understanding of the complex aetieology of insights into molecular mechanisms will lead to development of new therapeutics with improved efficiency and minimal side effects.

Keywords: Type I hypersensitivity, allergy, Th2 cells, corticosteroids, bronchodilators, mediator antagonists, immunotherapy, serine protease inhibitors, anti-oxidants, peptide immunotherapy.

INTRODUCTION

Allergy or type I hypersensitivity is the clinical manifestation of an immune response against potentially innocuous antigens called allergens. Allergens are potent inducers of Th2 cell responses leading to elevated levels of IgE antibodies

***Address correspondence to Naveen Arora:** Allergy and Immunology Section, CSIR-Institute of Genomics and Integrative Biology, Delhi University Campus, Mall Road, Delhi, India; Tel: +911127666156; Fax: +911127667471; Email: naveen@igib.res.in; navdelhi@hotmail.com

Atta-ur-Rahman (Ed)

specific to allergens. Allergic diseases are patient specific and include asthma, allergic rhinoconjunctivities, sinusitis, food allergies, angioedema, anaphylaxis, urticaria and atopic dermatitis [1]. Allergic diseases have reached epidemic proportions with current estimates stating that almost 25% of population in industrialised countries are suffering from allergy with increasing prevalence in last decade [2]. This places enormous financial burden on the community in terms of health care cost and loss of working days [3].

Allergic reaction is a complex interplay between environmental factors called allergens and various components of immune system. It can be roughly divided into two phases *viz.* sensitization and re-exposure phase. When a predisposed individual is exposed to an allergen, it is first taken up by professional antigen presenting cells, primarily dendritic cells. After allergen uptake, these cells migrate to draining lymph nodes and present the processed allergens (peptides) along with MHC class II molecules to naive T-cells. These naive T-cells differentiate into Th2 cells and upregulate expression of cluster of genes encoded on chromosome 5q31-33 *viz.* IL-3, IL-4, IL-5, IL-9, IL-13 and GM-CSF. These cytokines are involved in class switching of B cells to IgE (IL-4 and IL-13), recruitment of mast cells (IL-4, IL-5 and IL-13), maturation of eosinophils (IL-5 and GMCSF), basophils (IL-3 and IL-4), and hyper secretion of mucus. The IgE antibodies bind to the high affinity FcεRI receptors present on mast cells and basophils. This marks the end of sensitization phase. Subsequent encounter with the same allergen causes cross linking of bound IgE in a specific manner and triggers degranulation of mast cells and basophils releasing pre-formed inflammatory mediators like histamine, lipid mediators (prostaglandins and cysteinyl leukotrienes) and cytokines. They are responsible for early allergic responses (occur within 30 minutes), such as increase in vascular permeability, smooth muscle contraction and mucus production. Chemokines released by mast cells along with Th2 cytokines leads to the recruitment of macrophages, eosinophils and basophils that together comprises the late allergic responses. Fig. **1** briefly summarizes the allergic reaction and indicates the targets of current therapeutics.

INHALED CORTICOSTEROIDS

Of all the available treatments inhaled corticosteroids are the first line of therapy used for persistent asthma because they are the most potent and effective over a long term [4]. Corticosteroids readily cross the cellular membrane and binds to activate the cytoplasmic glucocorticoid receptors. After activation these receptors then translocate to the nucleus and modulate the transcriptional activity of target genes by gene transactivation and gene transrepression [5]. These receptors initiate the transcription of steroid sensitive genes by binding to glucocorticoid response elements (GREs) in their promoters. This leads to transcription of anti-inflammatory genes like annexin 1, IL-10, SLPI and inhibitor of nuclear factor–κB [6]. Inhaled corticosteroids (ICSs) suppress the Th2 mediated airway inflammation by inhibiting the expression of cytokines, mediators and adhesion molecules [7]. Cellular effect of corticosteroids includes reduction in inflammatory cells (eosinophils, mast cells and dendritic cells) and their mediators (including T-cell cytokines and macrophage cytokines).

Though ICS are the cornerstone in asthma management, their prolonged use or increased dose to achieve maximum improvement in asthma symptoms risks the patients to its potential side effects. Oral candidiasis, pharyngeal inflammation, sensation of thirst, laryngeal disorders, cough and dysphonia have been reported to be the local side effects associated with corticosteroid therapy [8-11]. Systemic side effects of ICSs include reduced bone mineral density, skin bruising, glaucoma, cataracts, and growth retardation in children. Corticosteroids are effective in suppressing Th2 cell–driven inflammation at least in part because they are very potent inhibitors of the Th2 regulating transcription factor GATA3.

BRONCHODILATORS

Bronchodialators relive and prevent bronchoconstriction and are effective in reducing asthma symptoms. They are important in management of asthma and allergy.

β_2-Agonists

β_2-adrenoreceptors are primarily present on bronchial smooth muscle cells and are also found on several inflammatory cells like eosinophils, neutrophils, lymphocytes, mast cells and macrophages. β_2-adrenoreceptor agonists are a group of sympathomimetic agents that act by stimulating β_2-receptors in the airway cells. β_2 adrenergic agonists affect airways by relaxing airway smooth muscles [12, 13]. They have been shown to effectively inhibit bronchoconstrictor mediator release from airway mast cells and also mediators from eosinophlis, macrophages, T-lymphocytes and neutrophils. β_2 agonists increases mucus secretion and mucociliary clearance and decreases cholinergic neurotransmission. They are grouped either as short acting (SABAs, 3-6 h duration of action) or long acting (LABAs, >12 h duration of action) β_2-adrenoreceptor agonists. SABAs have been the backbone of therapy in airway diseases. They have consistently produced effective bronchodilation and improved lung function. But because of their short period of action, SABAs are not preferred for long term maintenance medications. Instead they are generally reserved for rescue use. SABAs are essential as rescue medications to relieve symptoms, prevent exercise-induced asthma, and treat exacerbations. Usually in these acute settings, high doses can be given at short intervals. In contrast, there appears to be no benefit of regular use of SABAs in the maintenance therapy of asthma [14]. LABAs like salmeterol and formoterol play an important role in asthma therapy and are usually administered through combination inhalers with corticosteroids. LABA used without corticosteroid cover increased severe exacerbation and mortality. However, when used in combination with corticosteroids they do not pose any risk and therefore have been suggested to be used in combination therapy. Several once-daily β_2 agonists called ultra-LABAs such as carmoterol, vilanterol and olodaterol are in clinical development.

Muscarinic Antagonists (Anti-Cholinergics)

Muscarine receptors (M1, M2 and M3) are G-protein coupled receptors present on the airway smooth muscle cells that regulate vagally-induced bronchoconstriction and mucus production. Anti-cholinergics or muscarine receptor antagonists are synthetic quaternary ammonium derivatives of atropine that inhibit muscarine receptors and subsequent bronchoconstriction. They are also known to inhibit mucous secretion from bronchial submucousal glands [15]. Ipratropium, a short acting muscarine receptor is less effective in reliving bronchoconstriction as they block only the cholinergic component of bronchoconstriction as compared to

SABA and hence are not recommended as first-line treatment for intermittent and mild asthma. Addition of ipratropium to β_2-adrenergic agonist has been shown to be beneficial in mild asthma [16, 17]. Several other reports have concluded that in acute asthma, there is no benefit of addition of ipratropium [18, 19]. In allergic rhinitis, intranasly given ipratropium has been shown effective in controlling watery rhinorrhea [20]. Ipratropium bromide has been associated with dryness of mouth and a bitter taste [21]. No anti-muscarine antagonist has been approved to be used in asthma in USA.

MEDIATOR ANTAGONISTS

Anti-Leukotrienes

Cystienyl leukotrienes (LTC_4, LTD_4 and LTE_4) are proinflammatory mediators secreted by activated mast cells and eosinophils. They are synthesized *via* 5-lipoxygenase pathway and play an important role in several asthma phenotypes [22, 23]. Increased levels of $cysLTC_4$, $cysLTD_4$ and $cysLTE_4$ have been observed in active asthma and rhinitis. Antileukotrienes are the drugs that inhibit the synthesis of the leukotrienes or block their receptors. They have been shown to be effective in the treatment of asthma [24, 25]. Two approaches have been adopted to decrease leukotriene mediated inflammation, first by using Leukotriene synthesis inhibitors (LTSI) and second by using leukotriene receptor antagonists (LTRA). LTSI acts by blocking the synthesis of leukotrienes (both CystLT and LTB_4).They are grouped into two classes, 5-LO inhibitors and 5-LO activating protein inhibitors (FLAP) based on the site of action. 5-LO inhibitors act by binding 5-Lipoxygenase enzyme and subsequently preventing the synthesis of leukotriene A_4. Alternatively, leukotriene receptor antagonists like montelukast blocks leukotriene D_4 receptors [26].

Antileukotrienes have been shown to reduce the risk of asthma exacerbations, both in preschool [27] and older children [28, 29]. Montelukast, a leukotriene receptor antagonist is the most widely used leukotriene modulator for the treatment of asthma. Montelukast showed clinical efficacy in asthmatic patients, both as monotherapy and in combination with inhaled corticosteroids by improving allergic symptoms like lung function and exacerbation rates along with quality of life. Several studies provided evidence that addition of an LTRA can improve several aspects in patients with in patients of allergic asthma and rhinitis.

The most commonly described side effects are generally mild and comprise headache, anxiety, depression and gastrointestinal complaints. In addition, several reports have associated Churg-Strauss syndrome (CSS) with montelukast therapy [30, 31] however, they seem to be more related to withdrawal of corticosteroids. GINA guidelines recommend low-dose ICS or a leukotriene modifier as controller therapy for asthma management in adults and children older than 5 years. In childrens, CystLT inhibitors have a potential to be used in monotherapy but their main use is as a supplement to ICS.

Anti-Histamines

Histamine plays a key role in manifestation of allergic inflammatory reactions. It exerts its physiologic effects through interactions with H(1-4) histamine receptors out of which H1 receptor has been implicated in allergic diseases [32]. Mast cells and basophils are prominent sources of preformed histamine in humans. IgE cross linking by allergens on mast cells and basophils triggers histamine secretion by these cells and is responsible for development of early responses in allergic diseases by causing smooth muscle contraction, mucus hypersecretion and increasing vascular permeability leading to mucosal edema. First generation anti-histamines (*e.g.*, chlorpheniramine, diphenhydramine, promethazine and hydroxyzine) are among the most widely recommended drugs in the world. Though first generation anti-histamines provide symptomatic relief from allergy and common cold [33], they are associated with considerable side effects owing to their ability to crosss blood brain barrier [34]. They are also associated with anticholenergic, local anaesthetic and anti-5-HT effects. Second-generation H1-receptor antagonists provide excellent, safe, and effective alternatives to first-generation antihistamines. Two of the second generation anti-histamines terfenadine and astemizole caused potentially serious arrhythmia and cardiac toxicity. The third generation anti-histamines have not shown the potential side effects of their predecessors and are equally potent.

MONOCLONAL ANTIBODIES AND CYTOKINE BLOCKERS

Monoclonal antibodies developed against important molecular targets in allergic cascade have shown a potential in treatment of these diseases.

Anti-IL-5 mAb

IL-5, a Th2 cytokine is essential for the maturation and differentiation of eosinophils. About 50% of severe asthma exacerbations are eosinophilic in nature [35]. Several studies have demonstrated that minimising the airway eosinophilic numbers can reduce the risk of severe exacerbations [36]. Humanized monoclonal antibodies specific for human IL-5, reslizumab (Sch55,700) and mepolizumab (SB-240,563) have been studied in patients. Mepolizumab decreased median serum eosinophils from baseline by 100% but decreased the airway eosinophils by 55% and failed to alter T-cell functions in asthmatic subjects [37, 38]. Mepolizumab has shown to reduce severe asthma exacerbations in difficult to treat asthma patients (40-50% of asthma patients) in which higher doses of ICS or oral corticosteroids proved ineffective [39, 40]. Castro *et al.* showed that reslizumab is effective in eosinophlic asthma and it can be effective in patients with nasal polyps. Reslizumab was administered to patients with eosinophilic asthma that was poorly controlled by high dose of ICSs. Reslizumab improved symptoms and FEV1 and also decreased sputum eosinophils in these patients. It also improved asthma control questionnaire in patients with nasal polyps [41]. Use of anti-IL-5 antibodies have not been approved in any country for use in treatment of asthma.

Anti-IgE mAb

Omalizumab is a 95% humanized murine monoclonal antibody specific against human IgE. It binds to an epitope on the Fc fragment of IgE at (Cε3) that specifically binds to the α chain of the IgE receptor. Binding of omalizumab to IgE inhibits it's interaction with high affinity IgE receptors (FcεRI) present on mast cells, basophils and dendritic cells as well as low affinity (FcεRII) receptors present on several immune and inflammatory cells. Thus omalizumab blocks the IgE-mediated release of inflammatory mediators from mast cells and other inflammatory cells. Omalizumab binds only to free circulating IgE regardless of antigen type (perennial, seasonal or both in case of multiple allergic sensitizations) and does not bind to cell-bound IgE. Omalizumab readily decreases serum IgE levels and regulates expression of FcεRI on various cell types. In one study, omalizumab administration decreased 99% of free serum IgE levels within 2 hours, 90% decrease in human basophil responsiveness in 3 months of therapy and FcεRI expression on dendritic cells and monocytes within 7 days. Apart from allergic asthma, omalizumab showed clinical efficacy in several other IgE-driven conditions including rhinosinusitis, conjunctivitis and bronchopulmonary allergic aspergillosis. Omalizumab is also effective for the treatment of allergic rhinoconjunctivitis, but therapy has to begin long before the onset of pollen season. A number of studies have established safety and efficacy of omalizumab but some studies have also reported side effects like pain and bruising. Some reports have identified rare episodes of anaphylaxis in less than 0.1% of treated patients and may occur within 24 hours of administration [42, 43].

Other mABs

Cytokines play a key role in orchestrating chronic inflammation and remodelling airway structure [44]. Almost 50 cytokines have been implicated in asthma and most have been targeted in clinical studies with disappointing results [45]. A number of antibodies are under development to target the cytokines such as IL-4 and IL-13 which are thought to play an important role in allergic diseases. IL-4 and IL-13 both exert their effects by binding to IL-4Rα/IL-13Rα1 receptor complex. IMA 638 is humanized IgG antibody that binds to an epitope on IL-13 and blocks binding with IL-4Rα. In patients whose asthma symptoms have not been controlled by high doses of ICSs, IMA 638 treatment significantly reduced both early and late asthmatic responses after allergen challenge [46] Lebrikizumab, an anti-IL-13 antibody, showed a small 5% increase in FEV1 but no change in asthma symptoms [47]. A recombinant IL-4Rα receptor binding protein Pitrakinra, with some adverse effects, has shown to reduce allergen induced late responses and is under development for use as inhaled medication [48]. Though several strategies have been developed to block the cytokines, it might be difficult to inhibit an inflammatory response merely by cytokine blocker because they are highly redundant in nature. Another problem developing cytokine blockers is high cost and can be restricted to be used in severe asthma cases.

IMMUNOMODULATORS

Allergen Specific Immunotherapy

Immune tolerance is induced naturally in beekeepers and cat owners who are exposed to high levels of allergens. Similarly immune tolerance to antigens such as allergens can be induced artificially by administration of high doses of the respective allergens. Allergen specific immunotherapy is an immune modifying therapy that induces a tolerant state in pheripheral T-cells. Pheripheral T-cell tolerance is characterised mainly by activation induced death, anergy or immune response modification by regulatory T-cells (Tregs) [49]. Allergen specific immunotherapy involves repeated administration of sensitizing allergen either by subcutaneous injection (SCIT), orally (OT) or by sublingual application (SLIT). It has been recommended in allergic rhinitis [50], venom hypersensitivity, mild bronchial asthma [51] and drug allergies. Allergen specific immunotherapy has been used for over a century and currently is the only curative treatment available for allergy. After natural exposure to allergens, SIT decreases recruitment of inflammatory cells like eosinophils, basophils and mast cells at the site of exposure. Allergen-SIT increases the production of IgA2 and IgG4 antibodies and subsequently reduces the levels of allergen specific IgE antibodies. Conventional SCIT involves repeated subcutaneous injections of allergen extracts or recombinant allergens in an increasing dose regime till tolerance is induced and may take several days to months. Usual approach is a build up phase (consisting of weekly injections) followed by a maintenance phase (consisting of monthly injections). SCIT has been a proven treatment of allergy to insect venom and inhalant allergens like pollens, molds, house dust mites and cat hair [52] but not for food [53] and latex allergies [54] due to the high risk of anaphlylaxis. As SCIT involves repeated administration of allergens, it may lead to systemic side effects like anaphylaxis. Sublingual immunotherapy (SLIT) is a safer alternative to SCIT and was developed to tackle problems of allergen administration by injection and systemic anaphylactic reactions in patients. In SLIT, allergens are administered to the oral mucosa and involves placement of extract under tongue for 1-2 min and then swallowed. A systemic and meta-analysis review has shown that though SLIT is clinically efficacious and the treatment benefit is approximately half of that achieved with SCIT [55]. In past few years, intensive research has been focused to increase the safety and efficacy of allergen-SIT. Current allergen-SIT use whole allergen extracts and are standardize in terms of total allergenic activity or potency or concentration of one major allergen. Tolerability and efficacy of immunotherapy with whole-body mosquito (*C. quinquefasciatus*) was evaluated in randomised controlled trial for 1 year in patients with allergic rhinitis and bronchial asthma sensitized to mosquito and showed improvement in symptoms and airway reactivity with increased IgG4 antibodies [56]. A double blind placebo-controlled trial of mix and single allergen IT for 1 year in 99 patients showed that IT with two to three mix extract from the same allergen group is effective for insect hypersensitivity [57]. Natural allergen extracts are undefined heterogeneous mixtures of carbohydrates, proteins and organic compounds. Administration of these heterogeneous extracts may cause life threatening anaphylactic reactions as well as induce false positive reactions during allergy diagnosis and/or additional IgE sensitization in patients during therapy [57, 58]. These unwanted problems can be overcome with the use of natural allergen extracts. New approaches to allergen SIT are focused to increase its efficacy and to decrease side effects. These include use of purified allergens [59-61], recombinant allergens [62-64], hypoallergenic recombinant allergens, T-cell reactive peptides, allergoids (chemically modified allergens), fragments of major allergens and chimeric allergens. IT with an inactive serine protease has more profound effect than the active protease [57, 65]. Allergen SIT is currently the only available curative treatment for allergy and new approaches to reduce potential side effects are under investigation.

NOVEL THERAPEUTIC INTERVENTIONS

Serine Protease Inhibitors

Serine proteases have been implicated in pathophysiology of allergic diseases, particularly in allergic asthma. Serine proteases like cathepsin G, tryptase and elastase from mast cells, leukocytes are elevated in airways of the asthmatic subjects and play a key role in exacerbation of allergic diseases. Many aeroallergens are proteases in nature. Serine proteases from house dust mite, *Curvularia lunata*, *Epicoccum purpurascens* and *Periplaneta americana* have been identified as major allergens [62-68]. The proteolytic activity of these allergens has been shown to drive the allergic immune response towards Th2 [69-

72] and provided an adjuvant effect towards self and other allergens. Serine protease inhibitors have shown to exhibit anti-inflammatory effects by inhibition of activation of leukocytes and fibrogenolytic activity of tryptase generated during coagulation cascade and inflammatory process. Recently, serine and tryptase protease inhibitors have been shown to reduce antigen-induced airway hyperreactivity in allergic guinea pigs and sheep. Nefamostat melisate and FOY, synthetic inhibitors of trypsin like serine protease inhibitors inhibited mast cell activation in early phase and showed immunoregulatory effects in late phase of allergic inflammation [73]. Saw *et al.* showed that AEBSF a serine protease inhibitor attenuated ovalbumin induced airway inflammation in mice model of airway allergic disease [74]. Similarly overexpression of secretory leukocyte protease inhibitor (SLPI), a naturally occurring protease inhibitor protects against allergic asthma phenotypes [75]. Thus serine protease inhibitors can be evaluated as therapeutic option in combination with current anti-allergic medications as adjunct therapy or as alternative medication for allergic asthma patients.

Targeting Oxidative Stress

An imbalance between oxidants and antioxidants causes oxidative stress. Evidence suggests that allergic disorders like asthma, allergic rhinitis, atopic dermatitis, urticaria are mediated by oxidative stress. Increased levels of reactive oxygen and nitrogen species is the hallmark of oxidative stress. Oxidative stress not only occurs by intrinsic factors like excessive inflammation that occurs in allergic diseases but also by environmental exposure to cigarette smoke and air pollution. Some reports implicate NADPH oxidases associated with pollens to induce excessive oxidative stress, which further leads to allergic airway inflammation. Therapeutic interventions that can minimize the exposure to environmental oxidants or augment antioxidant defences might be beneficial as adjunct therapies in allergic diseases. Existing antioxidant defences can be modified by administration of exogeneous antioxidants (alpha-tocopherol, α-lipoic acid, N-acetylcysteine, ambroxol) which were effective in suppressing allergic airway inflammation and BHR in mouse model of asthma [76, 77]. Further it has been shown that administration of catalytic antioxidants like intraperitoneal administration of SOD in guinea pigs reduced airway hyperresponsiveness. Inhalation of mGST (mutated Glutathione S-transferase) mutated to reduce its IgE binding reduced airway inflammation in mice by limiting oxidative stress and Th2 response [78]. Further, it was also shown that mutated mGST when combined with reduced glutathione exhibited synergistic effect in ameliorating oxidative stress and airway inflammation [79].

Choline, a lipotropic factor, is used as a dietary supplement and has potential as a drug for immune inflammatory diseases like asthma, rhinitis and others. The repeated consumption of choline chloride *via* i.n., oral or i.p. routes do not cause toxicity in mice, which makes it safe bait for allergic therapeutics [80]. When administered *via* oral gavage or intranasal (i.n.) choline chloride reduced inflammatory parameters in mouse model of allergic airway inflammation [81]. Further studies revealed that choline exerted this anti-inflammatory property by reducing oxidative stress possibly by modulating redox state of the cell [82]. A randomized study of 76 asthmatics administered with choline for 6 months suppressed immune inflammation and oxidative stress. Also the results suggested that choline exerts anti-inflammatory effect on the airways and reduces BHR in asthmatics. Precise role of antioxidants and oxidative stress in allergic disorders requires further studies. As allergic diseases like asthma are multifactorial merely suppressing the oxidative stress might not be useful in resolution of allergic disorders but might be used as an adjunct therapy.

Peptides

Immunotherapy with whole body extracts poses a risk of systemic reactions or asthma exacerbations in patients. Purified allergenic native or recombinant proteins may cause adverse reactions due to cross linking of IgE on mast cells and basophils thereby triggering the release of inflammatory mediators. Short synthetic peptides from allergens engineered to reduce or diminish IgE crosslinking but having intact immunodominant T cell regions can be used for safe and effective immunotherapy. Sharma *et al.* demonstrated to identify B and T cell peptides in-silico using bioinformatics tools for Cur l 3 and confirmed the observation using *in vitro* experiments [83]. A homology model of Cur l 3 was made using bioinformtaics and the peptides were identified by different criteria like solvent accessibility, hydrophobicity, hydrophilicity *etc.* A study in mice model of allergic asthma showed that IT with Cur l 3 derived short synthetic peptides (with reduced IgE binding) was more pronounced compared with whole *Curvularia* extract or purified Cur l 3 [84]. In another study, short term immunotherapy with peptides derived from phospholipase 2 of bee venom demonstrated induction of allergen specific T cell tolerance [85]. Studies with peptides derived from Fel d 1 (cat allergen) and Api m1 (bee venom allergen) have shown improved tolerance in terms of skin reactivity or airway hyper-reactivity after immunization. Recent studies with Alt a 13 and *Curvularia lunata* ADH used *in silico* approaches for identifying B and T cells epitopes of allergens. *In vitro* evaluation of these epitopes has shown that short peptides derived from these allergens have a potential for safe and effective immunotherapy [86, 87]. Animal experiments are being carried out to confirm the observations.

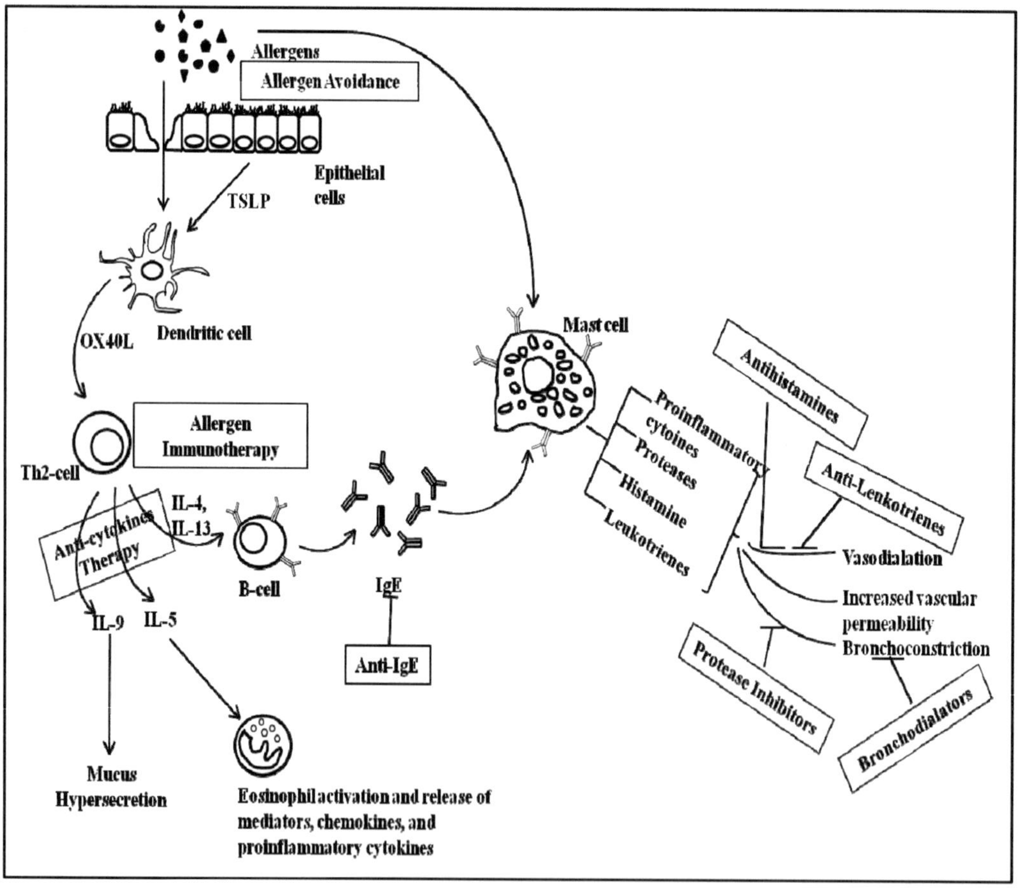

Figure 1: Targets of current anti-allergic therapeutics.

Table 1: Allergy therapeutics and their adverse effects.

Sr. No.	Type		Adverse Effect	Outcome	Refs.
1.	Corticosteroids		Suppresses hypothalamic-pituitary-adrenal axis		[88, 89]
			Skin thinning and bruising	Patients treated with high dose ICS had significantly thinner skin and increased risk of bruising	[90, 91]
			Reduction in bone mineral density	An inhaled steroid at a concentration of 0.67g/m2/day reduces BMD in prepubertal children.	[92]
2.	Bronchodilators		LABA used as monotherapy increased risk of death in patients of asthma	LABA should not be used as a monotherapy	[93]
3.	Mediator antagonists	Leukotriene antagonists	Churg Strauss Syndrome	Withdrawing corticosteroids gradually while replacing them with leukotriene antagonists increased the risk of Churg Strauss syndrome	[94-96]
		Anti-histamines	Sedation and psychomotor function impairment	Side effects are associated with first generation antihistamines and patients whose occupation require vigilance divided attention should use second generation antihistamines	[97]
4.	Monoclonal antibodies	Omalizumab	Local cutaneous reactions, Anaphylaxis	Anaphylaxis like reactions occurred in 0.2 % of the patients receiving Xolair for treatment of asthma	[42]
5.	Immunothera-py	SIT	Local allergic reactions (lump at injection site), Systemic side effects (Urticaria, asthma or anaphylaxis)		[98, 99]

CONCLUSIONS

In this chapter we have discussed various strategies and currently available therapeutic options for treatment of allergic diseases along with their potential side effects and risks involved as summarized in Table **1**. Extensive research on mechanisms resulting in initiation of allergic reactions and in-depth knowledge of molecular mechanisms involved in orchestrating these reactions will open up new opportunities to establish effective and safe therapies for allergic diseases.

ACKNOWLEDGEMENTS

SLK is a senior research fellow of Council of Scientific and Industrial Research. Authors thank CSIR network project for financial support.

CONFLICTS OF INTEREST

The authors declare that there are no conflicts of interest.

REFERENCES

[1] Galli SJ, Tsai M, Piliponsky AM. The development of allergic inflammation. Nature 2008; 454(7203); 445-54.

[2] Salib RJ, Drake-Lee A, Howarth PH. Allergic rhinitis: past, present and the future. Clin.Otolaryngol.Allied Sci. 2003; 28(4); 291-303.

[3] Masoli M, Fabian D, Holt S, Beasley R. The global burden of asthma: executive summary of the GINA Dissemination Committee report. Allergy 2004; 59(5); 469-78.

[4] Hanania NA, Chapman KR, Kesten S. Adverse effects of inhaled corticosteroids. Am.J.Med. 1995; 98(2); 196-208.

[5] Barnes PJ, Adcock IM. How do corticosteroids work in asthma? Ann.Intern.Med. 2003; 139(5 Pt 1); 359-70.

[6] Barnes PJ, Pedersen S, Busse WW. Efficacy and safety of inhaled corticosteroids. New developments. Am.J.Respir.Crit Care Med. 1998; 157(3 Pt 2); S1-53.

[7] Barnes PJ, Chung KF, Page CP. Inflammatory mediators of asthma: an update. Pharmacol.Rev. 1998; 50(4); 515-96.

[8] Toogood JH, Jennings B, Greenway RW, Chuang L. Candidiasis and dysphonia complicating beclomethasone treatment of asthma. J.Allergy Clin.Immunol. 1980; 65(2); 145-53.

[9] Babu S, Samuel P. The effect of inhaled steroids on the upper respiratory tract. J.Laryngol.Otol. 1988; 102(7); 592-4.

[10] Williams AJ, Baghat MS, Stableforth DE *et al.* Dysphonia caused by inhaled steroids: recognition of a characteristic laryngeal abnormality. Thorax 1983; 38(11); 813-21.

[11] Dubus JC, Marguet C, Deschildre A *et al.* Local side-effects of inhaled corticosteroids in asthmatic children: influence of drug, dose, age, and device. Allergy 2001; 56(10); 944-8.

[12] Barnes PJ. Effect of beta-agonists on inflammatory cells. J.Allergy Clin.Immunol. 1999; 104(2 Pt 2); S10-S17

[13] Barnes PJ. Beta-adrenergic receptors and their regulation. Am.J.Respir.Crit Care Med. 1995; 152(3); 838-60.

[14] Donohue JF. Safety and efficacy of beta agonists. Respir.Care 2008; 53(5); 618-22.

[15] Bellia V, Battaglia S, Matera MG, Cazzola M. The use of bronchodilators in the treatment of airway obstruction in elderly patients. Pulm.Pharmacol.Ther. 2006; 19(5); 311-9.
[16] Lanes SF, Garrett JE, Wentworth CE, III, Fitzgerald JM, Karpel JP. The effect of adding ipratropium bromide to salbutamol in the treatment of acute asthma: a pooled analysis of three trials. Chest 1998; 114(2); 365-72.
[17] Rodrigo GJ, Castro-Rodriguez JA. Anticholinergics in the treatment of children and adults with acute asthma: a systematic review with meta-analysis. Thorax 2005; 60(9); 740-6.
[18] Watson WT, Becker AB, Simons FE. Comparison of ipratropium solution, fenoterol solution, and their combination administered by nebulizer and face mask to children with acute asthma. J.Allergy Clin.Immunol. 1988; 82(6); 1012-8.
[19] Diaz JE, Dubin R, Gaeta TJ, Pelczar P, Bradley K. Efficacy of atropine sulfate in combination with albuterol in the treatment for acute asthma. Acad.Emerg.Med. 1997; 4(2); 107-13.
[20] Tran NP, Vickery J, Blaiss MS. Management of rhinitis: allergic and non-allergic. Allergy Asthma Immunol.Res. 2011; 3(3); 148-56.
[21] Tamaoki J, Chiyotani A, Tagaya E, Sakai N, Konno K. Effect of long term treatment with oxitropium bromide on airway secretion in chronic bronchitis and diffuse panbronchiolitis. Thorax 1994; 49(6); 545-8.
[22] Holtzman MJ. Arachidonic acid metabolism. Implications of biological chemistry for lung function and disease. Am.Rev.Respir.Dis. 1991; 143(1); 188-203.
[23] Lewis RA, Austen KF, Soberman RJ. Leukotrienes and other products of the 5-lipoxygenase pathway. Biochemistry and relation to pathobiology in human diseases. N.Engl.J.Med. 1990; 323(10); 645-55.
[24] Drazen JM, Israel E, O'Byrne PM. Treatment of asthma with drugs modifying the leukotriene pathway. N.Engl.J.Med. 1999; 340(3); 197-206.
[25] O'Byrne PM, Israel E, Drazen JM. Antileukotrienes in the treatment of asthma. Ann.Intern.Med. 1997; 127(6); 472-80.
[26] Diamant Z, Sampson AP. Anti-inflammatory mechanisms of leukotriene modulators. Clin.Exp.Allergy 1999; 29(11); 1449-53.
[27] Bisgaard H, Zielen S, Garcia-Garcia ML *et al.* Montelukast reduces asthma exacerbations in 2- to 5-year-old children with intermittent asthma. Am.J.Respir.Crit Care Med. 2005; 171(4); 315-22.
[28] Johnston NW, Mandhane PJ, Dai J *et al.* Attenuation of the September epidemic of asthma exacerbations in children: a randomized, controlled trial of montelukast added to usual therapy. Pediatrics 2007; 120(3); e702-e712
[29] Johnston NW, Johnston SL, Duncan JM *et al.* The September epidemic of asthma exacerbations in children: a search for etiology. J.Allergy Clin.Immunol. 2005; 115(1); 132-8.
[30] Carlesimo M, Mari E, Palese E, Pranteda G, Camplone G. Churg-Strauss and montelukast. Int.J.Immunopathol.Pharmacol. 2011; 24(4); 1079-82.
[31] Solans R, Bosch JA, Selva A, Orriols R, Vilardell M. Montelukast and Churg-Strauss syndrome. Thorax 2002; 57(2); 183-5.
[32] Beaton G, Moree WJ. The expanding role of H1 antihistamines: a patent survey of selective and dual activity compounds 2005-2010. Expert.Opin.Ther.Pat 2010; 20(9); 1197-218.
[33] Handley DA, Magnetti A, Higgins AJ. Therapeutic advantages of third generation antihistamines. Expert.Opin.Investig.Drugs 1998; 7(7); 1045-54.

[34] Oppenheimer JJ, Casale TB. Next generation antihistamines: therapeutic rationale, accomplishments and advances. Expert.Opin.Investig.Drugs 2002; 11(6); 807-17.

[35] Turner MO, Hussack P, Sears MR, Dolovich J, Hargreave FE. Exacerbations of asthma without sputum eosinophilia. Thorax 1995; 50(10); 1057-61.

[36] Green RH, Brightling CE, McKenna S *et al.* Asthma exacerbations and sputum eosinophil counts: a randomised controlled trial. Lancet 2002; 360(9347); 1715-21.

[37] Flood-Page PT, Menzies-Gow AN, Kay AB, Robinson DS. Eosinophil's role remains uncertain as anti-interleukin-5 only partially depletes numbers in asthmatic airway. Am.J.Respir.Crit Care Med. 2003; 167(2); 199-204.

[38] Leckie MJ, ten BA, Khan J *et al.* Effects of an interleukin-5 blocking monoclonal antibody on eosinophils, airway hyper-responsiveness, and the late asthmatic response. Lancet 2000; 356(9248); 2144-8.

[39] Haldar P, Brightling CE, Hargadon B *et al.* Mepolizumab and exacerbations of refractory eosinophilic asthma. N.Engl.J.Med. 2009; 360(10); 973-84.

[40] Nair P, Pizzichini MM, Kjarsgaard M *et al.* Mepolizumab for prednisone-dependent asthma with sputum eosinophilia. N.Engl.J.Med. 2009; 360(10); 985-93.

[41] Castro M, Mathur S, Hargreave F *et al.* Reslizumab for poorly controlled, eosinophilic asthma: a randomized, placebo-controlled study. Am.J.Respir.Crit Care Med. 2011; 184(10); 1125-32.

[42] Cox L, Platts-Mills TA, Finegold I *et al.* American Academy of Allergy, Asthma & Immunology/American College of Allergy, Asthma and Immunology Joint Task Force Report on omalizumab-associated anaphylaxis. J.Allergy Clin.Immunol. 2007; 120(6); 1373-7.

[43] Lin RY, Rodriguez-Baez G, Bhargave GA. Omalizumab-associated anaphylactic reactions reported between January 2007 and June 2008. Ann.Allergy Asthma Immunol. 2009; 103(5); 442-5.

[44] Barnes PJ. The cytokine network in asthma and chronic obstructive pulmonary disease. J.Clin.Invest 2008; 118(11); 3546-56.

[45] Hansbro PM, Kaiko GE, Foster PS. Cytokine/anti-cytokine therapy - novel treatments for asthma? Br.J.Pharmacol. 2011; 163(1); 81-95.

[46] Gauvreau GM, Boulet LP, Cockcroft DW *et al.* Effects of interleukin-13 blockade on allergen-induced airway responses in mild atopic asthma. Am.J.Respir.Crit Care Med. 2011; 183(8); 1007-14.

[47] Corren J, Lemanske RF, Hanania NA *et al.* Lebrikizumab treatment in adults with asthma. N.Engl.J.Med. 2011; 365(12); 1088-98.

[48] Wenzel S, Wilbraham D, Fuller R, Getz EB, Longphre M. Effect of an interleukin-4 variant on late phase asthmatic response to allergen challenge in asthmatic patients: results of two phase 2a studies. Lancet 2007; 370(9596); 1422-31.

[49] Verhagen J, Blaser K, Akdis CA, Akdis M. Mechanisms of allergen-specific immunotherapy: T-regulatory cells and more. Immunol.Allergy Clin.North Am. 2006; 26(2); 207-31, vi.

[50] Durham SR, Till SJ. Immunologic changes associated with allergen immunotherapy. J.Allergy Clin.Immunol. 1998; 102(2); 157-64.

[51] Lerch E, Muller UR. Long-term protection after stopping venom immunotherapy: results of re-stings in 200 patients. J.Allergy Clin.Immunol. 1998; 101(5); 606-12.

[52] Bousquet J, Lockey R, Malling HJ. Allergen immunotherapy: therapeutic vaccines for allergic diseases. A WHO position paper. J.Allergy Clin.Immunol. 1998; 102(4 Pt 1); 558-62.
[53] Hansen KS, Khinchi MS, Skov PS *et al.* Food allergy to apple and specific immunotherapy with birch pollen. Mol.Nutr.Food Res. 2004; 48(6); 441-8.
[54] Sutherland MF, Suphioglu C, Rolland JM, O'Hehir RE. Latex allergy: towards immunotherapy for health care workers. Clin.Exp.Allergy 2002; 32(5); 667-73.
[55] Wilson DR, Lima MT, Durham SR. Sublingual immunotherapy for allergic rhinitis: systematic review and meta-analysis. Allergy 2005; 60(1); 4-12.
[56] Srivastava D, Singh BP, Sudha VT, Arora N, Gaur SN. Immunotherapy with mosquito (Culex quinquefasciatus) extract: a double-blind, placebo-controlled study. Ann.Allergy Asthma Immunol. 2007; 99(3); 273-80.
[57] Srivastava D, Singh BP, Arora N, Gaur SN. Clinico-immunologic study on immunotherapy with mixed and single insect allergens. J.Clin.Immunol. 2009; 29(5); 665-73.
[58] Osterballe O. Side effects during immunotherapy with purified grass pollen extracts. Allergy 1982; 37(8); 553-62.
[59] Dhyani A, Singh BP, Arora N, Jain VK, Sridhara S. A clinically relevant major cross-reactive allergen from mesquite tree pollen. Eur.J.Clin.Invest 2008; 38(10); 774-81.
[60] Kukreja N, Sridhara S, Singh BP, Gaur SN, Arora N. Purification and immunological characterization of a 12-kDa allergen from Epicoccum purpurascens. FEMS Immunol.Med.Microbiol. 2009; 56(1); 32-40.
[61] Sudha VT, Arora N, Gaur SN, Pasha S, Singh BP. Identification of a serine protease as a major allergen (Per a 10) of Periplaneta americana. Allergy 2008; 63(6); 768-76.
[62] Sharma V, Singh BP, Gaur SN, Arora N. Molecular and immunological characterization of cytochrome c: a potential cross-reactive allergen in fungi and grasses. Allergy 2008; 63(2); 189-97.
[63] Shankar J, Singh BP, Gaur SN, Arora N. Recombinant glutathione-S-transferase a major allergen from Alternaria alternata for clinical use in allergy patients. Mol.Immunol. 2006; 43(12); 1927-32.
[64] Sharma V, Gupta R, Jhingran A *et al.* Cloning, recombinant expression and activity studies of a major allergen "enolase" from the fungus Curvularia lunata. J.Clin.Immunol. 2006; 26(4); 360-9.
[65] Srivastava D, Mehta AK, Arora N, Gaur SN, Singh BP. Proteolytically inactive per a 10 allergen of Periplaneta americana modulates Th2 response and enhances IL-10 in mouse model. J.Clin.Immunol. 2010; 30(3); 426-34.
[66] Bisht V, Arora N, Singh BP *et al.* Epi p 1, an allergenic glycoprotein of Epicoccum purpurascens is a serine protease. FEMS Immunol.Med.Microbiol. 2004; 42(2); 205-11.
[67] Gupta R, Sharma V, Sridhara S, Singh BP, Arora N. Identification of serine protease as a major allergen of Curvularia lunata. Allergy 2004; 59(4); 421-7.
[68] Tripathi P, Nair S, Singh BP, Arora N. Molecular and immunological characterization of subtilisin like serine protease, a major allergen of Curvularia lunata. Immunobiology 2011; 216(3); 402-8.
[69] Sudha VT, Arora N, Singh BP. Serine protease activity of Per a 10 augments allergen-induced airway inflammation in a mouse model. Eur.J.Clin.Invest 2009; 39(6); 507-16.
[70] Kukreja N, Sridhara S, Singh BP, Arora N. Effect of proteolytic activity of Epicoccum purpurascens major allergen, Epi p 1 in allergic inflammation. Clin.Exp.Immunol. 2008; 154(2); 162-71.

[71] Tripathi P, Kukreja N, Singh BP, Arora N. Serine protease activity of Cur l 1 from Curvularia lunata augments Th2 response in mice. J.Clin.Immunol. 2009; 29(3); 292-302.

[72] Goel C, Govindaraj D, Singh BP *et al.* Serine protease Per a 10 from Periplaneta americana bias dendritic cells towards type 2 by upregulating CD86 and low IL-12 secretions. Clin.Exp.Allergy 2012; 42(3); 412-22.

[73] Chen CL, Wang SD, Zeng ZY *et al.* Serine protease inhibitors nafamostat mesilate and gabexate mesilate attenuate allergen-induced airway inflammation and eosinophilia in a murine model of asthma. J.Allergy Clin.Immunol. 2006; 118(1); 105-12.

[74] Saw S, Kale SL, Arora N. Serine protease inhibitor attenuates ovalbumin induced inflammation in mouse model of allergic airway disease. PLoS.One. 2012; 7(7); e41107

[75] Marino R, Thuraisingam T, Camateros P *et al.* Secretory leukocyte protease inhibitor plays an important role in the regulation of allergic asthma in mice. J.Immunol. 2011; 186(7); 4433-42.

[76] Cho YS, Lee J, Lee TH *et al.* alpha-Lipoic acid inhibits airway inflammation and hyperresponsiveness in a mouse model of asthma. J.Allergy Clin.Immunol. 2004; 114(2); 429-35.

[77] Silva BF, Valenca SS, Lanzetti M *et al.* Alpha-tocopherol and ascorbic acid supplementation reduced acute lung inflammatory response by cigarette smoke in mouse. Nutrition 2006; 22(11-12); 1192-201.

[78] Tripathi P, Singh BP, Arora N. Mutated glutathione-S-transferase reduced airway inflammation by limiting oxidative stress and Th2 response. Free Radic.Biol.Med. 2008; 45(10); 1413-9.

[79] Tripathi P, Nair S, Singh BP, Arora N. Mutated glutathione S-transferase in combination with reduced glutathione shows a synergistic effect in ameliorating oxidative stress and airway inflammation. Free Radic.Biol.Med. 2010; 48(6); 839-44.

[80] Mehta AK, Arora N, Gaur SN, Singh BP. Acute toxicity assessment of choline by inhalation, intraperitoneal and oral routes in Balb/c mice. Regul.Toxicol.Pharmacol. 2009; 54(3); 282-6.

[81] Mehta AK, Gaur SN, Arora N, Singh BP. Effect of choline chloride in allergen-induced mouse model of airway inflammation. Eur.Respir.J. 2007; 30(4); 662-71.

[82] Mehta AK, Arora N, Gaur SN, Singh BP. Choline supplementation reduces oxidative stress in mouse model of allergic airway disease. Eur.J.Clin.Invest 2009; 39(10); 934-41.

[83] Sharma V, Singh BP, Gaur SN, Pasha S, Arora N. Bioinformatics and immunologic investigation on B and T cell epitopes of Cur l 3, a major allergen of Curvularia lunata. J.Proteome.Res. 2009; 8(6); 2650-5.

[84] Sharma V, Singh BP, Arora N. Cur l 3, a major allergen of Curvularia lunata-derived short synthetic peptides, shows promise for successful immunotherapy. Am.J.Respir.Cell Mol.Biol. 2011; 45(6); 1178-84.

[85] Fellrath JM, Kettner A, Dufour N *et al.* Allergen-specific T-cell tolerance induction with allergen-derived long synthetic peptides: results of a phase I trial. J.Allergy Clin.Immunol. 2003; 111(4); 854-61.

[86] Shankar J, Singh BP, Gaur SN, Arora N. Engineered Alt a 13 fragment of Alternaria alternata abrogated IgE binding without affecting T-cell stimulation. J.Clin.Immunol. 2009; 29(1); 63-70.

[87] Nair S, Kukreja N, Singh BP, Arora N. Identification of B cell epitopes of alcohol dehydrogenase allergen of Curvularia lunata. PLoS.One. 2011; 6(5); e20020

[88] Harrison TW. Systemic availability of inhaled budesonide and fluticasone propionate: healthy *vs.* asthmatic lungs. BioDrugs. 2001; 15(6); 405-11.

[89] Donnelly R, Williams KM, Baker AB *et al.* Effects of budesonide and fluticasone on 24-hour plasma cortisol. A dose-response study. Am.J.Respir.Crit Care Med. 1997; 156(6); 1746-51.

[90] Capewell S, Reynolds S, Shuttleworth D, Edwards C, Finlay AY. Purpura and dermal thinning associated with high dose inhaled corticosteroids. BMJ 1990; 300(6739); 1548-51.

[91] Mak VH, Melchor R, Spiro SG. Easy bruising as a side-effect of inhaled corticosteroids. Eur.Respir.J. 1992; 5(9); 1068-74.

[92] Allen HD, Thong IG, Clifton-Bligh P *et al.* Effects of high-dose inhaled corticosteroids on bone metabolism in prepubertal children with asthma. Pediatr.Pulmonol. 2000; 29(3); 188-93.

[93] Jaeschke R, O'Byrne PM, Mejza F *et al.* The safety of long-acting beta-agonists among patients with asthma using inhaled corticosteroids: systematic review and metaanalysis. Am.J.Respir.Crit Care Med. 2008; 178(10); 1009-16.

[94] Michael AB, Murphy D. Montelukast-associated Churg-Strauss syndrome. Age Ageing 2003; 32(5); 551-2.

[95] Kinoshita M, Shiraishi T, Koga T *et al.* Churg-Strauss syndrome after corticosteroid withdrawal in an asthmatic patient treated with pranlukast. J.Allergy Clin.Immunol. 1999; 103(3 Pt 1); 534-5.

[96] Green RL, Vayonis AG. Churg-Strauss syndrome after zafirlukast in two patients not receiving systemic steroid treatment. Lancet 1999; 353(9154); 725-6.

[97] Kay GG. The effects of antihistamines on cognition and performance. J.Allergy Clin.Immunol. 2000; 105(6 Pt 2); S622-S627

[98] Williams AP, Krishna MT, Frew AJ. The safety of immunotherapy. Clin.Exp.Allergy 2004; 34(4); 513-4.

[99] Abramson MJ, Puy RM, Weiner JM. Injection allergen immunotherapy for asthma. Cochrane.Database.Syst.Rev. 2010;(8); CD001186.

Send Orders for Reprints on reprints@benthamscience.net

CHAPTER 6

Main Food Allergic Therapies (Promising Ongoing Projects)

Marina Pérez-Gordo*, Carlos Pastor-Vargas and Bárbara Cases

Institute of Applied Molecular Medicine (IMMA) and San Pablo CEU University School of Medicine of Madrid, Jiménez Díaz Foundation (IIS-FJD) of Madrid, Research and Development Department of Inmunotek S.L, Madrid, Spain

Abstract: Food allergies have been increasing in prevalence over the last 10 years. Currently, about 2-8% of the population of Western countries suffers from some type of food allergy whose impact ranges from a mere inconvenience to a life threatening condition. While allergy immunotherapy has been successfully used to treat other allergies such as hay fever, it is nearly recent that it has begun to be used in the treatment of food allergy. Nowadays, avoidance therapy is the best measure for the prevention of any food allergic reaction, although can be difficult in cases of common foods such as milk, egg, soy, wheat and peanut. There are a number of promising emerging therapeutic modalities for food allergy, including allergen-specific and allergen non-specific immunotherapeutic approaches, that we would like to review in this chapter. Among allergen-specific immunotherapy we should distinguish oral immunotherapy (OIT), where gradually increasing amounts of allergens are directly swallowed; from sublingual immunotherapy (SLIT), where allergen dose is before placed under the tongue. In both cases, a desensitization process to specific foods is expected. Considering that the characterization of epitopes on food allergens is becoming the target for the development of novel diagnostic tools and for specific therapy, it is important to highlight the use of recombinant food proteins or peptides. With these proteins antigen-specific T cells stimulation is preserved without triggering mast cell activation. Allergen non-specific immunotherapy approaches are being developed for individuals with multiple food allergies. In this sense, the use of anti-IgE, for instance, could decrease the amount of IgE available to bind an allergen. The idea would be to obtain a suppressive effect on all or some part of Th2-mediated immunity. It has been also proven that the use of traditional Chinese herbs in rodent models of peanut allergy is translated in lower peanut-specific IgE and higher peanut-specific IgG2a. This and other alternative strategies addressed in the text are currently being tested in clinical trials. The aim of this chapter is to provide an overview of the ongoing projects in order to develop safe and effective treatments for food allergy.

Keywords: Food allergy, allergens, immunotherapy, ongoing projects, IgE-mediated reactions, cross reactivity, Th1/Th2 balance, hypoallergens, anti-IgE.

***Address correspondence to Marina Pérez-Gordo:** Department of Medicine of CEU San Pablo University and Institute of Applied Molecular Medicine (IMMA) of CEU San Pablo University, Madrid, Spain. Tel: +343724700 (ext. 4675); Fax: +3724000; Email: marina.perezgordo@ceu.es

Atta-ur-Rahman (Ed)

ALLERGY

Allergy is one of the immune tolerance-related diseases that arise as a direct consequence of a deregulated immune response. The allergic reaction or hypersensitivity reaction may be defined as an over reactive immune response to an antigen, often innocuous, known as allergen.

The concept of allergy was originally introduced in medical literature in 1906 by Clemens Von Pirquet, meaning "variation in reactivity". Restrictions on the type of immune response in patients were not established at the time. It was later in 1921 when Praunistz and Küstner, two Austrians doctors, published the results of the local passive transfer, injecting Küstner serum, which was allergic to fish, into Prausnitz skin, which was not allergic to it. A positive reaction was obtained 15 minutes after the fish extract was introduced *via* a local intradermal injection. This experiment laid the foundations for food-induced anaphylaxis, and more specifically for fish-induced anaphylaxis. But it was not until 1967 that the serum substance responsible for the reaction, named "reagine", was simultaneously identified as IgE antibody by Bennich and Johansson in Sweden [1] and by the married couple Ishizaka in the USA [2]. Therefore, it was proved that at least three components were involved in this immune affliction: An antigen as a trigger for the affliction (allergen), a serum factor which differentiates between healthy and allergic individuals (IgE) and a cellular component present in every individual (immune cells).

The predisposition toward the development of allergic reactions is called atopy and it reflects an increase in the synthesis of IgE specific antibodies against the allergen, which might cause clinical symptoms such as rhinitis, asthma, colic or diarrhea. Although allergic diseases usually begin in childhood, they may occur at any age; however, the predisposition for immune deviation and atopy appear to be clearly determined in early life [3]. As we know it today, allergy induction and maintenance is developed throughout two different stages which will vary according to the contact with the allergen; a first stage of sensitization and memory and a second stage of provocation, in which, due to a new exposure to the allergen, mast cells and basophiles are activated. There are two phases of an allergic reaction, an early phase (when preformed chemical mediators are released) and a late phase. If symptoms appears a few minutes after the exposure to the allergen, then we are talking about an immediate reaction, on the contrary, if this exposure is extensive and prolonged then we are talking about delayed reaction (see "Immunological basis" section).

Numerous studies have shown that atopic allergy is a multifactorial polygenic disease as it is determined by intrinsic factors, including genetic susceptibility, age and gender. Current studies on the genetics of food allergy have linked more than 10 genes to the genetic susceptibility of this allergy [3]. Regarding the age, the most affected range is between 5 and 40 years old, with a much higher incidence among 15-30 year old age range. In regard to gender, the impact on males is higher during childhood, while in a later stage women will be increasingly equally subject to it as males.

Extrinsic and environmental factors also play a very important role in allergies. Those factors are usually connected with lifestyle changes. Therefore, it has been postulated that environments which are extremely clean as well as the indiscriminate use of antibiotics might result in an immune system's altered evolution and in an absence of microorganisms that stimulate the Th1 response, leading to an overactive Th2 response, which in turn led to allergic disease. This theory, known as "hygiene hypothesis", was first proposed by Strachan 20 years ago, who studied the epidemiology of hay fever in a sample of 17,000 British children [4], and nowadays has been extended from the field of allergy to that of autoimmune diseases such as type 1 diabetes (T1D) or multiple sclerosis (MS) [5, 6].

There are other factors involved in the allergic process development such as alterations of the target organs, caused by extrinsic or intrinsic determining factors (Fig. **1**); viral infections which would operate as triggers and pollutant agents which would operate as adjuvants as they are able to concentrate allergen molecules on the surface, thus favoring its transport to the inside of the body [7].

The main nongenetic risk factors associated in the development of food allergy will be detailed further in the text ("Food Allergy" section).

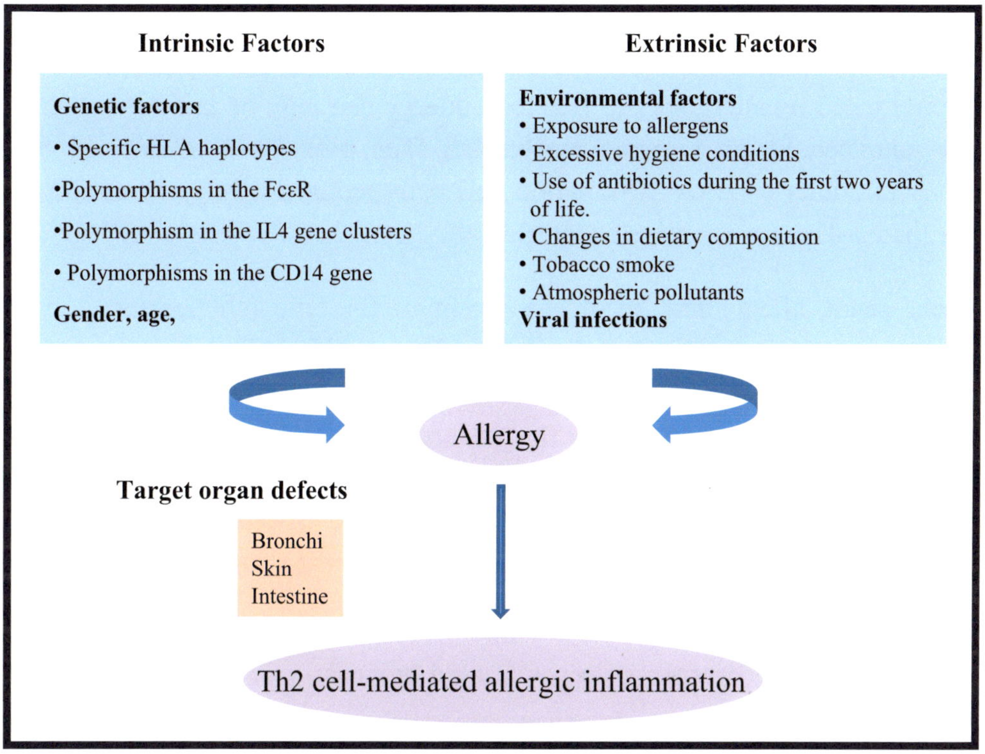

Figure 1: Mainly factors implicated in the development of atopy and Th2 cell-mediated allergic inflammation.

ADVERSE REACTIONS TO FOOD: CONCEPT AND CLASSIFICATION

The complexity of adverse reactions to food has led to a great confusion as to the terminology used to describe allergic and no-allergic reactions. Adverse reaction to food is a generic term which indicates a cause-effect relationship between feed intake and an abnormal response. In the case of a reproducible reaction, it may be caused by toxic or pharmacological phenomena, metabolism disorders or a specific immune response.

Allergy to food is a term used to describe an adverse reaction conditioned by an immune response, IgE or cell mediated type, to food antigens. A difference can be made between food allergy and food sensitization. In the latter case there is a demonstrable IgE response to food, but it does not necessarily correspond to the allergy clinical symptoms.

Adverse reactions to food are very common. A study conducted in Spain, for example, founded that this kind of reactions holds the fifth position among disorders treated by allergists [8]. But food allergy can only be understood as the allergy mediated by an immune mechanism. The prevalence of adverse food reactions in adults exceeds 30%, while IgE cell-mediated allergy is usually no greater than 3-4% in westernized countries [9].

In recent years, allergy has become a synonym for type I hypersensitivity or immediate hypersensitivity (IgE-mediated allergy). Hypersensitivity reactions make up a very heterogeneous group of immune disorders. In 1963, Gell and Coombs [10], in order to facilitate the understanding of the different types of immune reactions caused by diverse antigens, classified hypersensitivity reactions into 4 types (I, II, III, IV). In each one of the reactions, different kind of cells and soluble mediators may be involved sequentially (Table **1**) and this classification still remains current.

Table 1: The four types of hypersensitivity reactions and the immunologic mechanism implicated

Type	**Immunologic Mechanism**
Type I: Immediate hypersensitivity	IgE antibodies
Type II: Antibody-mediated	IgG o IgM mediated autoimmune
Type III: Immune complex-mediated	Antigens *vs.* IgE / IgM
Type IV: T-cell mediated	1. CD4+ cells (retarded hypersensitivity)
	2. CD8+ cells (cytolysis by T cells)

In 1984 the American Academy of Allergy and Immunology Committee on Adverse Reactions to Foods (AAAI) and National Institute of Allergy and Infectious Diseases, published the "NIH manual of Adverse Reactions to Foods" [11]. Terms such as food allergy and intolerance reactions were clearly distinguished in this manual (Fig. **2**).

Ten years later, in 1995, the European Academy of Allergy and Clinical Immunology Subcommittee on Adverse Reactions to Food (EAACI) submitted a Position Paper [12] suggesting a new classification of adverse reactions to food. This classification remained in force until 2001, when definitions of allergic

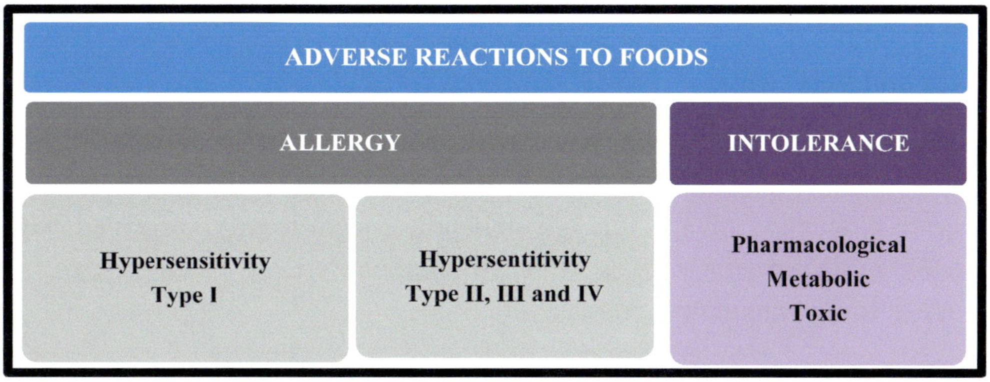

Figure 2: Classification of adverse reactions to foods.

reactions were reviewed by the EAACI Nomenclature Commission creating a Nomenclature Position Statement [13] and later on by the revision made by the World Allergy Organization (WAO) [14] to present a globally acceptable nomenclature for allergic diseases (Fig. **3**). According to these recommendations, any adverse reaction to food would fall within the definition of "food hypersensitivity". Whenever it can be proved that an immune mechanism is involved in the reaction, it may meet the definition of "food allergy". Should this immune mechanism be an IgE-dependent mechanism, the term "IgE-mediated food allergy" would be used. The rest of reactions which previously used to fall within the definition of "food intolerance" must now be named "non-allergic food hypersensitivity"

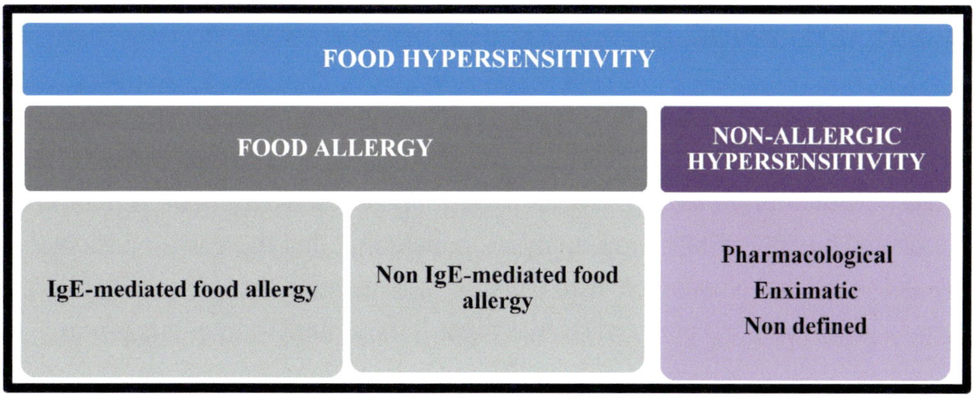

Figure 3: Classification of food hypersensitivity reactions (2001 EAACI Nomenclature Commission and 2003 WAO Revision).

FOOD ALLERGY

Concept and Prevalence

Food allergy, IgE mediated allergy or type I immediate hypersensitivity (Fig. **4**), is a medical anomaly, confirmed through *in vivo* or *in vitro* test, characterized by the higher production of specific IgE antibodies, significantly correlated with symptoms in the patient and/or with provocation test. It is considered an antigenic-specific immunologic disease.

The overall allergy incidence has increased substantially in recent years, affecting up to 30% of the population in developed countries [15]. It is estimated today that 5-6% of child population and 3 to 4% of the adult population is affected by it in industrialized countries [9, 16].

The prevalence of food allergy has also increased in the last several decades throughout the world. It is variable from one geographic area to another in terms of percentage and in the type of allergenic food source. Moreover, studies of allergy to a specific food have shown different clinical and immunologic patterns in different areas of the world [17].

Determining the prevalence of food allergy remains difficult. Rates varied widely between studies [18]. Prevalence rates determine on the basis of patient self-reporting are usually higher than those based on clinical history and testing. That is what Rona *et al.* [19] reported when studying prevalence of food allergy to cow's milk, hen's eggs, peanut, fish and shellfish. Similar variations were seen by Zuidmeer *et al.* [20], when reviewing the prevalence of food allergy to plants since 1990, including fruits, vegetables, legumes, tree nuts, wheat, cereals, soy and seeds. Prevalence estimates were categorized by food item and method used (food challenges, skin prick test, serum IgE, parent/self-reported symptoms), complemented by appropriate meta-analyses, concluding that there was considerable heterogeneity in the prevalence estimates of sensitization or perceived allergic reactions to plant food and between studies regardless of food item or age group.

In the clinical study Alergológica [8] conducted in Spain in 2005, fruits (30%) and tree nuts (25%) were pointed as the most common cause of allergy. They were followed by legumes (5%), cereals (5%), greens (3%) and vegetables (1%). Data from Vegetalia study [21] showed that peach is the first cause of allergy to plant foods, followed by melon and kiwi and, less frequently, by tree nuts, apple, other nuts and peanuts. This data stand in contrast with what happens in north and center of Europe, where apple is the most common cause of allergy to plant foods; and with data from Anglo-Saxon countries (USA, United Kingdom) where peanut allergy is the most prevalent.

It is thought that environmental reasons (pollen exposure, food habits) and genetic factors might conditioned the fact that geographical differences affect no just the frequency of occurrence but also the form in which allergy to certain kind of food is expressed. Therefore, allergy to apple or peach is relatively a common cause of severe allergic reactions in the south of Europe, while it causes mild symptoms in countries from the north and the center of the continent. Peanut is another clear example, in Anglo-Saxon countries it primarily affects in early childhood with severe symptoms, while in Spain the systemic reactions percentage is lower, affecting later in life and with even milder symptoms than in Nordic countries.

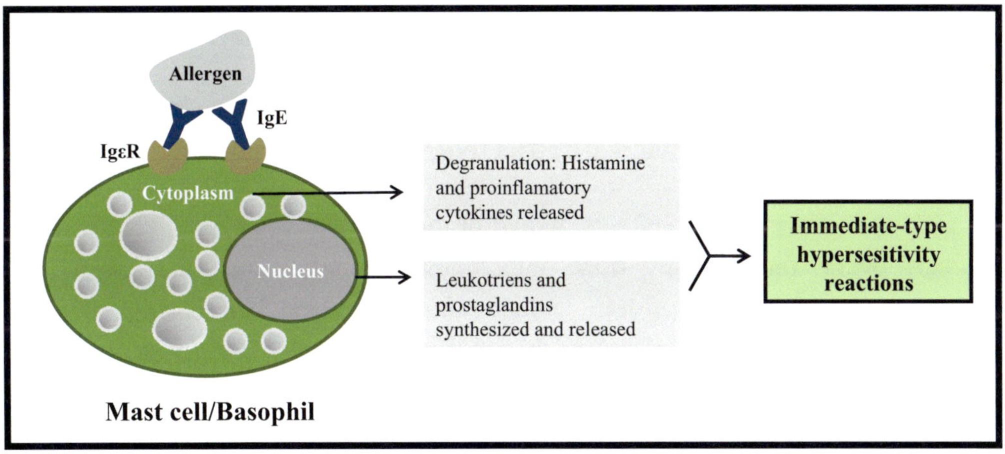

Figure 4: Representation of "IgE mediated allergy" or type 1 immediate hypersensitivity. This Hypersensitivity type is mediated by factors released by mast cells and basophils as a response to intracellular signals generated by the IgεR on the surface of such cells. These signals result when multiple IgE molecules, associated with the IgεR molecules, bind with high affinity to a protein allergen. Thus, immediate-type hypersensitivity is dependent upon the presence of multiple IgE binding sites (two sites shown here for example) on the surface of a protein allergen. *Adapted from: Huby RD, Dearman RJ and Kimber I. Why are some proteins allergens? Toxicological Sciences 55, 235-246 (2000)* [22].

Food is the greatest antigen challenge to the human immune system. The physiological response is the development of immunological tolerance. It has not been established yet which mechanisms lead to an IgE-mediated response to a food antigen, rather than tolerance response. It is known that individual's genetic susceptibility in the development of IgE-mediated responses (atopy) and exposure to food are two major factors. Food which frequently induces allergic reactions will therefore be conditioned by age, diet and existing conditions in different geographical areas.

Although food allergy has been well known for a long time, there was a great deal of controversy regarding its real frequency, its symptomatology and its best possible methods of diagnosis and treatment.

Before getting into the description of ongoing treatment therapies for food allergy, we will briefly describe the possible risk factors or theories that might partially explain the development of food allergy, some of them have been already mentioned above, and then we will focus on the immunological basis of food allergy and important concepts as cross-reactivity and cross-reactivity syndromes in order to better understand the diagnosis, treated later in the chapter.

Based on the reviewed of Lack G [23], the possible nongenetic risk factors for the development of FA could be summarized as follows:

1) *Allergen-exposure hypothesis*, which points out that food sensitization can occur through low-dose cutaneous exposure and that early consumption of food protein, induces oral tolerance. This is a recent shift in the conventional belief that early exposure to allergenic food proteins during pregnancy or lactation could lead to food allergy. The timing of food introduction seems to play an important role in the development of atopy and/or tolerance induction. It has been shown that in societies where peanuts are avoided in pregnancy and infancy, the prevalence of peanut allergy is higher [24]. In animal models it has been shown that an early high dose of oral protein antigen induces oral tolerance to the respective antigen. Based on this hypothesis, there is an interesting randomized controlled trial currently being performed

(LEAP study, Learning Early About Peanut Allergies), in which half the infants tested in their first 6 months of life are avoiding peanut and the other half are consuming it [25], that will surely give light to these questions. Moreover, a study from 2006 showed that delaying initial exposure to cereal grain after 6 months of life was associated with an increased risk of IgE-mediated food allergy [26]. However, this statement needs to be confirmed in different foods allergens.

2) *Vitamin D hypothesis*, with its two opposite forms: The vitamin D excess hypothesis, postulated by Wjst [27] which suggests that vitamin D is a risk factor for allergy based on its effects on the Th1/Th2 shift to Th2 dominance; and the vitamin D deficiency (VDD) hypothesis, postulated by Devereux *et al.* [28] which argues the opposite, based on the protective role that vitamin D plays in the maintenance of the mucosal barrier integrity.

The following theories or nongenetic risk factors would contribute to explain the development of allergy in general but there is still a lack of information to relate them directly with the development or induction of food allergy:

3) *Hygiene hypothesis*, and its revised version postulated by Noverr MC [4, 29] which suggest that early exposures to microbial pathogens could protect against subsequent atopic diseases. This hypothesis has been extensively studied in the development of eczema, which is frequently a manifestation of food allergy, but very little has been studied related directly to food allergy.

4) *Dietary fat hypothesis*, which suggests that the higher consumption of vegetable oils and the reduction on animal fats lead to the increase of allergies. This consumption tendency is translated into higher intakes of ω-6 and lower intakes of ω-3 fatty acids and therefore an increased production of prostaglandin E2 (PGE2), which can inhibit the production of Th1 cytokines (IFN-γ) by T lymhocytes, and promotes synthesis of Th2 cytokines. In this case, this has also been confirmed in the development of asthma rhinitis and eczema but there is a lack of information to support this theory with respect to food allergy.

5) *Antioxidant hypothesis*, which stresses the anti-inflammatory effects of antioxidants in allergic diseases such as asthma and hay fever but no such studies exist regarding food allergy.

Immunological Basis

The induction of allergic diseases requires sensitization of a predisposed individual to a specific antigen. IgE- mediated hypersensitivity reactions to foods may occur after exposure to an allergen *via* different routes such as nose, lungs, eyes, skin and intestine. Food allergens pass through the intestinal epithelium in its native form or partially digested and interact with the immune system cells [30]. Interaction with allergens results in processing of the allergen by antigen presenting cells (APC), including macrophages and dendritic cells (DC). These cells process the allergen protein into peptides and present the epitope bearing peptides *via* major histocompatibility complex (MHC) to particular T cell subsets. CD4+ Naive T cells responses differentiate into different T cell subsets depending on the cytokines, other molecules and cells present in the microenvironment, with IL-4 directing a T-helper-2-type response and interferon IFNγ a Th1 profile. Allergic diseases represent complex innate and adaptive immune responses to environmental antigens leading to inflammatory reactions with a Th-2 cell and allergen-specific IgE predominance [31, 32]. Subsequently, antigen presentation will lead to a rapid activation of Th-2 cells and the recruitment and activation of effector cells such as eosinophils and basophils (Fig. **5**).

Once a Th2 shift is established, the mechanism of allergic diseases consist of two main phases [33]. In the early phase, Th2 response is associated with activation of specific B cells that transform into plasma cells. The differentiation and clonal expansion of allergen-specific CD4+ Th2 cells, producing cytokines such as IL-4, IL-5, IL-9 and IL-13 [34], which, are essential in the induction of class switching to the ε immunoglobulin heavy chain in B cells and the production of allergen-specific IgE antibodies. In addition, novel cytokines with proinflammatory functions, such as IL- 25, IL-31 and IL-33, have recently been associated with Th2 response [35], inducing allergen-specific IgE, eosinophilia, mucus production and the recruitment of inflammatory cells to inflamed tissues.

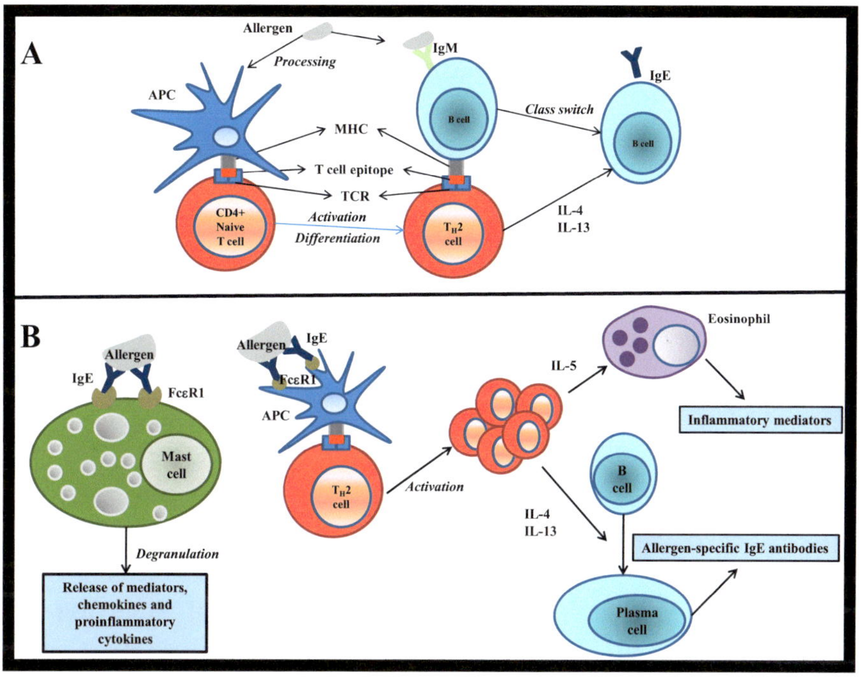

Figure 5: Immunological mechanisms of allergen-specific response. A: Sensibilitazion. B: Type I hypersensitivity reactions

Plasma cells produce and release into the serum an allergen-specific IgE capable of binding to the high affinity receptor FcεRI, on the surface of mast cells and basophils as well as to antigen presenting cells (APCs) allowing for an increased uptake of allergens and the release of mediators from these cells, which subsequently, generate symptoms of the allergic response [36]. The late phase is characterized by inflammation and tissue injury caused by effector cell action.

After re-exposure allergen-IgE immune complexes produce receptor crosslinking, which in turn results in the activation and release of mediators that cause the development of type I hypersensitivity reactions [37].

Food allergies may be IgE mediated, characterized by immediate symptoms and possible anaphylaxis, cell-mediated, with more delayed symptoms, or a combination of both. Although these different forms of food allergy have different clinical presentations, the pathophysiology of all of them is the same, with food antigen sensitization and Th2 shift of the immune system.

Food allergens pass through gastrointestinal tract and contact with the immune system through multiple mechanisms (Fig. **6**):

- Food antigen transport by intestinal epithelial cell junctions (Fig. **6A**).
- Invagination or endocytosis process (Fig. **6B**).
- Absorption mediated by specialized cells called M cells, strategically located on the Peyer's plates that allow the release of antigen directly into lymphatic cells (Fig. **6C**).
- Dendritic cells in lumen epithelium take food antigens (Fig. **6D**).

The ability to keep the integrity of allergenic determinants through the gastrointestinal tract is an important condition required for food proteins to produce an allergic reaction. Resistance to gastrointestinal digestion of food allergens is considered one dominant feature that reflects a food allergen's capacity to stimulate a specific immune response [38].

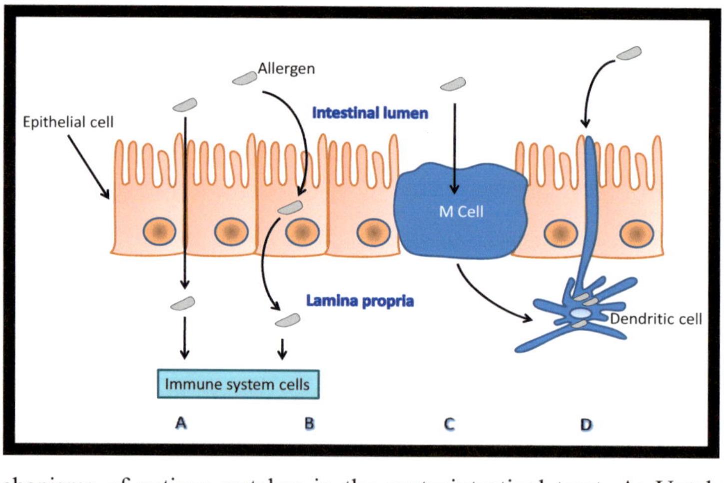

Figure 6: Mechanisms of antigen uptakes in the gastrointestinal tract. A: Uptake by intestinal epithelial cell junctions; B: Invagination or endocytosis process; C: Absorption mediated by M cells; D: Uptake by dendritic cells.

To date, most of the studies dealing with the influence of the gastro duodenal digestion on the potential allergenicity of foods have been carried out on isolated proteins [39]. In this sense, low gastric acid pH is crucial for activation and liberation of gastric and pancreatic proteases. These enzymes degrade proteins to small peptides, which can be ignored by the immune system or lead to tolerance. This implicates that the functional acidic stomach has a protective function against many digestion-labile proteins, which otherwise could present antigens or even allergens. Gastric pepsin activation and pancreatic enzymes released is determined by gastric acid levels. It is worth noting that when an antiulcer drug is used, the gastric acid is neutralized, therefore food allergens remain intact and allergic reactions may occur *via* the oral route [40].

T-REGULATORY CELLS

The central role of Th1/Th2 balance in the regulation of immune responses has been widely studied. However, during the past few years there has been significant progress in understanding the mechanisms by which abnormal T cell responses are generated in allergic diseases. These mechanisms were explained by the activity of a heterogeneous group of regulatory T cells (T-regs). Regulatory T cells play crucial roles in the induction of tolerance to antigens. Subsets of Treg cells with distinct phenotypes and mechanisms of action include the naturally occurring, thymus-selected CD4+CD25+FOXP3+ Treg cells and and the inducible Treg cells, which are generated in the periphery under various tolerogenic conditions. Among them, T-regulatory type 1 (Tr1) cells have been shown to play a major role in allergen tolerance [41]. In addition, subsets of CD8+T cells, $\gamma\delta$ T cells, dendritic cells, IL-10-producing B cells, natural killer (NK) cells and resident tissue cells, could contribute to suppressive and regulatory events [42, 43].

Induction of peripheral tolerance through the generation of Treg cells is the key event, with several functional modulations in the allergic immune response.

Treg cells contribute to the control of allergen-specific immune responses in 5 major ways [44]:

- Suppression of antigen-presenting cells that support the generation of effector Th2 and Th1 cells.

- Suppression of Th2 and Th1 cells.

- Regulatory function on B cells by suppression of allergen-specific IgE and induction of IgG4, IgA, or both.

- Suppression of mast cells, basophiles, and eosinophils.

- Interaction with resident tissue cells and remodeling.

Tr1 cells have been shown to play a major role in allergen tolerance and can be induced by allergen specific immunotherapy in humans. CD4+CD25+Foxp3+ Treg cells can directly suppress B cell Ig response and Ig class switch recombination [45]. In contrast, Tr1 cells also cross-talk to B cells through secreting IL-10 and TGF-β, which leads to regulation of antibody production. IL-10 has been described as essential in peripheral tolerance to allergens: inhibits IgE synthesis, reduces proinflammatory cytokine release in mast cells, induces IL-10 production in dendritic cells and stimulates the production of IgG4 and IgA [46].

TGF-β also contributes to peripheral tolerance to allergens synergistically with IL-10: reduces IgE synthesis, deletes functionality Th-1 cells, Th-2 and Th-17, participates in the differentiation of Th-2 cells in Th-9 and Th-17 and induces synthesis of IgA [47]. The discovery of Th9 cells and Th17 is relatively recent, being both involved in inflammatory processes [48, 49].

With regard to food allergy, it is interesting the function attributed to IL-10 and TGF-β in the production of IgA. IgA is an important regulatory factor in the mucosal immune system and it is secreted by plasma cells and reacts with antigens upon exposure of mucosal surfaces in the intestine to pathogens and food antigens [50].

IgA levels have been related to development of an allergic response. In fact, in animal models of food allergy, low IgA concentrations in the intestine have been associated with the development of allergy, suggesting the essential role of this immunoglobulin in peripheral tolerance. Peyer's patches consist of germinal centers comprised of B lymphocytes. Peyer's patches are directly involved in the synthesis of IgA, stimulated by the presence of IL-10 and TGF-β. Therefore, the loss of activity by Treg could lead to an increase in Th-2 allergic response, since both, healthy and allergic individuals, exhibit all 3 allergen specific subsets in different proportions, indicating that a change in dominant subset might lead to allergy development or recovery [44].

Cross Reactivity

Cross-reactivity (CR) occurs when an adaptive immune response to a particular antigen causes reactivity to other antigens that are structurally related to the inducer [51]. This phenomenon has consequences for the diagnosis and treatment of certain food allergies. It occurs with a primary sensitization to an allergen which induces antigen-specific IgE synthesis. These IgE antibodies may, subsequently, recognize antigens in similar proteins from another source. Such proteins share similar structure and common epitopes (fragments of 5-7 amino acids). Nevertheless, it is possible to react to an allergen showing clinical features of immediate hypersensitivity without there being previous exposure to such allergen. This occurs due to a pre-existing sensitization to a highly homologous allergen, although this is not always the case. Sometimes *in vivo* or *in vitro* recognition of cross-reacting allergens does not imply clinical symptoms. Due to cross-reactivity, a patient may be sensitized to two or more allergic sources and still may not show symptoms of any of them. Thus, CR should be regarded as an immunological event and not as a clinical one.

In order for cross-reactivity between two allergens to occur, both proteins should share partial homology, or even most, a single epitope should be recognized. Proteins with well-preserved molecular structure tend to present a phylogenetic sequence almost unaltered, therefore sequential and conformational epitopes are more likely to be shared. Cross-reactivity occurs when there is more than 35% of sequence similarity over a segment of 80 amino acids or complete identity with a peptide of 6-8 amino acids from an allergen (WHO. Codex ad Hoc Intergovernmental Task Force on Foods Derived from Biotechnology. Joint FAO/WHO Food Standards Program. Yokohama: World Health Organisation. 2003. http: //www.codexalimentarius.net/). However, CR has also been described between allergens sharing only 35% identity [52]. Even so, it is worth noting that CR between IgE and effector cells (mast cells and/or basophils) is unlikely to happen if sequential similarity is less than 70% [53].

Cross-reactive proteins which, being ubiquitous in nature, are present in taxonomically unrelated allergenic sources fall within the definition of panallergens.

Numerous associations both between sensitization to different foods and between foods and neumoallergens have been described, among which pollen-food reaction stands out. Many of these reactions are due to profilins and defense proteins (PRP, pathogenesis related proteins), including homologous proteins to birch pollen allergen, Bet v1 (PR-10) [54]. Less than 25% of patients with this syndrome are sensitized to Bet v 2 (birch profilin), although its contribution to symptoms remains not very well defined.

Tropomyosin is a panallergen present in food of animal origin. It is considered to be responsible for cross-reactivity between different shrimp spices, other crustaceans, insects, arachnids and parasites [55]. In the case of parvalbumin, a major allergen among different fish species, it is considered as fish and amphibian panallergen, and causes extensive CR among fish from different families [56], although not with the same intensity or likelihood than clinical reactivity [57].

It is a clinical problem to determine the frequency of sensitization (positive skin test and/or high specific IgE levels) to multiple foods that share homologous proteins and sometimes, can be very difficult to resolve. Even if molecular biological methods were and still are being used in order to investigate the nature of these allergens, clinical trials do not progress fast enough. It is also difficult to determine the risk of food allergic reaction to interrelated foods or to foods related with pollens, latex *etc.* Therefore, an assessment can only be made after taking a careful history, laboratory data and many times a provocation test of the suspected food allergen.

Based on a recent review from Garcia BE and Lizaso MT [53] the main cross-reactivity syndromes in food allergy are: latex-fruit syndrome; pollen-plant food syndromes and syndromes due to LTPs. In this chapter we are going to briefly describe each of them.

LATEX-FRUIT SYNDROME

This syndrome, affects up to 50% of latex-allergic patients and is based on th association between latex allergy and allergy to plant foods, such as, banana, avocado, chesnut and kiwi. Normally allergy to latex precedes food allergy and clinical symptoms are often severe.

The CR between latex and these plant foods is due mainly to the homology between the hevein (Hev b 6.02) of the latex with the hevein-like N-terminal domain of the class I chitinases of plants, which share 70% of sequence identity [58]. Several studies carried out recently highlight the necessity of further multi parametric studies based on a combination of clinical history, latex challenge test and diagnostics test to make an effective latex-fruit syndrome diagnosis [59].

POLLEN-PLANT FOOD ALLERGY SYNDROME

Many kinds of allergic reactions to various fruits and vegetables have been described in association with pollen allergy. They may vary among different geographical areas, as they are dependent on the allergenic local plants and on the food habits of the population under study. Pollen reacts like an allergen source, producing a primary respiratory sensitization which will lead later into an allergic reaction to cross-reacting foods, included in the regular diet.

Since pollinosis is the most prevalent respiratory allergy among adults, it is easy to understand that associated plant food allergy is the most common type of cross-reactive syndrome as well as the most frequent food allergy observed in adults. Although there are no epidemiological studies to carry out an accurate assessment of the prevalence rates, they seem to have increased over the past few decades (in parallel to the increase in pollen allergies) and they may vary depending on the kind of pollen inducing the primary sensitization. Pollinosis is more likely to be observed in patients mono-sensitized to birch pollen, followed by those mono-sensitized to *Artemisa* pollen, and it rarely occurs in patients with sensitization to the grasses. However, allergy frequency to plant food increases as sensitizations are associated to several of these pollen allergens. It is estimated that one third to two thirds of pollen allergic individuals in Europe present plant food allergy reactions [60].

In central and northern Europe, birch pollen has been identified as the most relevant one. Firstly, due to the number of people primary sensitized with it, and secondly, due to the existing cross-reactivity between *Betulaceae* members (hazel, alder) as well as between other species categorized in similar plant families such as *Fagaceae* members (beech, oak, chestnut). It has been shown that natural birch, alder, horn beam, hazel, and oak pollen contain allergens that share IgE epitopes with Bet v 1 and Bet v 2. The combination of Bet v 1 and Bet v 2 accounted therefore for 82% of the epitopes of *Fagaceae* pollen-specific IgE [54]. About 70% of patients allergic to birch pollen often have an oral allergy syndrome to certain fruits and vegetables such as apples, pears, peach, kiwi, celery, potatoes, carrots and nuts. This association between oral allergy syndrome to *Rosaceae* family and pollinosis is very common on northern and central Europe. Allergy to *Rosaceae* family fruits (especially to apples) is the most common fruit allergy linked to birch pollen allergy. However, this kind of fruit allergy does exist in birch-free areas, and it is indeed the most common food allergy among adolescents and young adults in Spain. According to the data emerging from the epidemiological study Alergológica, undertaken in 2005 in Spain, *Rosaceae* fruits are liable to cause allergy to 24% of the food allergic patients [8].

Based on these findings, various studies demonstrate that such food contains similar proteins to the birch pollen allergens, Bet v 1 and Bet v 2 [54, 61] therefore it pose a potential threat to patients with tree pollen allergies. It is well known that some of these foods can be safely eaten by sensitized patients, indicating thermolability of these allergens.

SYNDROME DUE TO LTPs

There was a study published in Spain in which researches found that allergy to *Rosaceae* fruits was not linked to pollinosis. The reason was shown to be a small thermo resistant protein of 9kDa, which appeared to be the major allergen of peach: Pru p 3, a lipid transfer proteins (LTP) [62]. LTPs are plant defense proteins that are highly conserved and present in all plant organs [63], which behave as full allergens, sensitizing by ingestion and often causing systemic reactions. They are major allergens of fruits from the *Rosaceae* family but accordingly to the Allergome database [64] they have been described as allergenic in other fruits such as kiwi, grape, orange, lemon or banana; in nuts (walnut, hazelnut, chestnut); legumes (peanut, lentil, haricot bean); other seeds as mustard; vegetables (tomato, lettuce, *etc.*); cereals (barley, wheat, *etc.*) as well as pollens and latex. Patients sensitized to multiple LTPs experience reactions that are often severe and, very frequently, the number of foods involved increases progressively

[53]. However, the higher levels of IgE observed are always those for Pru p 3 than for other LTPs.

FOOD ALLERGY: CLINICAL PRESENTATION AND DIAGNOSIS

Food allergy symptoms often observed among food allergic patients can be divided into different groups. These symptoms may be immediate or delayed (see immunological basis) [33, 65]:

1. Gastrointestinal symptoms, affecting the perioral zone with immediate symptoms such as pruritus and angioedema of tongue, lips and/ or palate; or the lower gastrointestinal tract, including immediate symptoms (abdominal pain, diarrhea, vomiting or reflux) or delayed symptoms (the previous mentioned and also hematochezia, irritability and food refusal).

2. Skin symptoms: pruritus, urticaria, angioedema, morbilliform eruption, erythema. These symptoms can be observed in both, immediate and delayed reactions.

3. Airway symptoms, divided into upper airway symptoms, where nasal congestion, rhinorrhea, sneezing and laryngeal edema are observed (immediate symptoms); and lower airway symptoms, including cough, dyspnea, wheezing (immediate or delayed reactions).

4. Ocular symptoms: pruritus, tearing and conjunctival erythema and/or edema in both, immediate and delayed reactions.

5. Cardiovascular symptoms (immediate reactions) such as tachycardia, hypotension, dizziness, fainting and even loss of consciousness.

6. Miscellanea: including symptoms such as uterine contractions or the sense of "impending doom".

Symptoms and severity depend on the amount of food ingested and on the way it has been ingested (weather it has been eaten well-cooked or raw or in the presence of other foods or medicaments). They also depend on other factors such as patient´s age and presence of other comorbid conditions (*i.e.,* asthma, dermatitis, *etc.*). The worst case of food allergy reaction involves systemic anaphylaxis, which can lead to patient´s death.

In order to manage food allergy it is very important to perform a good and reliable food allergy diagnosis, therefore the exact and particular food source responsible for the symptoms in the allergic patient and the immunologic mechanism implicated can be established.

Diagnosis begins with an exhaustive clinical history of the patient; this is of vital importance and helps to determine the origin of the problem. Clinical histories should include information about the suspected food of causing the allergic reaction, timing of reaction after ingestion and symptoms observed.

IgE Determinations

These analyses are appropriate when an IgE mediated reaction is suspected. IgE determinations include *in vitro* and *in vivo* analyses, but both need to be interpreted in the context of the clinical history.

IgE determinations can be carried out by different methods, such as RAST (Radioallergosorbent test) or ELISA (Enzyme-linked immunosorbent assay). Nowadays, ImmunoCAP (Thermoscientific-Phadia, Sweden) is the most common diagnostic tool in every allergology sevice.

One limitation of current tests for IgE determinations are cross-reactivity reactions: false positive results may occur between related proteins, for example among fish sensitized patients up to 40% of patients sensitized to one or more fish species show no symptoms after ingesting other species, even though they show positive skin prick tests or sIgE determinations to all of them [66].

Referring to the IgE levels detected by ImmunoCap, seven allergy categories can be addressed (Table **2**).

Table 2: Allergy classification according to IgE levels (ImmunoCap).

Class	kU/L	Antibody levels
0	<0.35	Negative
1	0.35-0.7	Positive, low
2	0.7-3.5	Positive, moderate
3	3.5-17.5	Positive, moderate to high
4	17.5-50	Positive, high
5	50-100	Positive, very high
6	>100	Positive, very high (máximum)

TOTAL AND SPECIFIC IgE DETERMINATIONS

IgE determinations are the first step in the identification of an atopic individual, but results must be carefully interpreted. High IgE titers mean a subjacent IgE mechanism, but not clinical relevance [67]. Variation in the IgE levels due to age or sex, as well as the time of the year or immunotherapy treatment have to be considered. Sometimes, there is an overlapping between atopic and non-atopic patients, but generally IgE levels above 1 kU/L means allergy to an specific allergen. Therefore, specific IgE determinations to specific foods are the next step to identify the likely allergen, although the high cost of these tests needs to be addressed.

Results may vary among different methods, and there has to be a compromise between sensitivity and specificity, because an increase of one of them means decrease of the other. In the case of food allergens there is a lower correlation between clinical history and specific IgE, compared to inhalant allergens. Specialized laboratories have standardized cutoffs for the determination of different foods IgE, but the definitive diagnosis of food hypersensitivity is achieved by means of provocation tests.

Prick Tests

They are widely used in the clinical practice to elucidate which allergenic source is responsible for the patients' reactions and are, in general, more sensitive than specific IgE determinations. The allergologist will apply a small volume of a commercial extract of the likely allergenic extract on the forearm of the patient and then scratch the skin with a lancet or needle. Due to the variability found among commercial extracts, and the loss of allergenicity observed in the case of fruits and vegetables due to their high content in labile proteins, Dreborg and Foucard introduced the Skin Prick-Prick tests, where fresh fruits or vegetables were scratched with the same lancet before scratching patient´s skin [68].

Histamine phosphate and saline solution are used as positive and negative controls of the tests, respectively. Results are commonly considered positive if a wheal larger than 3 mm of diameter is observed after approximately 15-30 min after the prick or just greater than the wheal produced by the negative control.

A positive skin prick test only indicates that there is an allergic sensitization, but not a clinically relevant hypersensitivity. Diagnostic should always be based on tests and clinical history together. In the same way, negative results (negative predicted value of 95%) allow exclusion of an IgE mediated reaction, but confirming probes should be performed.

Other skin tests performed on patients apply the suspected food allergens intradermically. But these tests are not reliable for diagnostics because of their extremely high false positive results rate. Furthermore, the use of intradermal tests is not recommended as they are associated with systemic reactions. Anyway, skin tests should not be performed if there is a risk of a subsequent life-threatening reaction for the patient.

Component-Resolved Diagnostics (CRD)

Component-resolved diagnostics, based on the use of isolated allergens, is a basic tool to achieve a correct and accurate diagnostic in allergic patients. It became possible in the last years, due to the great advances achieved in the molecular biology and allergen purification fields. CRD has a great importance in the investigation of the origin of the IgE-mediated allergies and the evaluation of cross-reactivities. In some cases, CRD may also help to predict severity of clinical reactions or the effect of a specific immunotherapy treatment [69].

- Microarrays

In the last years microarray technology allowed great improvements in diagnostics [67], identifying a large number of IgE binding proteins or glycoproteins at the same time using minimal volumes of sera [70-73], defining the patterns of sensitization of every allergic patient. Other points that have to be addressed, are that results obtained by microarray technology correlate with those obtained by solid-phase IgE determinations [65] and the fact that very low concentrations of proteins are fixed to the matrix, this mimics *in vivo* conditions, where allergens are not in excess to bind free IgE [74].

At the moment, the most advanced *in vitro* molecular diagnostic tool based in the microarray technique is the Immuno Solid-phase Allergen Chip (ISAC), developed by the same company as the ImmunoCap test (Thermoscientific, Phadia, Sweden). In its current version, it allows the detection of IgE levels to 112 different allergens from 51 allergenic sources, including foods, aeroallergens and venoms.

Other application of microarray is the detection of the IgE- binding epitopes on the allergenic molecules, making possible the IgE epitope mapping of a given protein, allowing the determination of different sensitization phenotypes among patients [75, 76] or the identification of different isoforms of the same protein showing different allergenic behavior [77].

Microarray technology has a great importance in food allergies. Very recently, several studies have been performed in patients suffering from different food allergies. For example, microarray combined with multivariate analysis routines improved the prognostic of patients to cow′s milk allergy [78].

Alessandri *et al.* probed through a microarray system, that IgE reactivity to ovomucoid, Gal d 1, is a very good predictor of hen's egg clinical allergy [79]. In other study, a novel diagnostic approach that can predict peanut allergy with high accuracy by combining the results of a peptide microarray immunoassay and bioinformatic methods has been recently developed [80].

In spite of this, in the clinical practice, evaluation of the patients should always be performed considering as well the clinical history and not only *in vitro* results.

Oral Challenges

Oral challenges are only justified in case all other diagnostic probes are negative. During oral challenges, small and increasing amounts of the suspected food are administered to the patient. This has to be carried out in a medical center or hospital, most of all when anaphylactic reactions are expected. Patients should not have eaten anything for at least 6 hours before the provocation, and drugs such as epinephrine has to be available. In order to minimize false negative results, corticoids, antihistamines and immunotherapy must to be avoided before the provocation.

There are different kinds of provocations:

- Double-Blind, Placebo-Controlled Food Challenge (DBPCFC).

This is the gold standard to confirm adverse reactions to foods, including allergy and results are highly reliable. It consists in a controlled exposure, where the patient ingests some beverages or capsules that include the likely allergen and some that do not (placebo). Flavor, smell and texture have to be concealed and neither patient nor medical supervisor knows whether the ingested food is the allergenic or not.

In order to compare challenges performed in different centers, it is important to establish validated protocols for different foods in adults and children. A pilot study was performed to standardize a validated vehicle and low-dose protocol for confirming food allergy to powdered hazelnut and celeriac ingredients in adults and children [81].

In this sense Vlieg-Boerstra and co-authors developed and validated recipes containing milk, soy, cooked egg, raw whole egg, peanut, hazelnut, and wheat for use in DBPCFCs in children [82] and more recently they have enlarged the validated recipes of cow's milk, peanut, egg hazelnut and cashew for these challenges in adults and children using larger amounts of allergenic foods than previously reported [83]. Other studies also developed a model for low-dose oral food challenge for the re-/introduction of milk or egg in young children [62].

Disadvantages of this kind of challenges are the possibility of life-threatening allergic reactions, the high economic resources and the time needed. For those reasons other challenges are frequently used to screen the foods:

- Single-blind.

Only the medical personnel are informed about the composition (with or without the likely allergen) of the food challenge. It becomes of especial interest if patients symptoms are unclear or not convincing for an allergy diagnosis. It is easier to perform and requires less medical infrastructure.

- Open challenges (or unblinded).

Patients ingest the likely allergen unmasked. These challenges are more practical and frequently used in the clinical practice, because they lack of several of the disadvantages described for DBPCFC [84].

Histamine and Serum Tryptase Determinations

Histamine and serum tryptase and derivates levels can help to elucidate if a patient has experienced an anaphylactic shock. These analyses are not frequent in the clinic practice; they are used more often in research investigations.

Basophil Stimulation Tests

It is based on the basophil degranulation after contacting an allergen in immediate-type hypersensitivities. Allergens trigger the formation of IgE by B cells and this leads to mediators release by basophils. Cells are labeled with different fluorescent dyes that can be detected using flow cytometry techniques that can distinguish activated and non-activated basophils. Results correlate well with skin prick tests.

There are several studies confirming the sensitivity and specificity of basophil stimulation test, for example, preliminary studies showed that basophil activation tests can even allow the determination of differences between basophil reactivity to heated milk tolerant and heated milk reactive among milk allergic patients [85].

Non IgE-Mediated Reactions Diagnostic

No standardized tests are currently available for the detection of non–IgE-mediated food allergies.

- Epicoutaneous patch: it is used for the diagnostic of allergic contact dermatitis, which is a delayed type of hypersensitivity of the skin. They are frequently used for testing milk and egg allergy. Even this tests is a very useful procedure, it is limited by the lack of standardization and clinical relevance in positive patch tests remains unclear [30, 86].

- Specific IgA, IgG or IgM determinations by ELISA, RAST, *etc.*

FOOD ALLERGY IMMUNOTHERAPIES

Previous Reports

Nowadays strict avoidance of the sensitizing agents is the most effective method to treat every allergic symptom, since there is no way to prevent or cure food allergy at the moment. Related to foods allergies, it has been demonstrated that removing the sensitizing components from the diet reduces the allergic symptoms of the patients, who develop allergenic tolerance after 1 or 2 years [87].

When an avoidance diet has been prescribed, serious problems or inconvenients can be observed, such as:

- **Nutritional problems:** primarily affecting children above all, it is necessary to bear the nutritional needs in mind and keep the patients and families informed.

- **Real avoidance problems:** avoiding allergenic foods is easier when patients are allergic only to one or few food sources or when these sources are easily identifiable. Sometimes allergenic nutrients are hidden in elaborated foods or used as additives (for example ovalbumin, milk proteins, *etc.*). It is necessary to ensure access to rescue medications, such as epinephrine, if accidental contact has been made.

- **Psychosocial and adaptation problems:** avoidance diets can lead to economical, emotional problems due to the efforts made by the patients. It has been observed that, in some of the cases, the restricted food is rejected by the patient when reintroduced.

Besides, there are symptomatic and palliative methods that provide symptomatic relief, if contact with the problematic source has been made.

Mast cell degranulation inhibitors are prevention drugs in cases of allergy, they bind the membranes of basophils and mast cells inhibiting the release of preformed (histamine, serine protease, *etc.*) and newly formed mediators (thromboxane, prostaglandin, leukotrienes, and platelet-activating factor) and cytokines. These drugs are ketotifen (inhibits degranulation of basophils and mast cells), anti-leukotrienes and inhaled or oral corticoids.

Symptomatic treatment of allergy can be achieved using anti histamines or bronchodilators, but these drugs don´t provide patient´s recovery:

- **Anti-histamines:** these are drugs that block the effect of the histamine released by mast cells during the allergic reaction (competitive antagonists of H1 receptors). The can be divided into two groups: First generation: can pass through the hemato-encephalic barrier (blood-brain barrier) and may cause drowsiness (chlorpheniramine, hydroxyzine, diphenhydramine, dimenhydrinate, *etc.*) and second generation, such as cetirizine, ebastine, desloratadine, which don´t pass the barrier and are not sedative.

- **Bronchodilators:** B2-adrenergic, used in cases of severe crisis (salbutamol, terbutaline, formoterol and salmeterol) and anticholinergic, which are atropine-derivated (ipratropium bromide and tiotropium) and used in mild symptoms cases, preventing airway narrowing when exposed to allergens.

These medications are available in oral or inhaled formulations and provide an improvement of the symptoms of the patients, but they can show unwanted side effects and need to be administered periodically as long as the patient is allergic. In this sense, vaccination is a high valued alternative to palliative drugs, since it can cure the disease.

Traditional Natural Extracts *vs* Recombinant Allergens

Immunotherapy with intact allergen extracts is a well-documented treatment for allergic diseases. However, it has been found to offer several disadvantages in terms of standardization and composition that can be avoided by other therapeutic approaches. Traditional natural extracts are prepared from natural allergen sources and usually contain undefined components that may promote allergic immune responses. New sensitizations may also occur since samples can become contaminated with allergens from other sources. There have been cases describing new IgE reactivities after immunotherapy with allergenic extracts [88]. Moreover, harmful adverse symptoms, which may range from local reactions to life-threatening conditions as anaphylactic shock, have been reported to be associated with this immunotherapy [89, 90].

Concerning to allergoids, which are natural allergen extracts chemically modified in order to reduce their allergenic activity and maintain their immunogenicity; their characterization remains as difficult as in the case of intact allergenic extracts. However, regarding to immunotherapy, allergoids allow the administration of higher doses of allergen extracts in a more rapid up-dosing scheme with a demonstrated clinical efficacy and increased safety, due to their reduced IgE binding capacity, maintaining dendritic cells and allergen-specific T-cell recognition [91, 92].

In contrast, recombinant allergens avoid the problems related to intact or chemically-modified allergenic extracts. The exact amount of allergen provided is well known, as well as its purity due to the use of standardized protocols and production procedures. The following table (Table **3**) from Valenta R *et al.* is very interesting as it summarizes the advantages of recombinant allergens *vs.* traditional allergen extracts [93].

Allergen Immunotherapy

Many food allergens have been characterized at a molecular level, and this knowledge, combined with an increasing appreciation of the nature of humoral and cellular immune responses resulting in allergy or tolerance, is leading to novel therapeutic approaches.

Table 3: Advantages of recombinant allergens over traditional allergen extracts [93].

Disadvantages of natural allergen extracts
• Contain numerous indefined components, some of which may promote allergic immune responses
• Lack or contain low amounts of important allergens
• Contain allergens with widely varying potencies and ratios
• Can be contaminated with unwanted materials or allergens from other sources
• Cannot be tailored to the patient's sensitization profile
• May induce new sensitizations
• Do not suit the international quality standards for vaccines
• Cannot be compared between different products, batches
• Do not allow the precise monitoring and investigation of mechanisms underlying treatment
Advantages of recombinant allergens
• Represent molecules with defined physicochemical and immunologic properties that can be modified to foster advantageous characteristics
• Amounts can be easily controlled on the basis of mass units
• Potencies and ratios can be exactly adjusted for each molecule
• Represent pure molecules
• Vaccines can be exactly tailored according to the patient´s sensitization profile
• Fit the international quality standards for vaccines
• Can be precisely compared to give consistent and reproducible products, batches
• Allow the precise monitoring and investigation of mechanisms underlying treatment
• Can be reproducibly modified to suit different treatment strategies

According to an excellent review from Sicherer SH and Sampson HA [94], two types of approaches can be distinguished, allegen-specific therapies and therapies that are not allergen-specific. This chapter is based on this differentiation, though with modifications. The main therapeutic approaches which are currently being explored worldwide will therefore be summarized here.

Allergen Specific Immunotherapy

Specific immunotherapy (SIT) is based on the gradual administration, usually subcutaneously, of increasing quantities of allergenic extract, in the hopes of desensitization (temporary loss of responsiveness due to continuous exposure which returns upon discontinuation) and/or promoting tolerance (permanent immunologic nonresponse) [16, 95].

The success of the treatment of several allergic diseases such as asthma, allergic rhinitis or insect-venom anaphylaxis, is in contrast with the deficiencies found in food allergy treatment. However, food-specific immunotherapy has been investigated as a potential treatment for food allergy.

It was first used in 1911 by Noon and Freeman to treat allergic rhinitis [96, 97] and stills remains one of the main therapies for allergy treatment [98]. The main immunological mechanisms taking place during immunotherapy are those directed to the development of oral tolerance. First of all, there is a deviation from a Th2 to a Th1-dominant immune response, characterized by a diminution of IL-4, IL-5 and IL-13 and an increase of IFN-γ production; secondly the generation of blocking antibodies, mostly IgG_4 isotype, that compete with IgE antibodies for antigen binding (a decreased of the IgE/IgG_4 ratio is expected within several months) [99]; and thirdly the generation of T regulatory cells, mainly Tr1 [100].

The first route of immunotherapy administration applied to food allergy was subcutaneously. Early attempts using injections with native peanut allergen resulted in unacceptably high rates of severe adverse reactions [101]. Since them subcutaneously immunotherapy (SCIT) has been controversial in the treatment of food allergy. However, its effectiveness has been shown in the case of birch pollen IT (immunotherapy), showing a decreased allergy to foods containing Bet v 1-homologous allergens [102]. The tendency of the immunotherapeutic approaches under study is to change the route of administration of proteins in order to avoid serious adverse effects. In this sense, oral and sublingual immunotherapies with standard food allergens are being investigated.

Oral immunotherapy (OIT), in which a food allergen is ingested in gradually increasing amounts over months, has been tested in egg, milk and peanut allergy. OIT appears to be safe and effective in desensitization of most patients. The first reference to OIT dates from 1908 [103]. After that, several open-label and randomized controlled studies were carried out and these have been recently summarized in an excellent review [104], but the first double-blind, placebo-controlled OIT study for food allergy was made 100 years later by Skripak *et al.* [105]. In this study twenty children were randomized to receive daily milk OIT in 3 phases. The majority of the patients manifested reactions during the post-OIT food challenge, highlightening that complete protection from allergic reactions was not achieved.

A year later Jones *et al.* [106] performed an uncontrolled open-label peanut OIT study in which desensitization was successfully reached in 81% of the patients after 4-22 months of maintenance therapy. Some other investigations in this direction showed lower satisfactory results [107, 108].

Although OIT efficacy in desensitization is clear, longer treatment and/or higher doses may be necessary in some patients. Moreover, there are associated side-effects that made approximately 15% of patients unable to continue OIT treatment [104]. Therefore, more studies are clearly required to assess safety and efficacy of OIT.

Sublingual immunotherapy (SLIT): constitutes another type of immunization where allergen dose is before placed under the tongue. SLIT with environmental allergens, evaluated for respiratory allergy, has been shown to induce regulatory T cells in early stages of the treatment and a shift to Th1 responses in later stages. There are few studies of SLIT with foods. It has been studied in hazelnut [109, 110], milk [111] and peach allergy [112], with promising results. In all of the cases, the mean threshold dose of ingested allergenic source resulting in allergic symptoms increased after a period of 5 to 6 months, decreased of specific SPT sizes, mild systemic reactions in a low percentage of patients and increasing levels of IgG_4 were also observed. Curiously, specific IgE levels did not change after SLIT in none of the studies, suggesting that other mechanisms may be involved in the induction of tolerance or desensitization counterbalancing IgE levels.

Like OIT, SLIT desensitizes patients but whether it induces permanent oral tolerance or not, remains unclear.

It is worth noting that immunologic changes observed during immunotherapy trials, such as smaller SPT wheals and/or higher IgG_4 levels among others, are similar to changes induced by a diet containing heated or baked milk and egg products. Studies suggest that children with milk or egg allergy might tolerate extensively heated forms of these foods, for example milk or egg baked into muffins [113, 114]. These studies point out that ingestion of denatured milk or egg may present a safer and more natural way of immunotherapy.

RECOMBINANT ALLERGEN-BASED VACCINES

Recombinant allergen-based vaccines do not contain unwanted components and are manufactured to suit the individual patient's sensitization profile. Nowadays, there are mainly two recombinant DNA approaches being used in the development of recombinant allergen-based vaccines [93].

The first one is based on the use of recombinant allergens that equal natural allergens. This approach is being used in the development of recombinant wild-type-based vaccines, as for example in a study of carrot allergy [115]. Reese G *et al.* proved that dimer composed of mutants of Dau c 1.0104 and Dau c 1.0201, major allergens of carrot and Bet-v 1 homologous, reduces human IgE reactivity by an average of 81%. The mutants were more antigenic than the wild-type forms, and the dimers induced higher IgG responses in mice than the monomers. These mutants' forms are considered promising vaccine candidates for the treatment of carrot allergy because of its high immunogenicity and drastically reduced allergenicity.

The second approach is the production of genetically modified recombinant allergens, in order to create reduced allergenic derivatives. It has been applied with great success in a multicenter, randomized, double-blind, placebo-controlled study of 124 patients with birch pollen allergy, using hypoallergenic derivatives of the major birch pollen allergen, Bet v 1 [116]. Active treatment with hypoallergenic formula induced protective IgG antibodies which inhibited allergen-induced release of inflammatory mediators. Moreover, a significant decreased in specific IgE levels during seasonal exposure to birch pollen in vaccinated patients was confirmed. This results together with the fact that cutaneous sensitivity was also reduced, makes vaccination with genetically modified allergen derivatives a reliable therapy to ameliorate allergic reactions.

In this sense, several studies have been carried out to treat peanut allergy (PNA), which nowadays is the major cause of fatal anaphylactic reactions to foods. It has been proven in murine models that administration of mutated peanut allergens combined with bacterial adjuvants (such as heat-liked *Listeria monocytogenes* HKLM, or heat-killed *E. coli*, HKE), enhace Th1-skewing effect and reduce the Th2-skewing effect. Li XM *et al.* showed that treatment with mAra h 1-3 (mutated major peanut allergens) plus HKLM not only reduced the incidence of anaphylactic symptoms considerably, but also reduced the severity of anaphylaxis [117]. In subsequent studies, the immunomodulatory effect of heat-killed *Escherichia coli* producing engineered (mutated) Ara h 1, 2, and 3 (HKE-MP123) administered rectally in a murine model of PNA was studied [118]. Three different doses were administered to mice to form three experimental groups. After the first challenge, IgE levels were significantly lower in all HKE-MP123 treated groups and proinflamamatory cytokines production by splenocytes of high dose HKE-MP123 treated mice were significantly reduced while IFN-γ and TGF-β production was considerably increased. Based on these results a Phase I clinical safety study is currently enrolling adult subjects with peanut allergy [119].

Talking about fish allergy implies talking about parvalbumin, a small (12 kDa) and thermo stable protein, belonging to a family of calcium binding proteins, which is the major cross-reactive allergen in fish. It is characterized by the presence of two helix-loop-helix metal binding domains termed EF-hands. In 2007 Swoboda I *et al.* [120], introduced mutations into the calcium binding domains of carp parvalbumin (Cyp c 1) by site directed mutagenesis and produced parvalbumin mutants in *E. coli.* Immunoblotting experiments performed with sera from 21 fish allergic patients showed that IgE reactivity was reduced by 95%. It was also shown in animal models that IgG antibodies could be raised by immunization with this mutant molecule which inhibited fish allergic patients' IgE binding to the wild type allergen. Thanks to this study, allergenicity of metal binding sites was confirmed and the double mutant created represented the basis for new forms of vaccination against fish allergy. In a recent study, mice challenged with rCyp c 1 0 1, recombinant carp parvalbumin, did not increased Th2 cytokine production in lymph node cells and splenocytes compared with its natural counterpart [121].

PEPTIDE IMMUNOTHERAPY

Despite clinical efficacy, current clinical practice with whole allergen extracts requires an extended period of treatment, 2 years or longer. The main reason for the long treatment period is caused by dose limitations related to the frequent occurrence of predominantly IgE-mediated adverse reactions. Adverse events are manifested as allergic reactions to the treatment and range from mild local reactions to severe systemic reactions including anaphylactic shock. Different strategies aimed at reducing the allergenicity of treatment preparations, whilst maintaining immunogenicity, have been described previously in this chapter. In this sense, the use of linear peptide sequences representing fragments of the native allergen is one approach to reduce allergenicity. Short peptides exhibit markedly reduced capacity to cross-link IgE and activate mast cells and basophils. In addition, allergen specific IgG antibodies are induced, which compete with IgE for allergen binding and thereby prevent an allergen-induced activation of effector cells as well as an IgE-mediated presentation of allergens to T cells. The advantages of allergy vaccines based on peptides derived from allergen sequences can be summarized in:

- High specificity and negligible ability to induced allergen-specific IgE responses.
- Should not induce T cell-mediated side effects.
- Safe application of a few high doses.
- Technology applicable for all allergens.

Further advantages include low production costs, ease of purification and good stability in lyophilized form without the need for cold storage. In contrast with others allergens, many foods and their allergens undergo heat processing before consumption and enzymatic digestion in the stomach and the gut. Because these modified allergens are not in their native conformation, they are more likely to induce immune responses to linearized amino acid sequence of food allergens. As a consequence, the humoral immune response to linear epitopes may be favored.

Experimental *in vivo* studies of peptide-induced tolerance have been reported in a number of disease areas including allergy, autoimmunity and transplantation. Indeed, new experimental immunotherapies have been explored in the development of cancer vaccines [122-124].

To develop based-peptide therapies, the first approach is the identification of responsible peptides for the allergic response: IgE-binding peptides and containing T-cell epitopes of allergens.

Therapies Based on IgE-Binding Epitopes

The IgE epitope mapping of allergens might reveal relevant information about antigen structure, the patient's immune response, and key dates for designing safer hypoallergenic immunotherapeutic. This approach is based on the identification of allergen peptides which are part of the major IgE binding sites on allergens but *per se* lack IgE and allergenic activity. In this sense, recent studies have suggested a potential role for IgE-binding epitopes sequential as biomarkers for characterizing phenotypes of food allergy. In particular, several candidate vaccines for the treatment of food allergy have been suggested on the basis of IgE epitope mapping data. In recent years, a high number of studies have been published in the field of epitope mapping in the most common allergy food sources: milk, peanut (reviewed in [76]), egg [125], fish [77], legumes [126] and shrimp [127].

These peptides which are typically between 20 and 35 amino acids in length can either be coupled chemically to a carrier protein or produced as recombinant fusion proteins with a carrier protein. The hapten–carrier principle can be used for the design of allergy vaccines lacking IgE and allergen-specific T cell reactivity. Immunization with carrier- bound allergen peptides induces and focuses IgG antibodies towards the IgE epitopes on allergens with the T cell help of the carrier protein and thus do not activate allergen-specific T cells. The allergen-specific IgG antibodies inhibit allergen-induced mast cell and basophil degranulation and thus immediate allergic symptoms [128]. Moreover allergen specific blocking IgG inhibits boosts of allergenic-specific IgE production by capturing allergens and thus decrease allergen-specific IgE, a mechanisms which may be important for the long-lasting effects on specific immunotherapy.

Viral carrier proteins have been suggested in order to generate a novel type of vaccine for the treatment of cat allergy allergens [129]. Recombinant fusion proteins consisting of the PreS domain of hepatitis B virus (HBV) containing nonallergenic Fel d 1 peptides were expressed in *Escherichia coli* and purified.

Authors demonstrated more than 1000-fold reduced allergenic activity of the fusion proteins and their ability to induce, on immunization, IgG antibodies that inhibit IgE binding of patients with cat allergy to Fel d 1.

Another approaches were developed using non allergen-derived carrier molecules as KLH (keyhole limpet haemocyanin), a protein from the giant sea mollusc *Megathura crenulata*. The peptide conjugates are then used to immunize animals (*e.g.* rabbits) in order to investigate, if they induce IgG responses against the corresponding allergen and if the IgG antibodies can block the binding of allergic patients IgE to the allergen as well as inhibit allergen-induced basophil activation. Several studies have been developed based in this approach using peptides from the major *Dermatophagoides pteronyssinus* allergen (Der p 2) [130] and the major allergen in olive pollen Ole e 1 [131]. In this study, five Ole e 1 peptides of approximately 30 amino acids were tested for IgE reactivity with sera from 67 olive pollen-allergic patients. Four of the five peptides showed very little or no IgE binding. These peptides appeared to be possible candidates for the development of a hypoallergenic olive pollen vaccine.

The strategy for generating a Der p 2-based vaccine was developed using five synthetic Der p 2-derived peptides that showed no relevant IgE reactivity and IgE-mediated allergenic activity. These peptides were identified using cultured peripheral blood mononuclear cells (PBMCs) from allergic patients, which induced lower T-cell proliferation and pro-inflammatory cytokine release than whole molecule Der p 2. Among these peptides, two were identified which, when coupled to a carrier molecule, induced allergen-specific IgG antibodies upon immunization, which were able to block allergic patients' IgE recognition and allergen induced basophil degranulation.

Focused on food allergy, Albrecht *et al.* selected the peanut allergen Ara h 2 and the shrimp tropomyosin Pen a 1, which have been described as containing sequential epitopes, as model allergens. Peptides identified as major sequence epitopes on Pen a 1 and Ara h 2 show low but detectable IgE binding in fluid phase. In contrast, IgE binding significantly increases when the epitope regions were grafted into the molecular framework of a nonallergenic molecule. This finding suggests that conformational and continuous epitopes may require a structural context for the precise epitope presentation, corroborating the hypothesis that a stable tridimensional structure seems to play an important role in terms of allergenicity, and thus, IgE-binding peptides are unlikely to act as full epitopes and cause clinical reactions [132].

Therapies Based on T Cell Epitopes Peptides

A different strategy for decrease IgE-mediated effects is based on the administration of allergen-derived T-cell reactive peptides. For the treatment of allergic disease, synthetic soluble peptides allow the delivery of T cell epitopes of the allergen in a tolerogenic form, whislt avoinding IgE-mediated allergic reactions. The mechanism behind the reduction of allergy symptoms using T cell epitopes is the ability of the peptides to induce immunologic tolerance. The properties of theses peptides should be:

- Contain dominant T-cell epitopes of allergens recognized by individuals with allergy.
- Different HLA-II molecules must present these peptides to target T cells in genetically diverse individuals.
- Without capacity to cross-link IgE and activate mast cells.
- Appropriate to therapeutic production.

This strategy has been more used in food allergy. There are studies based on T cell epitopes peptides in allergy to peanut, egg and milk.

Focused in peanut allergy, Prickett *et al.* [133] generated a library of overlapping peptides consisting of 20 amino acids with an offset of 11, corresponding to the primary sequence Ara h 2, the most widely recognized and potent allergen for individuals with peanut allergy. Using peripheral blood mononuclear cells (PBMCs) from patients with peanut allergy, this group reported the novel identification and characterization of 5 dominant T-cell epitopes of Ara h without binding peanut reactive serum IgE and propose these peptides as candidates for a therapeutic for peanut allergy.

A similar approach was used to define immunodominant T cell epitopes in αs1-casein, the most immunogenic casein protein involved in cow's milk allergy (CMA), and to evaluate whether specific epitope recognition and cytokine production are linked to allergy or tolerance. Responses in T cell derived from PBMCs were investigated in children with CMA, atopic children (tolerant to cow's milk) and non-atopic children. Casein-specific TCLs were used to determine T cell proliferation and cytokine production in response to whole as1-casein. In addition, overlapping synthetic peptides spanning the entire as1-casein molecule was used. Four main regions in the αs1-casein molecule were immunogenic to T cells. The sequence spanned by amino acid residues 133–156 was found to be immunodominant. These peptides were recognized by 52% of TCLs generated from patients and control subject. In contrast, no major differences were observed in epitope T recognition between tolerant and allergic subjects. The region covered by amino acid residues 55–96 was only recognized by T cells from children tolerant to cow's milk (atopic and non-atopic subjects).

Other allergens involved in CMA, as β-lactoglobulin (β-LG) have been studied. Pecquet *et al.* identified tolerogenic peptides (obtained by tryptic hydrolysis of the purified β-LG) that induce oral tolerance at the humoral and cellular levels [134]. Authors suggest that specific oral tolerance induction could be initiated using hypoallergenic formulas enriched in tolerogenic peptides when there is a risk in newborn infants.

In the context of egg allergy, Yang *et al.* [135] carried out a study aimed at the assessment of peptide-based immunotherapy (PIT) in a mouse model of food allergy, exploiting the reported T cell epitope map of ovalbumin (OVA), a major egg allergen [136]. Three peptides peptide sequences, reported as immunodominant T cell determinants of OVA, were administered to orally sensitized BALB/c mice *via* subcutaneous injections. The administration of a mixture of the three immunodominant T cell peptides promoted a robust reduction in anaphylactic responses, serum histamine and OVA-specific IgE levels, compared with placebo-treated mice. These variations were not observed in single peptide treated mice. Also, co-administration of mixture containing three OVA T cell determinants increased significantly mRNA expression of FOXP3 and TGF-β in intestinal tissues, compared with placebo-treated mice. TGF-β has been reported to act directly inhibiting the proliferation and differentiation of effector T cells [137] and FOXP3-expressing T cells have been well documented for their inhibitory effects on Th2-allergic responses [138]. Therefore, authors suggest that the repeated administration of synthetic peptides containing immunodominant T cell determinants, promoted *in vivo* allergy suppressive effects in this food allergy mouse model.

Another approach in therapies based in T cell epitopes peptides is to study panallergens instead of specific allergens from each source. As it has been mentioned before, panallergens are responsible for many cross-reactions between plant-derived foods and pollens. In this sense, lipid transfer proteins (LTPs), particularly peach Pru p 3, are the most relevant plant food allergens in the South of Europe. Tordesillas *et al.* [139] described two immunogenic T-cell epitopes in Pru p 3 (Pru p $3_{65–80}$ and Pru p $3_{25–35}$) using PBMCs and TCLs from peach-allergic patients and non peach-allergic controls stimulated with the allergen and with a set of overlapping peptides representing the full sequence of Pru p 3. Authors claim peptide named Pru p $3_{65–80}$ to be a good candidate to develop new vaccines for hypersensitivity reactions associated with LTP allergens.

Based on previous studies, therapies based on T cell epitopes appear to be one of the most important alternatives to the development of new treatments against food allergy. However, studies performed with synthetic allergen-derived T cell epitopes without IgE reactivity have reported adverse reactions. These findings have demonstrated the activation of T cells during SIT by IgE-independent mechanisms which can contribute to late phase and chronic allergic inflammation [140, 141]. This activation seemed to precede the induction of T cell tolerance and would be dose-related. T cell–mediated events, such as isolated late asthmatic reaction, are related to high doses of peptide by the activation of memory effector T cells. Recent data suggest that the side-effects can be avoided using lower peptide doses, which are still capable of inducing tolerance. Currently doses and application modes are investigated in order to reduce the adverse reactions in favor of tolerance induction. Clinical trials are ongoing to investigate underlying mechanism responsible for the beneficial effects of therapy with T cell peptides on IgE mediated immediate allergic symptoms [142].

OTHER APPROACHES

Several other approaches including molecules as chitosan, which is a cationic polysaccharide from crustacean's shells, are currently under study. This molecule is very interesting because due to its cationic nature is able to attach to negative surfaces, such as mucosal epithelia. It also has the capacity to encapsulate antigens, which facilitates its capitation by antigen presenting cells. There are studies that highlighting these interesting properties when applied with bacterial plasmid DNA vaccines, peptides or complete allergens.

The plasmid DNA strategy relies on the fact that endogenously produced antigen would not stimulate an allergic immune response. Oral immunization in mice with nanoparticules of chitosan/plasmid DNA encoding the peanut allergen Ara h 2, showed successful prevention of peanut allergy in a certain strain of mice [143]. According to pDNA efficacy, different results were observed in a different strain of mice, suggesting that the effect of pDNA-based immunotherapy may be strain-dependant and thus leading to variable outcomes in humans [144].

An alternative approach to DNA-based immunotherapy is to attach determinants that activate nonallergic immune responses to allergens. For example, unmethylated cytosine and guanine motifs (CpG motifs), that act as immune stimulatory sequences (ISSs) reducing IgE binding and enhancing Th1 responses. In one study mice were immunized intranasally with ISS-linked Ara h 2, four weeks later sensitized with peanut and then challenged with Ara h 2 five weeks later [145]. Treated mice showed mild symptomps and lower plasma histamine when compared to controls. The use of antigen-ISS immunization may prevent food allergy, but whether it will improve established food allergy or not remains unclear.

Non Specific Allergen Immunotherapy

In the last few years allergen nonspecific therapies have been investigated, although some of them have been studied *in vitro* and using animal models, there are others in which, in spite of the promising results obtained, further investigations in human clinical trials are required.

The use of alternative and complementary medicine for the treatment of food allergies is increasing in the last years; these methods include acupuncture, herbal medicine, probiotics, and the use of parasites, such as helminths.

ANTI-IgE THERAPY

This is based on a recombinant humanized monoclonal antibody directed against IgE. The first anti- IgE antibodies were antibodies of animal origin which could lead to an anaphylactic reaction. Thus, new Anti-IgEs were generated so that the new antibody is 95% human and 5% murine protein. Humanized monoclonal antibodies such as Omalizumab, of 149 kDa, were further demonstrated to have desirable anti-IgE properties. [146].

Omalizumab binds to free IgE, forming an inert molecule. Thus, prevents free IgE from attaching to mast cells, basophils and also to dendritic cells [147], blocking mediator and cytokine release, inhibiting antigen presentation by these cells [148]. This prevents early and late phase allergic reactions of skin and lungs, since it dramatically reduces free IgE levels for months. But the effect of Omalizumab is further improved as it down regulates FcεRI on mast cells, basophils and other effector cells [149, 150] and its effect is not specific, reducing levels of IgE directed at all allergens.

Omalizumab is mainly used for the treatment of severe asthma, although attempts at desensitization to different foods were performed, mainly to milk, peanut and fruits, in order to improve food intolerance and therefore, the quality of life of these patients, Although it has been demonstrated that only the symptoms improved, the histological changes suffered due to the allergic reaction did not change [151].

A case report of severe asthma and peach allergy treated with anti-IgE antibody Omalizumab controlled the asthma and allergic symptoms to fruits of the patient, concluding that in this case, omalizumab therapy was highly effective in achieving remission from both asthma and peach allergy [152].

In a study performed by Bedoret *et al.,* children with cow's milk allergy were treated with a rapid high-dose oral desensitization enabled by IgE reduction with

Omalizumab. Desensitization was associated with reduction in milk-specific IgE and a 15-fold increase in milk-specific IgG4, suggesting that high-dose oral allergen desensitization may be associated with deletion of allergen-specific T cells, without the apparent development of allergen-specific Foxp3(+) regulatory T cells [153].

Studies performed with patients allergic to nuts are the most striking, due to the severity of these allergies.

Omalizumab therapy can reduce both, increase of basophil CD203c levels at baseline and following rapid *ex vivo* stimulation in patients with nuts allergy. These results have also highlighted the potential of using basophil CD203c levels for baseline diagnosis and therapeutic monitoring in subjects with nut allergy [154].

Other human trial (double-blind, randomized, dose-ranging) was carried-out in 84 peanut allergic patients treated with Hu-901(humanized IgG1 monoclonal antibody against IgE). They experienced a significant decrease of symptoms and an increase of the threshold of tolerance compared with the placebo group, but a variable response was observed among patients [155]. In a Phase II dose-finding study of omalizumab in peanut anaphylaxis, authors state that the use of the drug in food allergy should be investigated more thoroughly and therefore should not be recommended at present for use in case of severe food allergy.

However, the clinical applicability of omalizumab and other anti-IgE drugs in allergic diseases is potentially vast. However, due to the high cost-effectiveness ratios for this newly developed agent, omalizumab is currently indicated only in patients with moderate to-severe asthma who have exhausted other conventional treatments for asthma. In future, further refinement of molecules will lead us to an even more improved and refined therapy for allergic diseases Further investigations of these drugs will lead to an improved therapy with reduced costs, making it more accessible to the public [156].

CHINESE HERBAL PREPARATION

Chinese herbal medicines are one of the major components in traditional Chinese medicine practice, and are prescribed in hospitals in China as either monotherapy or complementary therapy to conventional western therapy [157].

Several studies support its benefits in treating asthma and ongoing preclinical studies are very promising for the treatment of food allergy: the herbal mixture called FAHF-2 (food allergy herbal formula-2) has demonstrated excellent immunotherapy results in a murine model of peanut sensitization [158, 159]. To date, no investigation has been reported but the FAHF-2, this being the only case in which human trials have been validated [160].

FAHF-2 is a mixture of 9 chinese herb extracts, that administered as an early [159] or late treatment, blocks anaphylaxis in allergic mice by suppression of histamine release and Th2 responses and up-regulation of Th1 responses [161]. It has been demonstrated that IFN-γ and CD8+ T cells play a very important role in long term protection provided by the formula [162].

These effects were very similar to those observed in an *in vitro* study, performed with human cells, where immunomodulation was observed by a suppression of IL-5 production and increased IFN-γ production [82]. Other effects observed were the inhibition of FcεRI expression and inhibition of mast cell degranulation [163].

Very recently, safety and tolerability of FAHF-2 in patients with food allergy was evaluated in a randomized, double-blinded placebo-controlled dose escalation, phase 1 trial. It was observed a significantly decreased interleukin levels (IL-5) in those patients which received the formula. Several *in vitro* studies demonstrated an increase of interferon gamma and IL-10 levels in culture supernatant and in addition a decreased IL-5 [163].

Taking the aforementioned into account FAHF-2 appears to be a perfect candidate to treat food allergies in humans, but further investigations need to be performed, as well investigations with other herb mixtures and/or individual herbs, although results obtained in a murine model of multiple food allergies indicates that it is capable of modulating the allergic response [162].

TOLL-LIKE RECEPTORS

Microbial products act on pattern recognition receptors including Toll-like receptors (TLRs) to initiate rapid host immune response. With the aim of trying to understand how microbial signals reshape ongoing allergic responses to peanut,

Pochard *et al.* designed an *in vitro* system to study TLR signaling in dendritic cells showing that TLR activation leads to Th1 skewing, which is able to reduce Th2 responses [164]. It was proven in a mouse model of peanut allergy it was proven that oral administration of a synthetic TLR9 agonist resulted in decreased gastrointestinal inflammation and protection form peanut anaphylaxis [165].

PARASITIC HELMINTH THERAPY

Helminths are parasite worms that developed different mechanisms designed to produce a hyporesponsive immune system in the host. This means an asymptomatic infection, allowing the parasites to escape from the immune system and survive inside their hosts for a long time, completing their life cycle [166, 167].

Helminths induce a "modified Th2-type response", but they can lead to a protection against allergy, as shown in several clinical studies [168]. During an infection, the key players in Th2-type immunity are CD4+ Th2 cells. IL- 4, IL-5, IL-9, IL-10, and IL-13 as well as IgE are implicated. This leads to the activation of eosinophils, basophils and mast cells. This translates into helminth resistance, although the parasites have developed a strategy to survive by modulating and/or suppressing this response. They induce the production of different regulatory cells and anti-inflammatory cytokines, such as IL- 10, and induce specific inhibitory antibody isotypes (increased IgG4 and decreased IgE levels) [151, 167].

It has been proposed that the eradication of helminth infections in developed countries had increased the prevalence of diseases associated with inappropriate immune responses.

It has been observed that the persistence of the parasite in the host is not necessary to reduce allergic symptoms [169], which is very interesting for the development of new therapeutic strategies based in helminth-derived molecules.

Several helminth species have been proposed as therapies in allergies, but also in other diseases, such as inflammatory bowel disease or multiple sclerosis, among others.

One of the most largely studied helminth is *Trichuris suis*, of the nematode family. The natural host from these parasites is pig, where no systemic infection occurs. *T. suis* has been selected for numerous studies because it seems to be nonpathogenic for humans and there is a strong evidence of safety [170, 171].

Concerning to food allergies, these nematodes have been used in a study of peanut allergy; authors did not find strongly conclusive data, but the safety [172]. But, the protective effect of helminths has been demonstrated in the case of peanut allergy in a murine model of oral immunization, where results indicate that the parasite *Heligmosomoides polygirus* avoids IgE production and atopy [173].

Other species, such as *Trichuris trichura* or *Necator americanus* have been used in clinical trials in the United Kingdom or Australia, but as human pathogens, their use as immunological therapies is not strongly suggested.

Nowadays, different helminth-molecules have been identified, as well as their immunomodulatory role during the infection [174]. The most studied is the ES-62, a 62 kDa phosphorylcholine containing glycoprotein.

In spite of this, there are studies suggesting that this kind of infection can produce a exacerbation of the allergic symptoms instead of a protection against allergy [175-177]. Some authors proposed that the difference could lie in the exposure: heavy exposures to the parasite would lead to immune suppressive mechanisms whereas mild exposure would even promote the allergic inflammation [176].

PROBIOTICS

Changes in the gut microflora can produce different diseases, such as intestinal tract problems (lactose malabsorption, diarrhea, *etc.*), intolerances and immune system diseases, including food allergies. These alterations are very common among the population of developed countries, causing a large number of problems of mucosal immune tolerance.

Probiotics are ingested live microorganisms that cause beneficial effects on human health [178]. They can be bacteria, molds, or yeasts, but the majority of the times they are lactic acid bacteria [179]. In fact, probiotics with the greatest number of proven benefits are *Lactobacillus rhamnosus* strain GG and *Saccharomyces boulardii.*

Probiotics benefits are due to different mechanisms: they attach to cells membrane, avoiding pathogens binding to cell surface, promote cytokine secretion, produce lactic acid that inhibits the growth of pathogens and balance other commensal microorganisms [180].

Benefits of probiotics have been proven for many diseases such as diarrhea. Several studies are looking for a role for probiotics in the treatment of food allergies, and the results found are promising. But these effects, in spite of the promising results, need additional support for other diseases such as caries prevention, inflammatory bowel disease, *etc.* [181].

Besides probiotics, prebiotics (non-digestible oligosaccharides that stimulate the growth of probiotic bacteria) and synbiotics (pre- and probiotics administered together) effects are also being studied.

A recent study performed to compare diets supplemented with pro-, pre- and synbiotics in cow´s milk allergic mice sensitized to whey, concluded that mice fed with the synbiotics mixture showed highly reduced anaphylactic reactions compared to the pre- and probiotic fed mice, endorsing the potential of synbiotics in reducing the allergic reactions to food allergens [182].

The use of probiotics is increasing, as well as the new applications and its benefits, although we should be cautious since negative effects have also been reported, as more studies are being issued.

CONCLUSIONS

Food allergy is health concern with increasing prevalence. It is an immune deregulated disease characterized by inflammatory reactions with a T-helper-2-type (Th2) cell and allergen specific IgE predominance.

The epidemiology of food allergy is still under study. Although recent studies confirmed that there is a genetic factor implicated in the development of atopy and food allergy, there are environmental factors which play an important role in the risk of food allergy, such as dose and time of allergen exposure, feeding pattern, diet/nutrition, and/or microbial exposure, that remain unclear.

On the other hand, strict avoidance diet is the only treatment for food allergy which is 100% effective nowadays, with all the associated nutritional and psychosocial consequences. The increasing knowledge of immunological mechanisms associated to food allergy has enable researchers to develop novel therapeutic tools in order to find alternatives to the paradigm of dietary avoidance.

It has been observed that skewing of Th2 response to a Th1 response change completely the releasing profile of proinflamatory mediators and therefore the severity of the disease. It has also been confirmed that higher levels of blocking IgG antibodies is translated into a change in the IgE reactivity profile as they compete with IgE antibodies for antigen binding and therefore less activation of degranulating cells (mast cells and basophiles) occur. A decreased IgE/IgG ratio is associated with a gain of tolerance. However, whether this tolerance is permanent or whether it is short term desensitization needs still to be addressed.

In this sense, promising results such as oral immunotherapy alone or in combination with anti-IgE antibody, vaccines based on mutated hypoallergenic derivatives associated or not to immunostimulatory sequences (ISSs), Chinese herbal formula FAHF-2, *etc.* have been observed with allergen-specific and allergen non specific immunotherapy approaches All of them towards the same direction, reduce symptomatology and achieve long-term tolerance. Although some of these therapies are currently in clinical trials, it would take time to implement them into clinical practice as larger sample studies still need to be done as well as long term safety tests. However, the increasing research activity on food allergy together with the efforts of both clinician and basic scientists offer the hope that an effective treatment for food allergy may be close.

ACKNOWLEDGEMENTS

We would like to thank Victoria Vergara Asensio for providing editorial assistance, Dr. Cuesta-Herranz for valuable suggestions and all researchers working in the development of safe therapeutic strategies to treat food allergy.

CONFLICT OF INTEREST

The author(s) confirm that this chapter content has no conflict of interest.

REFERENCES

[1] Johansson SG, Bennich H. Immunological studies of an atypical (myeloma) immunoglobulin. Immunology 1967; 13: 381-394.

[2] Ishizaka K, Ishizaka T. Identification of gamma-E-antibodies as a carrier of reaginic activity. J Immunol 1967; 99: 1187-1198.

[3] Hong X WX. Early life precursors, epigenetics and the development of food allergy. Semin Immunopathol. 2012.

[4] Strachan DP Hay fever, hygiene, and household size. BMJ 18-11-1989; 299: 1259-1260.

[5] Okada H, Kuhn C, Feillet H, Bach JF. The 'hygiene hypothesis' for autoimmune and allergic diseases: an update. Clin Exp Immunol 2010; 160: 1-9.

[6] Bach JF The effect of infections on susceptibility to autoimmune and allergic diseases. N Engl J Med 19-9-2002; 347: 911-920.

[7] Knox RB, Suphioglu C, Taylor P, Desai R, *et al.* Major grass pollen allergen Lol p 1 binds to diesel exhaust particles: implications for asthma and air pollution. Clin Exp Allergy 1997; 27: 246-251.

[8] Fernandez RM. Food allergy in Alergologica-2005. J Investig Allergol Clin Immunol 2009; 19 Suppl 2: 37-44.

[9] Dupont C Food allergy: recent advances in pathophysiology and diagnosis. Ann Nutr Metab 2011; 59 Suppl 1: 8-18.

[10] Coombs RRA, Gell PGH. Classification of allergic reactions responsible for clinical hypersensitivity and disease.; in In: Coombs RRA (ed): Clinical Aspects of Immunology. 1968, pp 575-596.

[11] Guidelines for the Diagnosis and Management of Food Allergy in the United States: Report of the NIAID-Sponsored Expert Panel. 126(6), 1105-1118. 2010. J Allergy Clin Immunol.

[12] Ortolani C, Vighi G. Definition of adverse reactions to food. Allergy 1995; 50: 8-13.

[13] Johansson SG, Hourihane JO, Bousquet J, Bruijnzeel-Koomen C, *et al.* A revised nomenclature for allergy. An EAACI position statement from the EAACI nomenclature task force. Allergy 2001; 56: 813-824.

[14] Johansson SG, Bieber T, Dahl R, Friedmann PS, *et al.* Revised nomenclature for allergy for global use: Report of the Nomenclature Review Committee of the World Allergy Organization, October 2003. J Allergy Clin Immunol 2004; 113: 832-836.

[15] Dahl R, Andersen PS, Chivato T, Valovirta E, *et al.* National prevalence of respiratory allergic disorders. Respir Med 2004; 98: 398-403.

[16] Sicherer SH, Sampson H.A. Food allergy: recent advances in pathophysiology and treatment. Annu Rev Med 2009; 60: 261-277.

[17] Vereda A, van HM, Ahlstedt S, Ibanez MD, *et al.* Peanut allergy: Clinical and immunologic differences among patients from 3 different geographic regions. J Allergy Clin Immunol 2011; 127: 603-607.

[18] Burks AW, Tang M, Sicherer S, Muraro A, *et al.* ICON: food allergy. J Allergy Clin Immunol 2012; 129: 906-920.

[19] Rona RJ, Keil T, Summers C, Gislason D, *et al.* The prevalence of food allergy: a meta-analysis. J Allergy Clin Immunol 2007; 120: 638-646.
[20] Zuidmeer L, Goldhahn K, Rona RJ, Gislason D, *et al.* The prevalence of plant food allergies: a systematic review. J Allergy Clin Immunol 2008; 121: 1210-1218.
[21] Cuesta-Herranz J, Barber D., Blanco C, Cistero-Bahima A, *et al.* Differences among pollen-allergic patients with and without plant food allergy. Int Arch Allergy Immunol 2010; 153: 182-192.
[22] Huby RD, Dearman RJ, Kimber I. Why are some proteins allergens? Toxicol Sci 2000; 55: 235-246.
[23] Lack G. Epidemiologic risks for food allergy. J Allergy Clin Immunol 2008; 121: 1331-1336.
[24] Lack G. The concept of oral tolerance induction to foods. Nestle Nutr Workshop Ser Pediatr Program 2007; 59: 63-68.
[25] Leap: Learning early about peanut allergy. www leapstudy co uk.
[26] Poole JA, Barriga K, Leung DY, Hoffman M, *et al.* Timing of initial exposure to cereal grains and the risk of wheat allergy. Pediatrics 2006; 117: 2175-2182.
[27] Wjst M Another explanation for the low allergy rate in the rural Alpine foothills. Clin Mol Allergy 5-6-2005; 3: 7.
[28] Devereux G, Litonjua AA, Turner SW, Craig LC, *et al.* Maternal vitamin D intake during pregnancy and early childhood wheezing. Am J Clin Nutr 2007; 85: 853-859.
[29] Noverr MC, Huffnagle GB. The 'microflora hypothesis' of allergic diseases. Clin Exp Allergy 2005; 35: 1511-1520.
[30] Wang J, Sampson HA. Food allergy. J Clin Invest 2011; 121: 827-835.
[31] Akdis CA. Allergy and hypersensitivity: mechanisms of allergic disease. Curr Opin Immunol 2006; 18: 718-726.
[32] Akdis M, Burgler S, Crameri R, Eiwegger T, *et al.* Interleukins, from 1 to 37, and interferon-gamma: receptors, functions, and roles in diseases. J Allergy Clin Immunol 2011; 127: 701-721.
[33] Kay AB. Allergy and allergic diseases. First of two parts. N Engl J Med 4-1-2001; 344: 30-37.
[34] Akdis M. Healthy immune response to allergens: T regulatory cells and more. Curr Opin Immunol 2006; 18: 738-744.
[35] Akdis CA, Akdis M. Mechanisms of allergen-specific immunotherapy. J Allergy Clin Immunol 2011; 127: 18-27.
[36] Abbas AK, Lichtman AH, Pillai S. Cellular and Molecular Immunology, ed 6th. Philadelphia, WB Saunders Company, 2009.
[37] Kalesnikoff J, Galli S.J. New developments in mast cell biology. Nat Immunol 2008; 9: 1215-1223.
[38] Bannon GA. What makes a food protein an allergen? Curr Allergy Asthma Rep 2004; 4: 43-46.
[39] Moreno FJ. Gastrointestinal digestion of food allergens: effect on their allergenicity. Biomed Pharmacother 2007; 61: 50-60.
[40] Pali-Scholl I, Jensen-Jarolim E. Anti-acid medication as a risk factor for food allergy. Allergy 2011; 66: 469-477.
[41] Sakaguchi S, Yamaguchi T, Nomura T, Ono M. Regulatory T cells and immune tolerance. Cell 30-5-2008; 133: 775-787.

[42] Deniz G, Erten G, Kucuksezer UC, Kocacik D, *et al.* Regulatory NK cells suppress antigen-specific T cell responses. J Immunol 15-1-2008; 180: 850-857.
[43] Zhou J, Appleton SE, Stadnyk A, Lee TD, *et al.* CD8+ gammadelta T regulatory cells mediate kidney allograft prolongation after oral exposure to alloantigen. Transpl Int 2008; 21: 679-687.
[44] Akdis M, Blaser K, Akdis CA. T regulatory cells in allergy: novel concepts in the pathogenesis, prevention, and treatment of allergic diseases. J Allergy Clin Immunol 2005; 116: 961-968.
[45] Lim HW, Hillsamer P, Banham AH, Kim CH. Cutting edge: direct suppression of B cells by CD4+ CD25+ regulatory T cells. J Immunol 1-10-2005; 175: 4180-4183.
[46] O'Garra A, Barrat FJ, Castro AG, Vicari A, *et al.* Strategies for use of IL-10 or its antagonists in human disease. Immunol Rev 2008; 223: 114-131.
[47] Letterio JJ, Roberts AB. Regulation of immune responses by TGF-beta. Annu Rev Immunol 1998; 16: 137-161.
[48] Dardalhon V, Awasthi A, Kwon H, Galileos G, *et al.* IL-4 inhibits TGF-beta-induced Foxp3+ T cells and, together with TGF-beta, generates IL-9+ IL-10+ Foxp3(-) effector T cells. Nat Immunol 2008; 9: 1347-1355.
[49] Veldhoen M, Uyttenhove C, van SJ, *et al.* Transforming growth factor-beta 'reprograms' the differentiation of T helper 2 cells and promotes an interleukin 9-producing subset. Nat Immunol 2008; 9: 1341-1346.
[50] Corthesy B. Roundtrip ticket for secretory IgA: role in mucosal homeostasis? J Immunol 1-1-2007; 178: 27-32.
[51] Bonds RS, Midoro-Horiuti T., Goldblum R. A structural basis for food allergy: the role of cross-reactivity. Curr Opin Allergy Clin Immunol 2008; 8: 82-86.
[52] Breiteneder H, Mills EN. Molecular properties of food allergens. J Allergy Clin Immunol 2005; 115: 14-23.
[53] Garcia BE, Lizaso M.T. Cross-reactivity syndromes in food allergy. J Investig Allergol Clin Immunol 2011; 21: 162-170.
[54] Hoffman-Sommergruber K, Rewers M. Bet v 1-homologous allergens; in Mills E, Shewry P (eds): Plant food allergens. Oxford, UK, Blackwell Science Ltd., 2004, pp 125-140.
[55] Boquete M, Iraola V, Morales M, *et al.* Seafood hypersensitivity in mite sensitized individuals: is tropomyosin the only responsible allergen? Ann Allergy Asthma Immunol 2011; 106: 223-229.
[56] Perez-Gordo M, Cuesta-Herranz J, Maroto AS, *et al.* Identification of sole parvalbumin as a major allergen: study of cross-reactivity between parvalbumins in a Spanish fish-allergic population. Clin Exp Allergy 2011; 41: 750-758.
[57] Van DT, Elsayed S, Florvaag E, *et al.* Allergy to fish parvalbumins: studies on the cross-reactivity of allergens from 9 commonly consumed fish. J Allergy Clin Immunol 2005; 116: 1314-1320.
[58] Blanco C, Diaz-Perales A, Collada C, *et al.* Class I chitinases as potential panallergens involved in the latex-fruit syndrome. J Allergy Clin Immunol 1999; 103: 507-513.
[59] Nucera E, Rizzi A, Buonomo A, *et al.* The clinical meaning of positive latex sIgE in patients with food/pollen adverse reactions. Int J Immunopathol Pharmacol 2012; 25: 445-453.
[60] Blanco C, Almeide L, Castillo R, Sanchez-Monje R, Fernandez-Rivas M. Síndromes de la reactividad cruzada en la alergia a los alimentos; in Peláez-Hernández A, Dávila González I (eds): Tratado de Alergología. Tomo II. 2007, pp 915-938.

[61] Breiteneder H, Ebner C. Molecular and biochemical classification of plant-derived food allergens. J Allergy Clin Immunol 2000; 106: 27-36.

[62] Devenney I, Norrman G., Oldaeus G., Stromberg L.*et al.* A new model for low-dose food challenge in children with allergy to milk or egg. Acta Paediatr 2006; 95: 1133-1139.

[63] Marrion D, Douliez J, Gautier M, Elmorjani K: Plant lipid Transfer Proteins: Relationship between Allergenicity and Structural, Biological and Technological Properties; in Mills E, Shewry P (eds): Plant food allergens. Oxford UK, Blackwell Science Ltd., 2004, pp 57-69.

[64] Mari A, Rasi C., Palazzo P., Scala E. Allergen databases: current status and perspectives. Curr Allergy Asthma Rep 2009; 9: 376-383.

[65] Wohrl S, Vigl K., Zehetmayer S., Hiller R.*et al.* The performance of a component-based allergen-microarray in clinical practice. Allergy 2006; 61: 633-639.

[66] Pascual C, Martin E.M., Crespo J.F. Fish allergy: evaluation of the importance of cross-reactivity. J Pediatr 1992; 121: S29-S34.

[67] Bhalla PL, Singh M.B. Biotechnology-based allergy diagnosis and vaccination. Trends Biotechnol 2008; 26: 153-161.

[68] Dreborg S, Foucard T. Allergy to apple, carrot and potato in children with birch pollen allergy. Allergy 1983; 38: 167-172.

[69] Sanz ML, Blazquez A.B., Garcia B.E. Microarray of allergenic component-based diagnosis in food allergy. Curr Opin Allergy Clin Immunol 2011; 11: 204-209.

[70] Deinhofer K, Sevcik H., Balic N., Harwanegg C.*et al.* Microarrayed allergens for IgE profiling. Methods 2004; 32: 249-254.

[71] Lin J, Bardina L., Shreffler W.G. Microarrayed allergen molecules for diagnostics of allergy. Methods Mol Biol 2009; 524: 259-272.

[72] Hiller R, Laffer S., Harwanegg C., Huber M.*et al.* Microarrayed allergen molecules: diagnostic gatekeepers for allergy treatment. FASEB J 2002; 16: 414-416.

[73] Mari A, Alessandri C., Bernardi M.L., Ferrara R.*et al.* Microarrayed allergen molecules for the diagnosis of allergic diseases. Curr Allergy Asthma Rep 2010; 10: 357-364.

[74] Kim TE, Park S.W., Cho N.Y., Choi S.Y.*et al.* Quantitative measurement of serum allergen-specific IgE on protein chip. Exp Mol Med 31-5-2002; 34: 152-158.

[75] Lin J, Bardina L., Shreffler W.G., Andreae D.A.*et al.* Development of a novel peptide microarray for large-scale epitope mapping of food allergens. J Allergy Clin Immunol 2009; 124: 315-22, 322.

[76] Lin J, Sampson H.A. The role of immunoglobulin E-binding epitopes in the characterization of food allergy. Curr Opin Allergy Clin Immunol 2009; 9: 357-363.

[77] Perez-Gordo M, Lin J., Bardina L., Pastor-Vargas C.*et al.* Epitope mapping of Atlantic salmon major allergen by peptide microarray immunoassay. Int Arch Allergy Immunol 2012; 157: 31-40.

[78] Wulfert F, Sanyasi G., Tongen L., Watanabe L.A.*et al.* Prediction of tolerance in children with IgE mediated cow's milk allergy by microarray profiling and chemometric approach. J Immunol Methods 31-8-2012; 382: 48-57.

[79] Alessandri C, Zennaro D., Scala E., Ferrara R.*et al.* Ovomucoid (Gal d 1) specific IgE detected by microarray system predict tolerability to boiled hen's egg and an increased risk to progress to multiple environmental allergen sensitisation. Clin Exp Allergy 2012; 42: 441-450.

[80] Lin J, Bruni F.M., Fu Z., Maloney J.*et al.* A bioinformatics approach to identify patients with symptomatic peanut allergy using peptide microarray immunoassay. J Allergy Clin Immunol 2012; 129: 1321-1328.

[81] Cochrane SA, Salt L.J., Wantling E., Rogers A.*et al.* Development of a standardized low-dose double-blind placebo-controlled challenge vehicle for the EuroPrevall project. Allergy 2012; 67: 107-113.

[82] Vlieg-Boerstra BJ, Bijleveld C.M., van der Heide S., Beusekamp B.J.*et al.* Development and validation of challenge materials for double-blind, placebo-controlled food challenges in children. J Allergy Clin Immunol 2004; 113: 341-346.

[83] Vlieg-Boerstra BJ, Herpertz I., Pasker L., van der Heide S.*et al.* Validation of novel recipes for double-blind, placebo-controlled food challenges in children and adults. Allergy 2011; 66: 948-954.

[84] Asero R, Fernandez-Rivas M., Knulst A.C., Bruijnzeel-Koomen C.A. Double-blind, placebo-controlled food challenge in adults in everyday clinical practice: a reappraisal of their limitations and real indications. Curr Opin Allergy Clin Immunol 2009; 9: 379-385.

[85] Wanich N, Nowak-Wegrzyn A., Sampson H.A., Shreffler W.G. Allergen-specific basophil suppression associated with clinical tolerance in patients with milk allergy. J Allergy Clin Immunol 2009; 123: 789-794.

[86] Devos SA, Van Der Valk P.G. Epicutaneous patch testing. Eur J Dermatol 2002; 12: 506-513.

[87] Cianferoni A, Muraro A. Food-induced anaphylaxis. Immunol Allergy Clin North Am 2012; 32: 165-195.

[88] Moverare R, Elfman L., Vesterinen E., Metso T.*et al.* Development of new IgE specificities to allergenic components in birch pollen extract during specific immunotherapy studied with immunoblotting and Pharmacia CAP System. Allergy 2002; 57: 423-430.

[89] Scranton SE, Gonzalez *E.G.*, Waibel K.H. Incidence and characteristics of biphasic reactions after allergen immunotherapy. J Allergy Clin Immunol 2009; 123: 493-498.

[90] Bernstein DI, Wanner M., Borish L., Liss G.M. Twelve-year survey of fatal reactions to allergen injections and skin testing: 1990-2001. J Allergy Clin Immunol 2004; 113: 1129-1136.

[91] Heydenreich B, Bellinghausen I., Lorenz S., Henmar H.*et al.* Reduced *in vitro* T-cell responses induced by glutaraldehyde-modified allergen extracts are caused mainly by retarded internalization of dendritic cells. Immunology 2012; 136: 208-217.

[92] Gallego MT, Iraola V., Himly M., Robinson D.S.*et al.* Depigmented and polymerised house dust mite allergoid: allergen content, induction of IgG4 and clinical response. Int Arch Allergy Immunol 2010; 153: 61-69.

[93] Valenta R, Niederberger V. Recombinant allergens for immunotherapy. J Allergy Clin Immunol 2007; 119: 826-830.

[94] Sicherer SH, Sampson H.A. Food allergy. J Allergy Clin Immunol 2010; 125: S116-S125.

[95] Qu C, Srivastava K., Ko J., Zhang T.F.*et al.* Induction of tolerance after establishment of peanut allergy by the food allergy herbal formula-2 is associated with up-regulation of interferon-gamma. Clin Exp Allergy 2007; 37: 846-855.

[96] Noon L Prophylactic inoculation against hay fever. Lancet 1911; 1: 1572-1573.

[97] Freeman J. Vaccination against hay fever, report of results during the last years. Lancet 1, 1178-1180. 1914.

[98] Compalati E, Penagos M., Tarantini F., Passalacqua G.*et al.* Specific immunotherapy for respiratory allergy: state of the art according to current meta-analyses. Ann Allergy Asthma Immunol 2009; 102: 22-28.

[99] Strait RT, Morris S.C., Finkelman F.D. IgG-blocking antibodies inhibit IgE-mediated anaphylaxis *in vivo* through both antigen interception and Fc gamma RIIb cross-linking. J Clin Invest 2006; 116: 833-841.
[100] Shim JY, Kim B.S., Cho S.H., Min K.U.*et al.* Allergen-specific conventional immunotherapy decreases immunoglobulin E-mediated basophil histamine releasability. Clin Exp Allergy 2003; 33: 52-57.
[101] Nelson HS, Lahr J., Rule R., Bock A.*et al.* Treatment of anaphylactic sensitivity to peanuts by immunotherapy with injections of aqueous peanut extract. J Allergy Clin Immunol 1997; 99: 744-751.
[102] Bolhaar ST, Tiemessen M.M., Zuidmeer L., van L.A.*et al.* Efficacy of birch-pollen immunotherapy on cross-reactive food allergy confirmed by skin tests and double-blind food challenges. Clin Exp Allergy 2004; 34: 761-769.
[103] Schofield A. A case of egg poisoning. Lancet 1, 716. 1908.
[104] Vickery BP, Burks W. Oral immunotherapy for food allergy. Curr Opin Pediatr 2010; 22: 765-770.
[105] Skripak JM, Nash S.D., Rowley H., Brereton N.H.*et al.* A randomized, double-blind, placebo-controlled study of milk oral immunotherapy for cow's milk allergy. J Allergy Clin Immunol 2008; 122: 1154-1160.
[106] Jones SM, Pons L., Roberts J.L., Scurlock A.M.*et al.* Clinical efficacy and immune regulation with peanut oral immunotherapy. J Allergy Clin Immunol 2009; 124: 292-300, 300.
[107] Clark AT, Islam S., King Y., Deighton J.*et al.* Successful oral tolerance induction in severe peanut allergy. Allergy 2009; 64: 1218-1220.
[108] Blumchen K, Ulbricht H., Staden U., Dobberstein K.*et al.* Oral peanut immunotherapy in children with peanut anaphylaxis. J Allergy Clin Immunol 2010; 126: 83-91.
[109] Enrique E, Pineda F., Malek T., Bartra J.*et al.* Sublingual immunotherapy for hazelnut food allergy: a randomized, double-blind, placebo-controlled study with a standardized hazelnut extract. J Allergy Clin Immunol 2005; 116: 1073-1079.
[110] Enrique E, Malek T., Pineda F., Palacios R.*et al.* Sublingual immunotherapy for hazelnut food allergy: a follow-up study. Ann Allergy Asthma Immunol 2008; 100: 283-284.
[111] de BD, Dupont C. Sublingual immunotherapy for cow's milk protein allergy: a preliminary report. Allergy 2006; 61: 1238-1239.
[112] Fernandez-Rivas M, Garrido F.S., Nadal J.A., Diaz de Durana M.D.*et al.* Randomized double-blind, placebo-controlled trial of sublingual immunotherapy with a Pru p 3 quantified peach extract. Allergy 2009; 64: 876-883.
[113] Huang F, Nowak-Wegrzyn A. Extensively heated milk and egg as oral immunotherapy. Curr Opin Allergy Clin Immunol 2012; 12: 283-292.
[114] Nowak-Wegrzyn A, Bloom K.A., Sicherer S.H., Shreffler W.G.*et al.* Tolerance to extensively heated milk in children with cow's milk allergy. J Allergy Clin Immunol 2008; 122: 342-7, 347.
[115] Reese G, Ballmer-Weber B.K., Wangorsch A., Randow S.*et al.* Allergenicity and antigenicity of wild-type and mutant, monomeric, and dimeric carrot major allergen Dau c 1: destruction of conformation, not oligomerization, is the roadmap to save allergen vaccines. J Allergy Clin Immunol 2007; 119: 944-951.
[116] Niederberger V, Horak F., Vrtala S., Spitzauer S.*et al.* Vaccination with genetically engineered allergens prevents progression of allergic disease. Proc Natl Acad Sci U S A 5-10-2004; 101 Suppl 2: 14677-14682.

[117] Li XM, Srivastava K., Huleatt J.W., Bottomly K.*et al.* Engineered recombinant peanut protein and heat-killed Listeria monocytogenes coadministration protects against peanut-induced anaphylaxis in a murine model. J Immunol 15-3-2003; 170: 3289-3295.

[118] Li XM, Srivastava K., Grishin A., Huang C.K.*et al.* Persistent protective effect of heat-killed Escherichia coli producing "engineered," recombinant peanut proteins in a murine model of peanut allergy. J Allergy Clin Immunol 2003; 112: 159-167.

[119] Nowak-Wegrzyn A, Sampson H.A. Future therapies for food allergies. J Allergy Clin Immunol 2011; 127: 558-573.

[120] Swoboda I, Bugajska-Schretter A., Linhart B., Verdino P.*et al.* A recombinant hypoallergenic parvalbumin mutant for immunotherapy of IgE-mediated fish allergy. J Immunol 15-5-2007; 178: 6290-6296.

[121] van der Ventel ML, Nieuwenhuizen N.E., Kirstein F., Hikuam C.*et al.* Differential responses to natural and recombinant allergens in a murine model of fish allergy. Mol Immunol 2011; 48: 637-646.

[122] Terazaki Y, Yoshiyama K., Matsueda S., Watanabe N.*et al.* Immunological evaluation of personalized peptide vaccination in refractory small cell lung cancer. Cancer Sci 2012; 103: 638-644.

[123] Uemura H, Fujimoto K., Mine T., Uejima S.*et al.* Immunological evaluation of personalized peptide vaccination monotherapy in patients with castration-resistant prostate cancer. Cancer Sci 2010; 101: 601-608.

[124] Hattori T, Mine T., Komatsu N., Yamada A.*et al.* Immunological evaluation of personalized peptide vaccination in combination with UFT and UZEL for metastatic colorectal carcinoma patients. Cancer Immunol Immunother 2009; 58: 1843-1852.

[125] Jarvinen KM, Beyer K., Vila L., Bardina L.*et al.* Specificity of IgE antibodies to sequential epitopes of hen's egg ovomucoid as a marker for persistence of egg allergy. Allergy 2007; 62: 758-765.

[126] Vereda A, Andreae D.A., Lin J., Shreffler W.G.*et al.* Identification of IgE sequential epitopes of lentil (Len c 1) by means of peptide microarray immunoassay. J Allergy Clin Immunol 2010; 126: 596-601.

[127] Ayuso R, Sanchez-Garcia S., Lin J., Fu Z.*et al.* Greater epitope recognition of shrimp allergens by children than by adults suggests that shrimp sensitization decreases with age. J Allergy Clin Immunol 2010; 125: 1286-1293.

[128] Niederberger V, Horak F., Vrtala S., Spitzauer S.*et al.* Vaccination with genetically engineered allergens prevents progression of allergic disease. Proc Natl Acad Sci U S A 5-10-2004; 101 Suppl 2: 14677-14682.

[129] Niespodziana K, Focke-Tejkl M., Linhart B., Civaj V.*et al.* A hypoallergenic cat vaccine based on Fel d 1-derived peptides fused to hepatitis B PreS. J Allergy Clin Immunol 2011; 127: 1562-1570.

[130] Chen KW, Focke-Tejkl M., Blatt K., Kneidinger M.*et al.* Carrier-bound nonallergenic Der p 2 peptides induce IgG antibodies blocking allergen-induced basophil activation in allergic patients. Allergy 2012; 67: 609-621.

[131] Twaroch TE, Focke M., Civaj V., Weber M.*et al.* Carrier-bound, nonallergenic Ole e 1 peptides for vaccination against olive pollen allergy. J Allergy Clin Immunol 2011; 128: 178-184.

[132] Albrecht M, Kuhne Y., Ballmer-Weber B.K., Becker W.M.*et al.* Relevance of IgE binding to short peptides for the allergenic activity of food allergens. J Allergy Clin Immunol 2009; 124: 328-36, 336.

[133] Prickett SR, Voskamp A.L., Dacumos-Hill A., Symons K.*et al.* Ara h 2 peptides containing dominant CD4+ T-cell epitopes: candidates for a peanut allergy therapeutic. J Allergy Clin Immunol 2011; 127: 608-615.

[134] Pecquet S, Bovetto L., Maynard F., Fritsche R. Peptides obtained by tryptic hydrolysis of bovine beta-lactoglobulin induce specific oral tolerance in mice. J Allergy Clin Immunol 2000; 105: 514-521.

[135] Yang M, Yang C., Mine Y. Multiple T cell epitope peptides suppress allergic responses in an egg allergy mouse model by the elicitation of forkhead box transcription factor 3- and transforming growth factor-beta-associated mechanisms. Clin Exp Allergy 2010; 40: 668-678.

[136] Yang M, Mine Y. Novel T-cell epitopes of ovalbumin in BALB/c mouse: potential for peptide-immunotherapy. Biochem Biophys Res Commun 9-1-2009; 378: 203-208.

[137] Chen W, Jin W., Hardegen N., Lei K.J.*et al.* Conversion of peripheral CD4+CD25- naive T cells to CD4+CD25+ regulatory T cells by TGF-beta induction of transcription factor Foxp3. J Exp Med 15-12-2003; 198: 1875-1886.

[138] Stock P, DeKruyff R.H., Umetsu D.T. Inhibition of the allergic response by regulatory T cells. Curr Opin Allergy Clin Immunol 2006; 6: 12-16.

[139] Tordesillas L, Cuesta-Herranz J., Gonzalez-Munoz M., Pacios L.F.*et al.* T-cell epitopes of the major peach allergen, Pru p 3: Identification and differential T-cell response of peach-allergic and non-allergic subjects. Mol Immunol 2009; 46: 722-728.

[140] Haselden BM, Kay A.B., Larche M. Immunoglobulin E-independent major histocompatibility complex-restricted T cell peptide epitope-induced late asthmatic reactions. J Exp Med 21-6-1999; 189: 1885-1894.

[141] Oldfield WL, Kay A.B., Larche M. Allergen-derived T cell peptide-induced late asthmatic reactions precede the induction of antigen-specific hyporesponsiveness in atopic allergic asthmatic subjects. J Immunol 1-8-2001; 167: 1734-1739.

[142] Larche M T cell epitope-based allergy vaccines. Curr Top Microbiol Immunol 2011; 352: 107-119.

[143] Roy K, Mao H.Q., Huang S.K., Leong K.W. Oral gene delivery with chitosan--DNA nanoparticles generates immunologic protection in a murine model of peanut allergy. Nat Med 1999; 5: 387-391.

[144] Li X, Huang C.K., Schofield B.H., Burks A.W.*et al.* Strain-dependent induction of allergic sensitization caused by peanut allergen DNA immunization in mice. J Immunol 1-3-1999; 162: 3045-3052.

[145] Kattan JD, Srivastava KD, Li XM, Sampson HA. Intranasal treatment with CpG oligonucleotides provides protection from anaphylaxis in a murine model of peanut allergy. J.Allergy Clin.Immunol. [111], S206. 2003.

[146] Shields RL, Whether W.R., Zioncheck K., O'Connell L.*et al.* Inhibition of allergic reactions with antibodies to IgE. Int Arch Allergy Immunol 1995; 107: 308-312.

[147] Vichyanond P Omalizumab in allergic diseases, a recent review. Asian Pac J Allergy Immunol 2011; 29: 209-219.

[148] Mirkina I, Schweighoffer T., Kricek F. Inhibition of human cord blood-derived mast cell responses by anti-Fc epsilon RI mAb 15/1 *vs.* anti-IgE Omalizumab. Immunol Lett 15-4-2007; 109: 120-128.

[149] MacGlashan DW, Jr., Bochner B.S., Adelman D.C., Jardieu P.M.*et al.* Down-regulation of Fc(epsilon)RI expression on human basophils during *in vivo* treatment of atopic patients with anti-IgE antibody. J Immunol 1-2-1997; 158: 1438-1445.

[150] MacGlashan D Loss of receptors and IgE *in vivo* during treatment with anti-IgE antibody. J Allergy Clin Immunol 2004; 114: 1472-1474.

[151] Anthony RM, Rutitzky L.I., Urban J.F., Jr., Stadecker M.J.*et al.* Protective immune mechanisms in helminth infection. Nat Rev Immunol 2007; 7: 975-987.

[152] Suzuki S, Matsuura T., Kimura T., Tazaki T.*et al.* [A case of severe asthma and peach allergy that improved with omalizumab therapy: a case report]. Arerugi 2012; 61: 215-223.

[153] Bedoret D, Singh A.K., Shaw V., Hoyte *E.G.et al.* Changes in antigen-specific T-cell number and function during oral desensitization in cow's milk allergy enabled with omalizumab. Mucosal Immunol 2012; 5: 267-276.

[154] Gernez Y, Tirouvanziam R., Yu G., Ghosn E.E.*et al.* Basophil CD203c levels are increased at baseline and can be used to monitor omalizumab treatment in subjects with nut allergy. Int Arch Allergy Immunol 2011; 154: 318-327.

[155] Leung DY, Sampson H.A., Yunginger J.W., Burks A.W., Jr.*et al.* Effect of anti-IgE therapy in patients with peanut allergy. N Engl J Med 13-3-2003; 348: 986-993.

[156] Sampson HA, Leung D.Y., Burks A.W., Lack G.*et al.* A phase II, randomized, doubleblind, parallelgroup, placebocontrolled oral food challenge trial of Xolair (omalizumab) in peanut allergy. J Allergy Clin Immunol 2011; 127: 1309-1310.

[157] Song Y, Qu C., Srivastava K., Yang N.*et al.* Food allergy herbal formula 2 protection against peanut anaphylactic reaction is *via* inhibition of mast cells and basophils. J Allergy Clin Immunol 2010; 126: 1208-1217.

[158] Kattan JD, Srivastava K.D., Zou Z.M., Goldfarb J.*et al.* Pharmacological and immunological effects of individual herbs in the Food Allergy Herbal Formula-2 (FAHF-2) on peanut allergy. Phytother Res 2008; 22: 651-659.

[159] Srivastava KD, Kattan J.D., Zou Z.M., Li J.H.*et al.* The Chinese herbal medicine formula FAHF-2 completely blocks anaphylactic reactions in a murine model of peanut allergy. J Allergy Clin Immunol 2005; 115: 171-178.

[160] Wisniewski JA, Li X.M. Alternative and complementary treatment for food allergy. Immunol Allergy Clin North Am 2012; 32: 135-150.

[161] Qu C, Srivastava K., Ko J., Zhang T.F.*et al.* Induction of tolerance after establishment of peanut allergy by the food allergy herbal formula-2 is associated with up-regulation of interferon-gamma. Clin Exp Allergy 2007; 37: 846-855.

[162] Srivastava KD, Qu C., Zhang T., Goldfarb J.*et al.* Food Allergy Herbal Formula-2 silences peanut-induced anaphylaxis for a prolonged posttreatment period *via* IFN-gamma-producing CD8+ T cells. J Allergy Clin Immunol 2009; 123: 443-451.

[163] Wang J, Patil S.P., Yang N., Ko J.*et al.* Safety, tolerability, and immunologic effects of a food allergy herbal formula in food allergic individuals: a randomized, double-blinded, placebo-controlled, dose escalation, phase 1 study. Ann Allergy Asthma Immunol 2010; 105: 75-84.

[164] Pochard P, Vickery B., Berin M.C., Grishin A.*et al.* Targeting Toll-like receptors on dendritic cells modifies the T(H)2 response to peanut allergens *in vitro*. J Allergy Clin Immunol 2010; 126: 92-97.

[165] Zhu FG, Kandimalla E.R., Yu D., Agrawal S. Oral administration of a synthetic agonist of Toll-like receptor 9 potently modulates peanut-induced allergy in mice. J Allergy Clin Immunol 2007; 120: 631-637.

[166] Maizels RM, Yazdanbakhsh M. Immune regulation by helminth parasites: cellular and molecular mechanisms. Nat Rev Immunol 2003; 3: 733-744.

[167] Allen JE, Maizels R.M. Diversity and dialogue in immunity to helminths. Nat Rev Immunol 2011; 11: 375-388.

[168] Smits HH, Everts B., Hartgers F.C., Yazdanbakhsh M. Chronic helminth infections protect against allergic diseases by active regulatory processes. Curr Allergy Asthma Rep 2010; 10: 3-12.

[169] Rodrigues LC, Newcombe P.J., Cunha S.S., Alcantara-Neves N.M.*et al.* Early infection with Trichuris trichiura and allergen skin test reactivity in later childhood. Clin Exp Allergy 2008; 38: 1769-1777.

[170] Fleming JO, Isaak A., Lee J.E., Luzzio C.C.*et al.* Probiotic helminth administration in relapsing-remitting multiple sclerosis: a phase 1 study. Mult Scler 2011; 17: 743-754.

[171] Bager P, Kapel C., Roepstorff A., Thamsborg S.*et al.* Symptoms after ingestion of pig whipworm Trichuris suis eggs in a randomized placebo-controlled double-blind clinical trial. PLoS One 2011; 6: e22346.

[172] Jouvin MH, Kinet J.P. Trichuris suis ova: Testing a helminth-based therapy as an extension of the hygiene hypothesis. J Allergy Clin Immunol 2012; 130: 3-10.

[173] Bashir ME, Andersen P., Fuss I.J., Shi H.N.*et al.* An enteric helminth infection protects against an allergic response to dietary antigen. J Immunol 15-9-2002; 169: 3284-3292.

[174] Cantacessi C, Young N.D., Nejsum P., Jex A.R.*et al.* The transcriptome of Trichuris suis first molecular insights into a parasite with curative properties for key immune diseases of humans. PLoS One 2011; 6: e23590.

[175] Joubert JR, van Schalkwyk D.J., Turner K.J. Ascaris lumbricoides and the human immunogenic response: enhanced IgE-mediated reactivity to common inhaled allergens. S Afr Med J 15-3-1980; 57: 409-412.

[176] Dold S, Heinrich J., Wichmann H.E., Wjst M. Ascaris-specific IgE and allergic sensitization in a cohort of school children in the former East Germany. J Allergy Clin Immunol 1998; 102: 414-420.

[177] Palmer LJ, Celedon J.C., Weiss S.T., Wang B.*et al.* Ascaris lumbricoides infection is associated with increased risk of childhood asthma and atopy in rural China. Am J Respir Crit Care Med 1-6-2002; 165: 1489-1493.

[178] Salminen S, Bouley C., Boutron-Ruault M.C., Cummings J.H.*et al.* Functional food science and gastrointestinal physiology and function. Br J Nutr 1998; 80 Suppl 1: S147-S171.

[179] Khani S, Hosseini H.M., Taheri M., Nourani M.R.*et al.* Probiotics as an alternative strategy for prevention and treatment of human diseases: a review. Inflamm Allergy Drug Targets 2012; 11: 79-89.

[180] Kailasapathy K, Chin J. Survival and therapeutic potential of probiotic organisms with reference to Lactobacillus acidophilus and Bifidobacterium spp. Immunol Cell Biol 2000; 78: 80-88.

[181] Goldin BR, Gorbach S.L. Clinical indications for probiotics: an overview. Clin Infect Dis 1-2-2008; 46 Suppl 2: S96-100.

[182] Schouten B, van Esch B.C., Hofman G.A., van Doorn S.A.*et al.* Cow milk allergy symptoms are reduced in mice fed dietary synbiotics during oral sensitization with whey. J Nutr 2009; 139: 1398-1403.

Send Orders for Reprints on reprints@benthamscience.net

CHAPTER 7

Vitamins in the Therapy of Inflammatory and Oxidative Diseases

Neena Philips*, Mathew Samuel, Harit Parakandi, Halyna Siomyk, Michael Ret, Sesha Gopal, Hui Jia and Hossam Shahin

School of Natural Sciences, Fairleigh Dickinson University, Teaneck, NJ 07666, USA

Abstract: The pathophysiology of several diseases, including allergy and asthma, is linked to increased reactive oxygen or nitrogen species and inflammatory cytokines. These oxidative and inflammatory mediators in turn alter the organization and functioning of the extracellular matrix (ECM). Hence anti-oxidative and anti-inflammatory vitamins may alleviate the pathology.

The etiological factors that produce inflammation and oxidative stress are intrinsic and environmental. The inflammatory and oxidative process consists of the breakdown of membrane lipids to generate important inflammatory mediators (prostaglandins, platelet activating factor) that activate immune cells, degranulate eosinophils, and mediate vascular alterations. The vascular changes are also from tissue damage, which induces plasma mediators by the kinin, fibrinolytic, and clotting pathways. The activated immune cells secrete three predominant inflammatory cytokines, tumor necrosis factor-α (TNF-α), interleukin-1 (IL-1), and interleukin-6 (IL-6). Collectively, the lipid mediators, plasma mediators and inflammatory cytokines facilitate infiltration of immune cells into tissue, their activation and respiratory burst to release reactive oxygen and nitrogen species: all of which cause breakdown of the structural extracellular matrix proteins, including collagen and elastin, and the stimulation of proteolytic enzymes such as elastases and collagenases. In addition, these mediators activate the inflammatory transcription factor NF-κB to act at the gene level.

Vitamins, such as ascorbate, lutein, and nicotinamide, exhibit anti-inflammatory and anti-oxidative properties and effects. Ascorbate is a potent antioxidant physiologically *via* the scavenging of reactive oxygen species (ROS), reactive nitrogen species and lipid hydro peroxides. Ascorbate also regenerates other cellular antioxidants such as vitamin E, glutathione (GSH) and beta-carotene from their radical species. Lutein (a non-vitamin A carotenoid) accumulates in the macula of the eye, where it prevents macular degeneration through the scavenging of ROS. Nicotinamide inhibits inflammatory cytokines and plasma mediators, and in addition generates nicotinamide adenine dinucleotide for energy production. In addition, research in our laboratory suggests beneficial regulation of the ECM by these vitamins.

***Address correspondence to Neena Philips:** Fairleigh Dickinson University, Teaneck, NJ 07666, USA; Tel: 201 692 6494; Fax: 201 692 7349; E-mail: nphilips@fdu.edu; neenaphilips@optonline.net

Ascorbate, lutein, and nicotinamide as supplements in the therapy of allergy or allergy may be beneficial in the prevention of the fragmentation of the collagen/elastin network, edema, vascular alterations, and inflammation in the lungs and skin.

Keywords: Inflammation, collagen, elastin, matrixmetalloproteinases, signal-transduction, nicotinamide, lutein, ascorbate, skin, lung.

INTRODUCTION

The biochemistry and molecular biology of inflammatory lung and skin diseases, such as asthma, eczema, emphysema, chronic obstructive pulmonary disease (COPD), acne, dermatitis or photoaging, are based on the cellular response to chronic inflammation and oxidative stress. The cellular response to inflammation and oxidative stress is through the activation of several signal transduction pathways, which in turn activate the expression of proteases that remodel the extracellular matrix (ECM) and thereby compromise the tissue structure and function. Anti-oxidant and anti-inflammatory vitamins may alleviate inflammatory diseases.

This chapter is a review of (i) inflammation and oxidative stress; (ii) ECM proteins and their remodeling; (ii) mediating signal transduction pathways; and (iv) vitamins (nicotinamide, lutein, ascorbate) that could alleviate inflammatory lung and skin pathology.

INFLAMMATION AND OXIDATIVE STRESS

The mediators of inflammation and oxidative stress overwhelm the cellular antioxidant capacity to protect tissue from damage (Figs. **1** and **2**).

Inflammation

While acute inflammation is a response to tissue repair, chronic inflammation is associated with pathology. The inflammatory mediators are released from leukocytes, damaged tissue, and endothelial lining of blood vessels. They include the plasma mediators (bradykinin, plasmin, fibrin); lipid mediators (prostaglandins, leukotrienes and platelet activating factor); and the inflammatory cytokines (interleukin-1 (IL-1), interleukin-6 (IL-6), and tumor necrosis factor- α

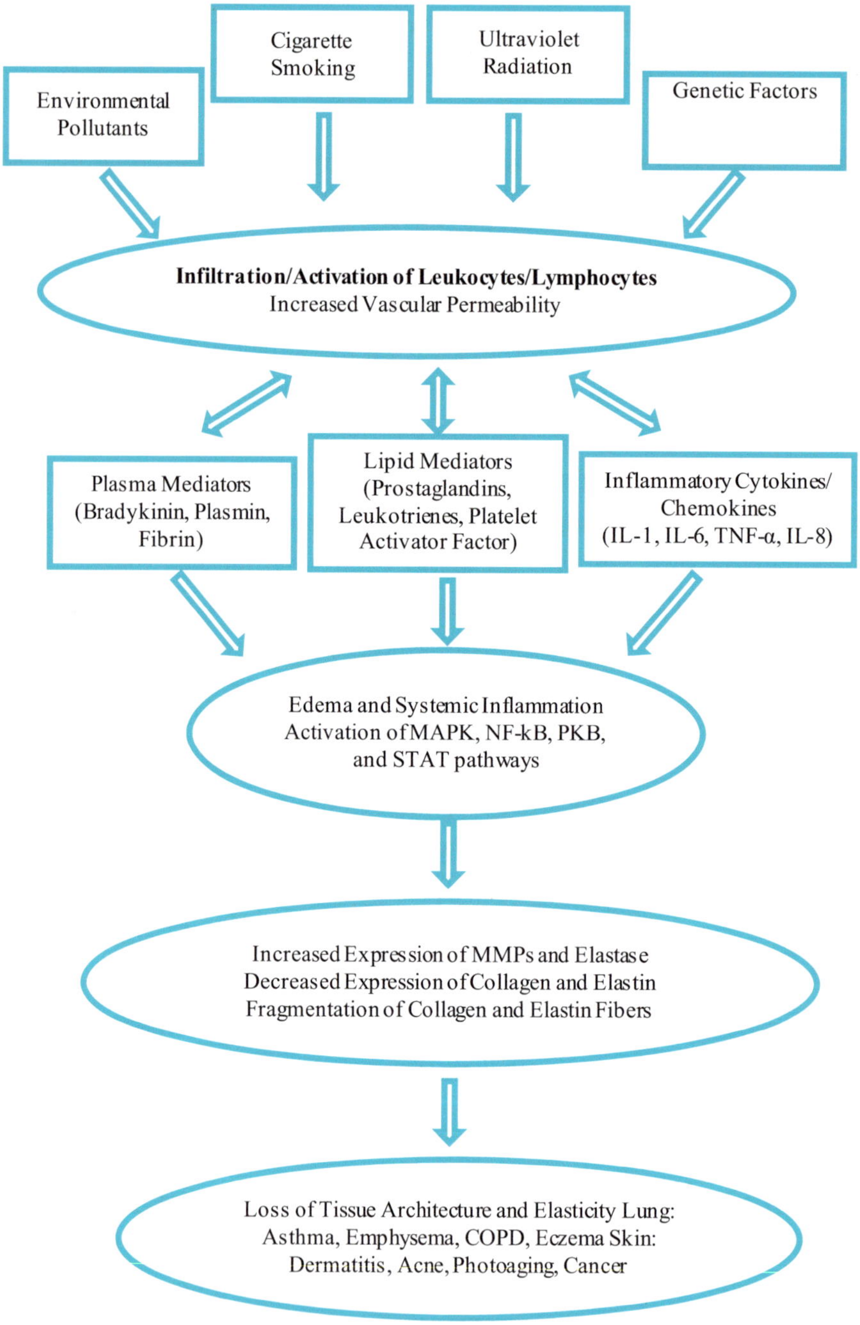

Figure 1: Inflammation in the mediation of the loss of tissue architecture and function. TNF-α: tumor necrosis factor-α, IL: interleukin, MAPK: mitogen activated protein kinase, NF: nuclear factor, PKB: protein kinase B, STAT: signal transduction and activation of transcription, MMP: matrixmetalloproteinase.

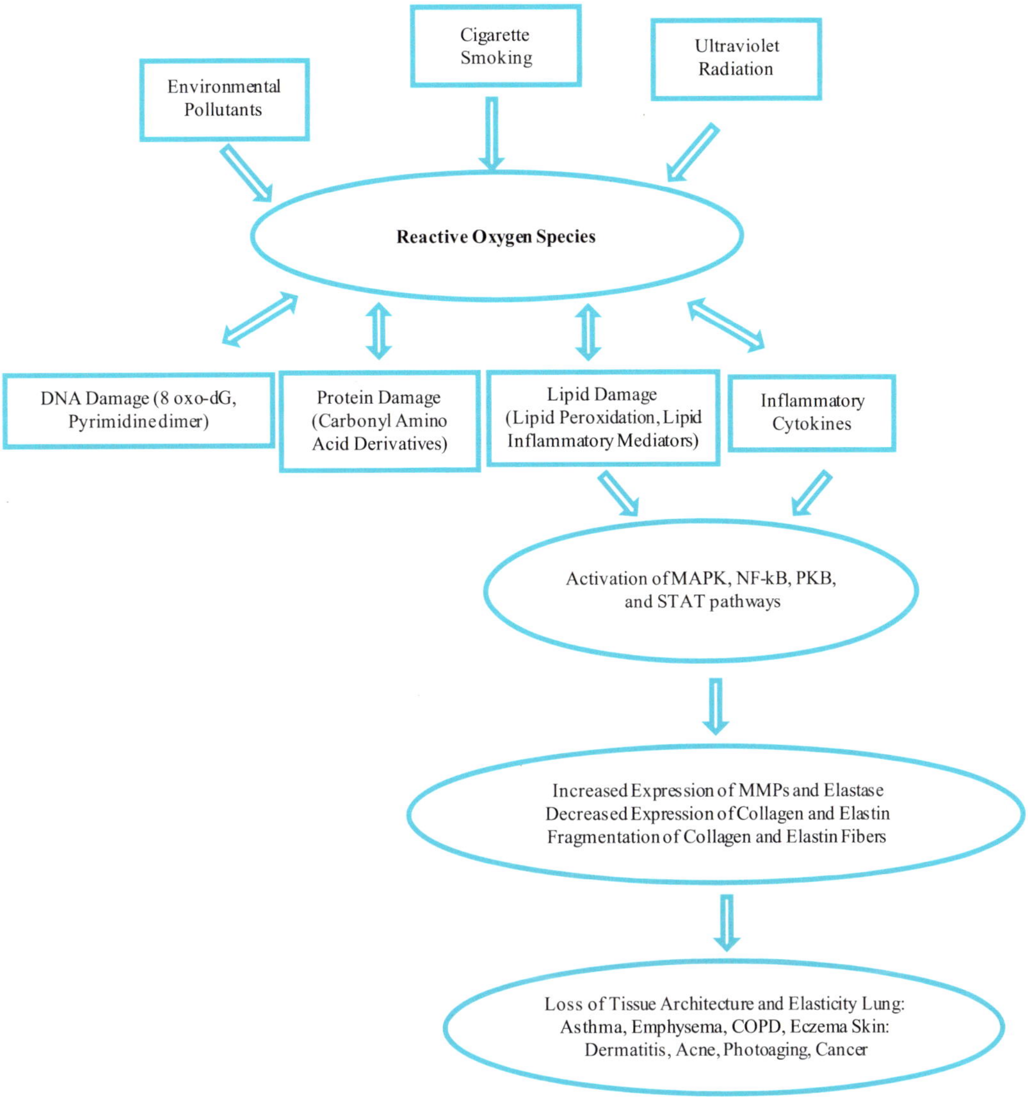

Figure 2: Oxidative stress in the mediation of the loss of tissue architecture and function. TNF-α: tumor necrosis factor-α, IL: interleukin, MAPK: mitogen activated protein kinase, NF: nuclear factor, PKB: protein kinase B, STAT: signal transduction and activation of transcription, MMP: matrixmetalloproteinase.

(TNF-α)). The mediators collectively increase vascular permeability, leukocyte chemotaxis, activation of the classical complement pathway, and the release of histamines from mast cells [1]. The chemotaxis of leukocyte is through the activation of its integrins that bind to the induced endothelial cell intercellular adhesion molecule-1 (ICAM-1) to invaginate into the tissue [2]. The inflammatory cytokines are also responsible for systemic inflammation; they causes the liver to switch from the expression of albumin and transthyretin to the expression of acute phase proteins such as the C-reactive protein, serum amyloid A, and fibrinogen [1]. The counteractive transforming growth factor-β (TGF-β) promotes the proliferation of fibroblasts and deposition of the extracellular matrix (ECM) for tissue repair; however it causes fibrosis with chronic inflammation [1].

The bronchiolar epithelium in COPD contains increased numbers of macrophages and mast cells, and airway inflammation limits airflow in asthma [3, 4]. Inflammation in skin is largely from ultraviolet (UV) radiation, which induces prostaglandins, histamine release and phospholipase activity [5]. The solar UV UVB radiation (290-320 nm) penetrates up to the dermis and activates the tissue leukocytes to generate prostaglandins and inflammatory cytokines [6].

Oxidative Stress

The tissue infiltered leukocytes produce reactive oxygen species (ROS) and reactive nitrogen species; as well as peroxidases that amplify oxidative events in asthma [1]. In addition, ROS is produced from the passage of electrons to oxygen during the process of aerobic electron transport and oxidative phosphorylation for ATP synthesis. The ROS in turn activate the expression of inflammatory cytokines. Hence, an amplified cascade results from the production of ROS by inflammation, and the formation of inflammatory mediators by ROS.

The cellular ROS include superoxide, hydroxyl radicals, hydrogen peroxide, and singlet oxygen, produced by the mitochondria and the tissue infiltration of leukocytes. The ROS cause direct harm to DNA, proteins and lipids. The DNA damage is observed as 8-oxo-7, 8-dihydro-2'-deoxyguanosine (8-oxo-dG) that generates a GC to TA transversion mutation during replication, and as pyrimidine dimers [6, 7]. UV radiation also damages mitochondrial DNA, which could lead to senescence and increased oxidative stress [8]. The oxidative damage to proteins is detected as carbonyl amino acid derivatives [9]. The oxidative damage to lipids results in lipid peroxidation and the generation of lipid inflammatory mediators, and oxidation products such as malonaldehyde [10, 11].

One of the major causes of oxidative stress of the skin is exposure to ultraviolet (UV) radiation. The solar UVC radiation (200-290nm) is absorbed by the atmospheric ozone but could penetrate the upper skin surface, and UVB radiation causes DNA damage [6]. UVA radiation (320-400nm) penetrates deeper into the dermis and causes oxidative damage through the generation of ROS, which is its predominant mechanism [6]. The oxidative damage causes cell-cycle arrest and apoptosis, and in the skin it leads to erythema and premature aged appearance.

In cellular oxidative damage, the ROS outbalance the cellular antioxidant system. The counteracting cellular antioxidants include enzymes such as catalase and glutathione peroxidase, and small molecules such as glutathione, ascorbate, α-tocopherol, and carotene [9]. Glutathione has been reported to control cellular pro-inflammatory processes [4].

EXTRACELLULAR MATRIX

The predominant structural ECM proteins, which provide tissue integrity and function, are collagen and elastin. The ECM is remodeled primarily by the matrixmetalloproteinases and elastases, in physiology and pathology.

Collagen

Collagens are central to the formation of fibrillar, microfibrillar, basement membrane, and other structures of the ECM. There are about 28 types of collagen. They are homo or hetero trimeric triple helical proteins. The triple helix is formed by repeating Gly-X-Y motifs, with X and Y being proline or hydroxyproline [2]. The unique properties of the different collagens are based on the lengths of the triple helical segments, interruptions to the triple helix, and amino acid modifications. Collagens may be classified as fibrillar collagens (types I, II, III, V), fibril associated collagens (types VI, IX), sheet forming and anchoring collagens (types IV, VII, XV), transmembrane collagens (types XIII, XVII), and host defense collagens [2]. The basement membrane is composed largely of type IV collagen, and the interstitial collagen fibers consist of the type I (90%), III, V, and VII collagens [9]. Collagen is synthesized primarily by the fibroblasts. Skin aging is associated with fibroblast senescence, and reduced synthesis and increased degradation of collagen fibers [12-15].

Elastin

The elastin fibers provide stretch-recoil properties to tissues and are vital to tissue function of resilience, expansion and contraction. They are composed predominantly of an elastin core (90%) and surrounded by fibrillin microfibrils [16].

Elastin is expressed as soluble hydrophobic tropoelastin, rich in proline, valine, lysine, alanine, glycine, leucine and isoleucine. It is targeted to the cell surface, transferred to the microfibril scaffold, and cross linked by lysyl oxidase and transglutamise [17-19]. Lysyl oxidase catalyzes the deamination of the lysine residues in elastin to form desmosines, and transglutaminase crosslinks elastin to the microfibrils [17-19].

Elastogenesis is directed by the microfibils, which are composed of fibrillin (FBN). There are three known FBNs (FBN 1-3), though FBN-1 is the most abundant in mature tissue and FBN2 is associated with elastin [20, 21]. The FBNs are cysteine rich highly disulphide bonded glycoproteins, with calcium binding epidermal growth factor like domains and structured repeats [18]. They are secreted in pro-forms, processed extracellularly by furine/PACE like activities, and assembled as parallel bundles of head to tail monomers followed by calcium binding and organization into microfibrils [18, 22, 23]. The assembly of the microfibrils is with the aid of heparin, heparan sulphate and fibronectin, and it associates with other glycoproteins such as microfibril associated glycoproteins and fibrillins [18, 22]. The microfibrils sequester transforming growth factor-β (TGFβ) in its latent form, and interact with the cell surface integrins through their RGD (Arg-Gly-Asp) domains [24, 25].

The elastic fibers are destroyed in pathology. The fragmentation of the elastic fiber system results in disorganized elastotic material, with altered architecture, and resultant loss of tissue elasticity. The oxidative damage to elastin includes protein oxidation, pathological cross-links, advanced glycation end products (AGE), increased tissue stiffness, calcification, L-aspartate to D-aspartate racemization, and mechanical fatigue [26-30].

Elastin is a major component of the adult lung, and is essential for alveogenesis [31]. Defects in the alveolar elastic fibers are associated with pathology such as emphysema [31]. The reduced lung elasticity (with aging as well as pathology like emphysema and COPD) results in reduced forced expiratory volume, reduced forced vital capacity, dilatation of the alveolus, and increased alveolar wall thickness; all of which could result in lung failure [32-35].

The loss of proper elastic fibers manifests as deep rough wrinkles in photoaged skin [28]. UV radiation depletes the microfibrillar network in the epidermal-dermal layer and the dermis, which contributes to the aberrant elastic fibers and wrinkles in photo aged skin [36, 37]. Elastin is also reduced with intrinsic aging and results in the loss of skin firmness and resiliency [12, 13, 38, 39].

The remodeling of the elastin fibers is by the serine protease neutrophil elastase, and the matrixmetalloproteinases (MMP) [40, 41]. The constitutive expression of the MMPs results in the fragmentation of elastin fiber proteins with age. The fragmentation is accelerated by the increased expression of elastases and MMPs in response to inflammation and oxidative stress; associated with emphysema, COPD, and photoaged skin [42-44].

Matrixmetalloproteinases/Elastases

The MMPs or matrixins are central to the remodeling of the ECM. The MMPs are expressed as prepro-enzymes and secreted as inactive pro-MMPs [45]. Most of the MMPs are composed of a propeptide domain with a unique cysteine that links it to the catalytic zinc in the inactive form, a catalytic domain with a zinc binding motif, and a C-terminal hemopexin like domain that is essential for its catalytic activity [46-48]. Proteases, such as plasmin, activate MMPs through proteolysis of the pro-peptide domain [48].

The MMPs have been classified on the basis of their substrate specificity: the interstitial collagenases (*e.g.,* MMP-1) cleave the fibrillar collagens, the gelatinases (MMP-2, 9) cleave the basement membrane collagens and elastin, the stromelysines (MMP-3, 10) degrade the basement membrane proteins, the membrane-type MMPs with a transmembrane domain act on pro-MMPs and fibrillar collagens, and the other MMPs include the matrilysin (MMP-7) and metalloelastase (MMP-12) that degrade the basement membrane proteins and elastin [45-48].

MMPs have also been classified on the basis of their promoters: group I MMPs (MMP-1, 3, 7, 9, 10, 12, 13, 19 and 26) contain TATA box and activator protein-1 (AP-1 site), group II MMPs (MMP-8, 11, 21) without the AP-1 site; and group III (MMP-2, 14, 28) without the TATA box and AP-1 site [49].

The pro-and active forms of MMPs are inhibited by the tissue inhibitors of MMPs or TIMPs [48, 50]. The TIMPs (TIMP-1, 2, 3, 4) bind unspecifically to MMPs, though TIMP-1 has preference for MMP-1 and TIMP-2 for MMP2 [48]. Conversely, MMP-2 is activated by TIMP-2 in collaboration with MT1-MMP [48]. The genes for TIMPs 1-4 have been mapped to chromosomes X, 17, 22, and 3 [50]. TIMP-1 and TIMP-3 are inducible, TIMP-2 is constitutive, and TIMP-4 is restricted in their expression to specific tissues [50]. The structure of TIMPs consists of an N-terminal conserved region essential to binding to the active site of MMPs, 6-loops, and a junction between the N-and C-terminal domains [50]. Most of the tissue destruction is from the increased expression or activation of MMPs and reduced expression of TIMPs. Further, the basal levels of MMPs are higher in aged skin relative to young skin [51].

SIGNAL TRANSDUCTION PATHWAYS

The receptors activated in inflammatory and oxidative stress response, include those of TNF-α, IL-1, PAF and insulin, and the pathways that are activated include the mitogen activated protein kinase (MAPK), the NF-kB/p65, the Akt/Protein kinase B (PKB), and the JAK/STAT (Signal Transduction and Activation of Transcription) [1, 2, 6, 9, 52].

MAPK Pathway

The MAPK pathway is comprised of the extracellular signal-regulated kinase 1/2 (ERK1/2), c-Jun-N-terminal-kinase, and p38 proteins. The activation of MAP kinase pathway, through the receptor tyrosine kinase, results in the activation of transcription factor AP-1 [9]. The transcription factor AP-1 stimulates the transcription of several MMPs that collectively degrade the ECM, such as MMP-1 that degrades interstitial collagenase, MMP-2/9 that further degrade interstitial collagen and the basement membrane, and MMP-3 that degrades the type IV collagen and activates pro-MMP1 [42]. Further, AP-1 inhibits the transcription of type I collagen gene [9]. Hence, the damage to the ECM and tissue integrity is from the reduced expression of the structural ECM proteins as well as enhanced degradation by MMPs. The JNK and p38 pathways play a major role in the UVA radiation mediated increase in AP-1 and COX-2 expression, and are targets for chemoprevention of skin aging and cancer [53].

NF-κB Pathway

The NF-κB pathway is activated through the activation of cytoplasmic I-kB kinase by infection, cellular stress, and inflammatory cytokines. Active I-kB kinase phosphorylates and degrades I-kB, the inhibitor of NF-kB (p65/p50 heterodimeric protein) transcription factor [2].The release of NF-kB, from its inhibitor (I-kB), results in its translocation to the nucleus to activate nitric oxide synthase (for the production of nitric oxide to kill infection and dilate blood vessels), the inflammatory cytokines, cyclooxygenase (COX-2, for the synthesis of prostaglandins), and anti-apoptotic proteins (to prevent cell death in response to the cellular stress) [2, 52].

The NF-kB activation is redox sensitive, and its activation is associated with UV radiation (UVA and UVB) mediated oxidative modification of cellular membrane components, [42, 54]. The activation of NF-kB is associated with the activation of histone acetylase (HAT) in inflammatory lung diseases [55, 56]. The anti-inflammatory effects of corticosteroids include the recruitment of histone deacetylases (HDAC) to inhibit HAT [57].

PKB Pathway

Active PKB or Akt, a serine threonine kinase, phosphorylates and inactivates pro-apoptotic proteins BAD and FOXO 3A through their sequestration by protein 14-3-3 [58].The sequestration of BAD allows for the anti-apoptotic Bcl2/Bcl-xl to inactivate the mitochondrial membrane ion channel protein BAX, prevent the release of cytochrome C into the cytoplasm to bind to Apaf-1, and thereby prevent the stimulation of the caspase cascade for apoptosis [2, 58, 59].

STAT Pathway

The cytokines secreted by leukocytes and lymphocytes influence each other and the activities of numerous cells involved in the immune response, such as B-cell,

T-cells, natural killer cells, macrophages, granulocytes, and hematopoietic stem cells [1]. Many of the cytokines bind to their cytokine receptors on cell surfaces to activate JAK kinase that activates STAT transcription factors through phosphorylation [2].The phosphorylation of STAT results in its dimerization and translocation into the nucleus to modulate gene expression [2]. The different cytokines activate different STAT proteins; STAT5 induction by erythropoietin in erythroid progenitor cells activates Bcl-x_L to prevent apoptosis, and allows for cell proliferation [2].

Inflammation and oxidative stress stimulates diverse intracellular pathways and the end result of cell proliferation, differentiation or apoptosis are dependent on the strength and duration of each signaling molecule [2]. Further, the diverse cytokines exhibit synergy, redundancy, pleiotrophy or antagonism in their regulation of cellular activities [1]. There is also cross-talk between oxidative-stress and inflammatory mediators. Hydrogen peroxide and TNF-α induce histone acetylation and subsequently AP-1 and NF-kB transcription factors [4, 60]. These transcription factors stimulate IL-8 gene, and reduce glutathione (GSH) levels in alveolar epithelial cells [4, 60].

VITAMINS IN THE MANAGEMENT OF INFLAMMATORY DISEASES

Corticosteroids have been traditionally used to treat inflammatory disorders. It crosses the cell membrane, binds to its receptor/transcription factor, and translocates into the nucleus to induce the transcription of the NF-kB inhibitor (IkB) to reduce inflammation [1]. The active ingredient of the nonsteroidal anti-inflammatory drug (NSAIDs) is salicylate, which inhibits the cyclooxygenase enzymes (COX-1 and COX-2) and thereby the synthesis of prostaglandins and thromboxanes [1]. The newer NSAIDs are specific COX-2 inhibitors, which reduce inflammation without causing GI tract damage [1].

The etiology of inflammatory diseases is inflammation and oxidative stress. Hence a beneficial preventive or supplemental regimen to lung or skin health is vitamins, which provide antioxidant and anti-inflammatory benefits. Three such vitamins are ascorbate, lutein and nicotinamide, which have been investigated in our laboratory.

Ascorbate

Ascorbate (Vitamin C) is essential for collagen formation, and serves as an antioxidant and anti-carcinogenic supplement. The food sources of ascorbate include fruits and vegetables, and a chemically identical L-ascorbate in synthesized in association with recombinant DNA technology [61].

Ascorbate is most known for its role in collagen formation and the prevention of scurvy. Ascorbate increases the transcription of collagen genes and the stability of the formed mRNA [62]. It is a cofactor for collagen and elastin hydroxylases that hydroxylates proline residues, essential for the collagen helix formation and secretion. A deficiency of ascorbate leads to reduced collagen expression, and an unstable collagen structure that undergoes increased cellular degradation [62, 63]. The extracellular matrix derived from human pulmonary fibroblasts contains twice as much collagen after ascorbate pretreatment [64]. Increased deposition of the extracellular matrix has been postulated to the encapsulation of tumors. The mechanism to the induction of collagen by ascorbate may also be through its stimulation of TGF-β, which stimulates collagen [12, 38].

Ascorbate acts as an antioxidant by donating an electron to a free radical and thereby inactivating it [65]. The resulting ascorbyl radical has low reactivity from resonance stabilization of the unpaired electron and is physiologically converted to ascorbate or dehydroascorbate. Ascorbate is transported into cells by the sodium-dependent vitamin C transporter or in its reduced form (dehydroascorbate) by the glucose transporters [66]. Mutations in glucose transporters result in defective collagen and elastin, from the lack of intracellular ascorbate [67]. Ascorbate acts as a potent antioxidant in the body by scavenging all of the cellular ROS or RNS, through its reducing properties, increasing ascorbate transporters, and generating antioxidants such as glutathione, vitamin E and β-carotene [65, 68, 69]. The direct inhibition of the oxidation of ABTS® (2, 2'-azino-di-[3-ethylbenzthiazoline sulphonate]) to ABTS® · + by metmyoglobin is used as an index of the antioxidant potential of agents (Cayman Chemical, Antioxidant assay kit). Ascorbate inhibits ABTS oxidation, indicative of its antioxidant activity (Fig. **3**).

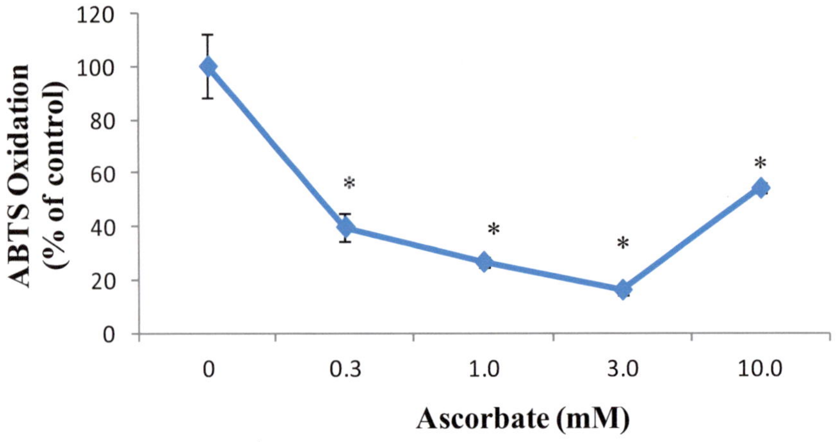

Figure 3: Direct significant inhibition of ABTS oxidation by ascorbate at 0.3 to 10 mM (*: $p<0.05$).

Oxidative stress from smoking or inflammatory diseases causes the depletion of ascorbate in the lungs [65]. The antioxidant nature of ascorbate is observed in lung repair in a mice emphysema model, with the stimulation of antioxidant enzymes (SOD, catalase) and the inhibition of inflammatory cytokines (TNF-α) [70]. Skin atrophy, with reduced hydroxyproline, and degeneration of collagen/eleastin, occurs in (CuZnSOD)-deficient mice and is reversed by ascorbate treatment, inferring the removal of superoxide radicals [71].

The antioxidant activity of ascorbate also retards the growth of gastric, mammary and renal tumors, through its chemical property, the inhibition of the intracellular oxidants or the oxidation of estrogen to active metabolites, and inhibits the invasiveness of gastric, oral and pulmonary cancers, as well as fibrosarcoma and melanoma [72-77]. Ascorbate reduces oxidative stress and protects DNA from ROS mediated mutations by reducing superoxides in a gastric carcinoma rat model [75]. It acts in synergy with vitamin K in the inhibition of tumors *in vitro* and *in vivo* [78]. The lower concentrations of ascorbate significantly inhibit renal, melanoma, and endometrial cancer cell viability; with stimulation of apoptotic proteins (p53, p21, Bax, caspase-3) in melanoma cells [79, 80]. The regulation of cell growth by ascorbate is by apoptotic and non-apoptotic mechanisms [81]. The increase in the expression of p53 and its downstream p21 activates the pro-apoptotic Bax that induces caspases and apoptosis [2, 82].

Ascorbate reduces inflammatory diseases through the removal of oxidants generated as a result of inflammation [83]. Ascorbate through its essence for collagen formation and its antioxidant activity is a beneficial supplement in the management of inflammatory and oxidative-stress associated diseases.

Lutein

Lutein, a carotenoid, has sunscreen, antioxidant, and anti-inflammatory properties. It protects the eye, skin, and is anticarcinogenic.

Carotenoids have been used for systemic photoprotection because of its antioxidant activity. The carotenoids occur naturally mostly in green or yellow leafy vegetables and fruits [84-88]. They have a sunscreen effect through the absorption of some of the wavelengths of visible sunlight, and the reduction of the chemiluminescence signal of UV radiation [89, 90]. Increased maternal consumption of carotenoids lowers the development of eczema and atopic dermatitis in offspring [91, 92]. Vitamin A as β-carotene has potent antioxidative ability independently or in combination with vitamin C, α-tocopherol (vitamin-E), zinc, and selenium [93-95]. Lutein (xanthophyll carotenoid) is a non-provitamin A carotenoid, which is structurally related to ß-carotene, and has better antioxidant properties than β-carotene; through the stimulation of the antioxidant enzymes catalase and superoxide dismutase or membrane protection from attack by free radicals [96-98].

The leading cause of blindness in the aged is age-related macular degeneration (AMD) [87]. Lutein and zeaxanthin, lutein's coexistent isomer, accumulate in the fovea centralis/macula lutea of the human retina and prevent AMD [84-87, 90, 99]. Lutein/zeaxanthin filter the high-energy wavelengths of solar radiation, and as antioxidants protect the eye by quenching reactive oxygen species [84-87, 90]. A lutein binding protein (SR-B1) has been identified in the retina, for the uptake of lutein, and its transport in the blood by high-density lipoprotein (HDL) has connected the regulation of SR-B1 and HDL levels with AMD [100]. Lutein has an anti-inflammatory effect through the suppression of NF-kB, iNOS, and COX-2 in several ocular inflammatory models as well as in a cellular oxidative stress model [100, 101].

Lutein accumulates in the skin, to provide anti-oxidant and anti-inflammatory protection, as well as to filter solar radiation [90, 102]. Lutein inhibits the expression of MMP-1 (transcriptionally) and MMP-2 in dermal fibroblasts, indicating prevention of interstitial collagen degradation as well as the remodeling of the basement membrane [38]. It reverses some of the loss in cellular viability and membrane integrity in UV radiation exposed skin cells [38]. The effects of lutein are similar to those of superoxide dismutase (SOD), in dermal fibroblasts, indicating the inhibition of cellular ROS as one of its mechanism [38]. The antioxidative capacity of lutein is represented below (Fig. **4**).

Carotenoids have cancer protective effects following metabolism [86]. Lutein in combination with zeaxanthin inhibits photoaging and photocarcinogenesis [103, 104]. The combination inhibits tissue infiltration of mast cells, acute edema, and epidermal thickening or hyperproliferation in a mice photoaging model; and reduces tumor multiplicity and volume in a mouse photocarcinogenesis model [103, 104]. Diets rich in phytonutrients, including lutein, improve skin health reduce the markers of UV damage such as lipid peroxidation, DNA damage, erythema, and MMP expression [105]. There is an inverse correlation between lutein in diet and melanoma risk [106]. Lutein's anticarcinogenic properties have also been reported in several other cancers, such as hepatoma, breast and colon cancer [86, 103, 107-109]. Lutein and other carotenoids have been documented in reducing lung cancer risks [110].

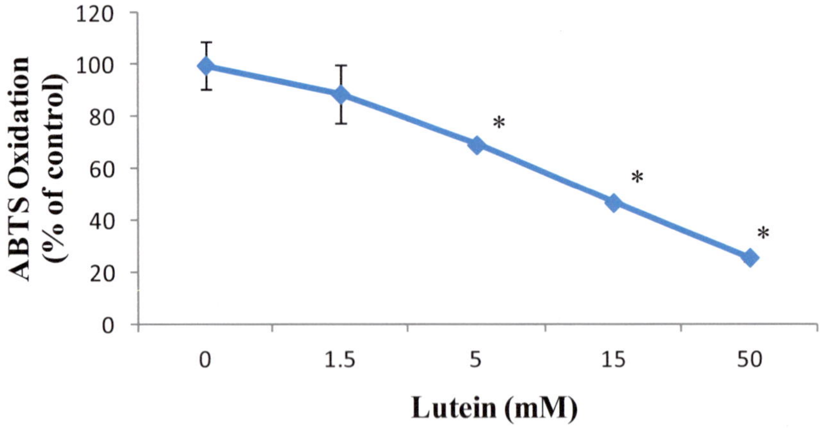

Figure 4: Direct significant inhibition of ABTS oxidation by lutein at 5 to 50mM (*: $p<0.05$).

The sunscreen, antioxidant and anti-inflammatory properties make lutein a recommended supplement in the prevention of oxidative stress and inflammatory diseases.

Nicotinamide

Nicotimamide is essential to cellular metabolism, cellular stress response, cell survival, and inactivation of the oxidative and inflammatory MAPK and NF-kB pathways.

Nicotinamide (pyridine-3-carboxamide) is the amide derivative of niacin or Vitamin B_3, obtained from diet as niacin or nicotinic acid, or through synthesis from tryptophan [11, 58, 111]. It is a precursor to the coenzymes nicotinamide adenine dinucleotide (NAD^+) and its phosphorylated form $NADP^+$, which are essential to catabolism for ATP synthesis and to anabolism for the synthesis of biomolecules. Nicotinamide promotes glucose uptake by stimulating the translocation of GLUT 4 glucose transporters from the cytoplasm to the membrane. It does so by phosphorylating and inactivating the AS160 protein, which sequesters the GLUT 4 transporters in vesicles in the cytoplasm.

NAD^+ protects cells from cellular stress by regulating sirtulin 1 (SIRT 1), a histone deacetylase, and by serving as a substrate for poly (ADP-ribose) polymerase (PARP) [11, 58, 112]. SIRT 1 facilitates cellular stress response, and PARP plays a role in DNA repair and genomic stability [11, 58, 112]. Nicotinamide also facilitates cell survival through the activation of protein kinase B (PKB or Akt) [58, 59].

Nicotinamide inactivates the MAPK and NF-kB pathways [59, 113]. It inhibits the phosphorylation of the signal mediators (MAP kinases, IkB kinase) and thereby the expression of inflammatory cytokines and lipid mediators [59, 113, 114]. Further, nicotinamide or NADPH can quench ROS, inhibit NADPH oxidase that causes accumulation of ROS, regenerate reduced glutathione, and inhibit lipid peroxidation and photosensitization induced cell toxicity [111, 115]. Nicotinamide caused a dose dependent inhibition of ABTS oxidation (Fig. **5**).

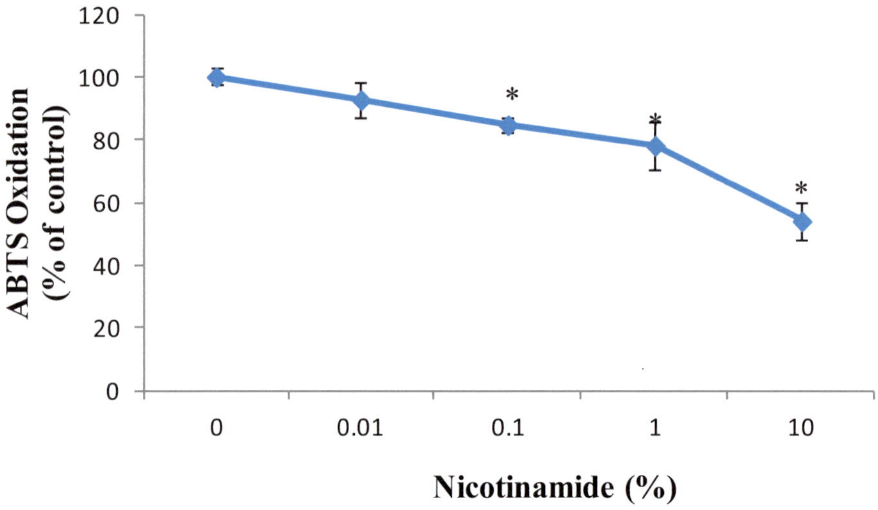

Figure 5: Direct significant inhibition of ABTS oxidation by nicotinamide at 0.1 to 10 % of a 50mg/ml nicotinamide solution (*: $p<0.05$).

Nicotinamide has been incorporated into skin care creams. It has sunscreen properties, and improves facial appearance through the reduction of hyperigmented spots, redness and wrinkles [116, 117]. We have investigated the mechanism to the beneficial effects of nicotinamide in dermal fibroblasts (unpublished data). Nicotinamide stimulates the expression of collagen (types I, III, V), elastic fiber components (elastin, fibrillin), and inhibits the expression and activities of MMPs (unpublished data).

Nicotinamide through its essence to cellular metabolism, cellular stress response, cell survival, and inactivation of the oxidative and inflammatory MAPK and NF-kB pathways improves the structural integrity and functioning of the ECM and thereby could to the health of the lungs and skin.

CONCLUSIONS

A circular loop of inflammation and oxidative stress is central to inflammatory diseases. Inflammation is caused by activation of leukocytes, and associated inflammatory mediators such as the plasma mediators (bradykinin, plasmin, fibrin); lipid mediators (prostaglandins, leukotrienes and platelet activating factor); and the inflammatory cytokines (IL-1, IL-6, IL-8, and TNF-α). Oxidative stress and oxidative damage to cellular components are largely from increased formation of reactive oxygen species (superoxide, hydroxyl radicals, hydrogen peroxide, and singlet oxygen), and reduced cellular antioxidants (glutathione, SOD, catalase, β-carotene, ascorbate). The consequence is the activation of signaling pathways (MAPK, NF-kB/p65, Akt/ PKB, and JAK/STAT), and altered expression of genes that lead to atrophy of the structural ECM (collagen and elastin) through the increased expression and activity of proteases (MMPs and elastases).

A preventive or supplemental regimen to skin, lung or systemic health is the removal of inflammation and oxidative stress. Vitamins with their antioxidant and anti-inflammatory properties would support a preventive and treatment role. A metanalysis of data on vitamins in chronic diseases indicate the need of the measurement of serum levels of vitamins as well as vitamin supplementation in the prevention of diseases such as coronary heart disease, retinal vascular occlusive disease, Alzheimer's, cirrhosis, osteoporosis, diabetes and cancer [118-123]. A metanalysis of data from 1966 to 2002 on 9 vitamins, including folate, vitamin B6, vitamin B12, vitamin C, and lycopene associate reduced risk of coronary heart disease with the B vitamins, and prostate cancer with lycopene [118]. Additional metanalysis indicate that folate and vitamin B12 prevent retinal vascular occlusive disease, consumption of fruits and vegetables prevent coronary heart disease, and vitamin C prevents age related macular degeneration [119-121]. The observational data indicate inverse relationships between vitamins and oxidative damage, vitamin C and coronary heart disease, and β-carotene and lung cancer [122]. A metanalysis of nicotinamide treatment for insulin dependent diabetes mellitus has shown beneficial effects of nicotinamide through the preservation of pancreatic beta cells [123]. Collectively, it is inferred that vitamins protect against chronic diseases.

Three vitamins that have been reported as beneficial in our laboratory are ascorbate, lutein, and nicotinamide. Ascorbate is a must for collagen formation and has antioxidant activity, including the regeneration of other antioxidants. Lutein has been proven to prevent macular degeneration, and has sunscreen, antioxidant, anti-inflammatory, and ECM strengthening properties. Nicotinamide is essential to cellular metabolism, cellular stress response, cell survival, and inactivates the oxidative and inflammatory MAPK and NF-kB pathways while stimulating the structural ECM for tissue structure and function.

ACKNOWLEDGEMENTS

Declared none.

CONFLICT OF INTEREST

The author(s) confirm that this chapter content has no conflict of interest.

REFERENCES

[1] Kindt TJ, Goldsby RA, Osborne BA. Leukocyte activation and migration. In Kuby Immunology. 6th ed. W. H. Freeman and Company 2007; pp 327-347

[2] Lodish H, Berk A, Kaiser CA, *et al.* Cell Signaling, Integrating cells into tissue. In Molecular Cell Biology. 6th ed. W.H Freeman and Company 2008; pp 665-712, 801-846

[3] de Boer WI, van Schadewijk A, Sont JK, *et al.* Transforming growth factor beta1 and recruitment of macrophages and mast cells in airways in chronic obstructive pulmonary disease. Am J Respir Crit Care Med 1998; 158: 1951-7.

[4] Rahman I. Antioxidant therapeutic advances in COPD. Ther Adv Respir Dis 2008; 2: 351-74.

[5] Hruza LL, Pentland AP. Mechanisms of UV-induced inflammation. Invest Dermatol 1993; 100: 35S-41S.

[6] Nichols JA, Katiyar SK. Skin photoprotection by natural polyphenols: anti-inflammatory, antioxidant and DNA repair mechanisms. Arch Dermatol Res 2010; 302: 71-83.

[7] Melnikova VO, Ananthaswamy HN. Cellular and molecular events leading to the development of skin cancer. Mutation Research 2005; 571: 91–106.

[8] Krutmann J. The role of UVA rays in skin aging. Eur J Dermatol 2001; 11: 170-1.

[9] Callaghan TM, Wilhelm KP. A review of ageing and an examination of clinical methods in the assessment of ageing skin. Part I: Cellular and molecular perspectives of skin ageing. Int J Cosmet Sci 2008; 30: 313-22.

[10] Briganti S, Picardo M. Antioxidant activity, lipid peroxidation and skin diseases. J Eur Acad Dermatol Venereol 2003; 17: 663-9.

[11] Surjana D, Halliday GM, Damian DL. Role of nicotinamide in DNA damage, mutagenesis, and DNA repair. J Nucleic Acids 2010; pii: 157591.

[12] Philips N, Conte J, Chen Y, *et al.* Beneficial regulation of matrixmetalloproteinases and its inhibitors, fibrillar collagens and transforming growth factor-β by P. leucotomos, directly or in dermal fibroblasts, ultraviolet radiated fibroblasts, and melanoma cells. Arch. Derm Res 2009; 301:487-495.

[13] Philips N, Samuel M, Arena R, *et al.* Direct inhibition of elastase and matrixmetalloproteinases, and stimulation of biosynthesis of fibrillar collagens, elastin and fibrillins by xanthohumol. J. Cosmet. Sci 2010; 61: 125-32.

[14] Philips N, Samuel P, Parakandi H, *et al.* Beneficial regulation of fibrillar collagens, heat shock protein-47, elastin fiber components, transforming growth factor–β, vascular endothelial growth factor and oxidative stress effects by copper in dermal fibroblasts. Connective Tissue Res 2012; 53: 373-8.

[15] Wlaschek M, Tantcheva-Poór I, *et al.* Solar UV irradiation and dermal photoaging. J Photochem Photobiol B 2001; 63: 41-51.

[16] Mecham RP, Davis EC. Elastic fiber structure and assembly. New York: Academic Press 1994.

[17] Keeley FW, Bellingham CM, Woodhouse KA. Elastin as a self-organizing biomaterial: use of recombinantly expressed human elastin polypeptides as a model for investigations of structure and self-assembly of elastin. Philos Trans R Soc B Biol Sci 2002; 357: 185-9.

[18] Kielty CM, Sherratt MJ, Shuttleworth CA. Elastic fibres. J Cell Sci 2002; 115: 2817-28.

[19] Rock MJ, Cain SA, Freeman LJ, *et al.* Molecular basis of elastic fiber formation: critical interactions and a tropoelastin-fibrillin-1 cross-link. J Biol Chem 2004; 279: 23748-58.

[20] Zhang H, Hu W, Ramirez F. Developmental expression of fibrillin genes suggests heterogeneity of extracellular microfibrils. J Cell Biol 1995; 129: 1165-76.

[21] Ramirez F, Pereira L. The fibrillins. Int J Biochem Cell Biol 1999; 31:255–259.

[22] Kinsey R, Williamson MR, Chaudhry S, *et al.* Fibrillin-1 microfibril deposition is dependent on fibronectin assembly. J Cell Sci 2008; 121: 2696-704.

[23] Robert L. Elastin, past, present and future. Pathol Biol 2002; 50: 503-11.

[24] Bax DV, Bernard SE, Lomas A, *et al.* Cell adhesion to fibrillin-1 molecules and microfibrils is mediated by alpha(5)beta(1) and alpha(v)beta(3) integrins. J Biol Chem 2003; 278: 34605-16.

[25] Hubmacher D, Tiedemann K, Reinhardt DP. Fibrillins: from biogenesis of microfibrils to signaling functions. Curr Top Dev Biol 2006; 75: 93-123.

[26] Sims TJ, Rasmussen LM, Oxlund H, Bailey AJ. The role of glycation cross-links in diabetic vascular stiffening. Diabetologia 1996; 39: 946-51.

[27] Bailey AJ. Molecular mechanisms of ageing in connective tissues. Mech Ageing Dev 2001; 122: 735-55.

[28] Yaar M, Gilchrest BA. Photoageing: mechanism, prevention and therapy. Br J Dermatol 2007; 157: 874-87.

[29] O'Rourke MF, Hashimoto J. Mechanical factors in arterial aging: a clinical perspective. J Am Coll Cardiol 2007; 50: 1-13.

[30] Robert L, Robert AM, Fulop T. Rapid increase in human life expectancy: will it soon be limited by the aging of elastin? Biogerontology 2008; 9: 119-33.

[31] Wendel DP, Taylor DG, Albertine KH, Keating MT, Li DY. Impaired distal airway development in mice lacking elastin. Am J Respir Cell Mol Biol 2000; 23: 320-6.

[32] Knudson RJ, Clark DF, Kennedy TC, Knudson DE. Effect of aging alone on the mechanical-properties of normal adult human lung. J Appl Physiol 1977; 43: 1054-62.

[33] Meyer KC, Rosenthal NS, Soergel P, Peterson K. Neutrophils and low-grade inflammation in the seemingly normal aging human lung. Mech Ageing Dev 1998; 104: 169-81.

[34] Snider GL, Kleinerman JL, Thurlbeck WM, Bengali ZH. The definition of emphysema: report of a National Heart, Lung-and Blood Institute, Division of Lung Diseases workshop. Am Rev Respir Dis 1985; 132:182-5.

[35] Verbeken EK, Cauberghs M, Mertens I, Clement J, Lauweryns JM, Vandewoestijne KP. The senile lung-comparison with normal and emphysematous lungs. 1. Structural aspects. Chest 1992; 101:793-9.

[36] Watson RE, Griffiths CE, Craven NM, Shuttleworth CA, Kielty CM. Fibrillin-rich microfibrils are reduced in photoaged skin. Distribution at the dermal-epidermal junction. J Invest Dermatol 1999; 112: 782-7.
[37] Watson RE, Ball SG, Craven NM, *et al.* Distribution and expression of type VI collagen in photoaged skin. Br J Dermatol 2001; 144: 751-9.
[38] Philips N, Keller T, Hendrix C, Hamilton S, Arena R, Tuason M, Gonzalez S. Regulation of the extracellular matrix remodeling by lutein in dermal fibroblasts, melanoma cells, and ultraviolet radiation exposed fibroblasts. Arch Dermatol Res 2007; 299: 373-9.
[39] Philips N, Hwang H, Chauhan S, Leonardi D, Gonzalez S. Stimulation of cell proliferation, and expression of matrixmetalloproteinase-1 and interluekin-8 genes in dermal fibroblasts by copper. Connective Tissue Res 2010; 51: 224-9.
[40] Chakraborti S, Mandal M, Das S, Mandal A, Chakraborti T. Regulation of matrix metalloproteinases: an overview. Mol Cell Biochem 2003; 253: 269-85.
[41] Kielty CM, Woolley DE, Whittaker SP, Shuttleworth CA. Catabolism of intact fibrillin microfibrils by neutrophil elastase, chymotrypsin and trypsin. FEBS Lett 1994; 351:85-9.
[42] Fisher GJ, Datta SC, Talwar HS, Wang ZQ, Varani J, Kang S, Voorhees JJ. Molecular basis of sun-induced premature skin ageing and retinoid antagonism. Nature 1996; 379: 335-9.
[43] Viegi, G, Scognamiglio, A, Baldacci, S, Pistelli, F, Carrozzi, L. Epidemiology of chronic obstructive pulmonary disease (COPD) Respiration 2001; 68: 4-19.
[44] Robbesom AA, Koenders M, Smits NC, Hafmans T, Versteeg EMM, Bulten J, Veerkamp JH, Dekhuijzen PNR, Kuppevelt TH. Aberrant fibrillin-1 expression in early emphysematous human lung: a proposed predisposition for emphysema. Mod Pathol 2008; 21: 297-307.
[45] Nagase H, Woessner JF. Matrix Metalloproteinases. J Biol Chem 1999; 274: 21491-94.
[46] Bode W, Gomis-Rüth FX, Stöckler W. Astacins, serralysins, snake venom and matrix metalloproteinases exhibit identical zinc-binding environments (HEXXHXXGXXH and Met-turn) and topologies and should be grouped into a common family, the 'metzincins'. FEBS Lett 1993; 331: 134-40.
[47] Gomis-Rüth FX, Gohlke U, Betz M, *et al.* The helping hand of collagenase-3 (MMP-13): 2.7 A crystal structure of its C-terminal haemopexin-like domain. J Mol Biol 1996; 264: 556-66.
[48] Herouy Y. Matrixmetalloproteinases in skin pathology. Int J Mol Med 2001; 7: 3-12.
[49] Yan C, Boyd DD. Regulation of matrix metalloproteinase gene expression. J Cell Physiol 2007; 211: 19-26.
[50] Verstappen J, Von den Hoff JW. Tissue Inhibitors of Metalloproteinases (TIMPs): Their Biological Functions and Involvement in Oral Diseases. Crit. Rev. Oral Biol Med J Dent Res 2006; 85: 1074-84.
[51] Zeng ZS, Huang Y, Cohen AM, Guillem JG. Prediction of colorectal cancer relapse and survival *via* tissue RNA levels of matrix metalloproteinase-9. J Clin Oncol 1996; 14: 3133-40.
[52] Meeran SM, Katiyar SK. Proanthocyanidins inhibit mitogenic and survival-signaling *in vitro* and tumor growth *in vivo*. Front Biosci 2008; 13: 887-97.
[53] Bachelor MA, Bowden GT. UVA mediated activation of signaling pathways involved in skin tumor promotion and progression. Semin Cancer Biol 2004; 14: 131-8.
[54] Vile GF, Tanew-Ilitschew A, Tyrrell RM. Activation of NF-kappa B in human skin fibroblasts by the oxidative stress generated by UVA radiation. Photochem Photobiol 1995; 62: 463-8.

[55] Adcock IM, Ito K, Barnes PJ. Histone deacetylation: an important mechanism in inflammatory lung diseases. COPD 2005; 2: 445-55.
[56] Li, T, Huang H, Huang B, Huang B, Lu J. Histone acetyltransferase p300 regulates the expression of human pituitary tumor transforming gene (hPTTG). J Genet Genomics 2009; 36: 335-42.
[57] Mroz RM, Noparlik J, Chyczewska E, Braszko JJ, Holownia A. Molecular basis of chronic inflammation in lung diseases: new therapeutic approach. J Physiol Pharmacol 2007; 58: 453-60.
[58] Maiese K, Chong ZZ, Hou J, Shang YC. The vitamin nicotinamide: translating nutrition into clinical care. Molecules 2009; 14: 3446-85.
[59] Ahn KS, Moon KY, Lee J, Kim YS. Downregulation of NF-kappaB activation in human keratinocytes by melanogenic inhibitors. J Dermatol Sci 2003; 31: 193-201.
[60] Rahman I, Gilmour PS, Jimenez LA, MacNee W. Oxidative stress and TNF-alpha induce histone acetylation and NF-kappaB/AP-1 activation in alveolar epithelial cells: potential mechanism in gene transcription in lung inflammation. Mol Cell Biochem 2002; 234-235: 239-48.
[61] Glick R, Pasternack JJ. Synthesis of commercial products by recombinant microorganisms. In Molecular biotechnology: Principles and applications of recombinant DNA .ASM Press 2003; pp 507-512.
[62] Greesin S, Murad, Pinnell S. Ascorbic acid stimulates collagen production without altering intracellular degradation in cultured human skin fibroblasts. Biochem. Biophys 1985; 866: 272-4.
[63] Davidson JM, LuValle PA, Zoia O, Quaglino D Jr, Giro M. Ascorbate differentially regulates elastin and collagen biosynthesis in vascular smooth muscle cells and skin fibroblasts by pretranslational mechanisms. J Biol Chem 1997; 272: 345-52.
[64] Soucy PA, Werbin J, Heinz W, Hoh JH, Romer LH. Microelastic properties of lung cell-derived extracellular matrix. Acta Biomater 2011; 7: 96-105.
[65] Naidu KA. Vitamin C in human health and disease is still a mystery? An overview. Nutr J 2003; 2: 7.
[66] Harrison FE, May JM. Vitamin C function in the brain: vital role of the ascorbate transporter SVCT2. Free Radic Biol Med 2009; 46: 719-30.
[67] Segade F. Glucose transporter 10 and arterial tortuosity syndrome: the vitamin C connection. FEBS Lett 2010; 584: 2990-4.
[68] Darr D, Combs S, Dunston S, Manning T, Pinnell S. Topical vitamin C protects porcine skin from ultraviolet radiation-induced damage. Br J Dermatol 1992; 127: 247-53.
[69] May JM. The SLC23 family of ascorbate transporters: ensuring that you get and keep your daily dose of vitamin C. Br J Pharmacol 2011; 164: 1793-801.
[70] Valenca SS, Bezerra FS, Souza BR, Paiva RO, Costa AMA, Porto LC. Supplementation with vitamins C and E improves mouse lung repair. J Nutritional Biochem 2008; 19: 604-11.
[71] Murakami K, Inagaki J, Saito M, *et al.* Skin atrophy in cytoplasmic SOD-deficient mice and its complete recovery using a vitamin Cderivative. Biochem Biophys Res Commun 2009; 382: 457-61.
[72] Liehr JG, Wheeler WJ. Inhibition of estrogen-induced renal carcinoma in Syrian hamsters by vitamin C. Cancer Res 1983; 43: 4638-42.
[73] Liu J, Nagao N, Kageyama K, Miwa N. Antimetastatic and anti-invasive ability of phospho-ascorbyl palmitated through intracellular ascorbate enrichment and the resultant antioxidant action. Oncol Res 1999; 11: 479-87.

[74] Lutsenko SV, Feldman NB, Severin SE. Cytotoxic and antitumor activities of doxorubicin conjugates with the epidermal growth factor and its receptor-binding fragment. J Drug Target 2002; 10: 567-71.

[75] Oliveira CP, Kassab P, Lopasso FP, Souza HP, Janiszewski M, Laurindo FR, *et al.* Protective effect of ascorbic acid in experimental gastric cancer: reduction of oxidative stress. World J Gastroenterol 2003; 9: 446-8.

[76] Potdar PD, Kandarkar SV, Sirsat SM. Modulation by vitamin C of tumour incidence and inhibition in oral carcinogenesis. Funct Dev Morphol 1992; 2: 167-72.

[77] Tsao CS. Inhibiting effect of ascorbic acid on the growth of human mammary tumor xenografts. Am J Clin Nutr 1991; 45: 1274S-2780S.

[78] Noto V, Henryk S, Taper S, Jiang YH, Jannsens J, Bonte J, De Loecker W. Effects of sodium ascorbate (vitamin C) and 2-methyl-1,4-naphthoquinone (vitamin K) treatment on humor tumor cell *in vitro*. I. Synergism of combined vitamin C and K action. Cancer 1989; 63: 901-909.

[79] Philips N, Keller T, Holmes C. Reciprocal effects of ascorbate on cancer cell growth and the expression of matrix metalloproteinases and transforming growth factor-beta. Cancer Letters 2007; 256: 49-55.

[80] Philips N, Dulaj L, Upadhya T. Growth inhibitory mechanism of ascorbate and counteraction of its matrix metalloproteinases-1 and transforming growth factor-beta stimulation by gene silencing or P. leucotomos. AntiCancer Res 2009; 29: 3233-8.

[81] Lin SY, Lai WW, Chou CC, Kuo HM, Li TM, Chung GJ, Yang JH. Sodium ascorbate inhibits growth *via* the induction of cell cycle arrest and apoptosis in human malignant melanoma A375.S2 cells. Melanoma Res 2006; 509-19.

[82] Zhang H. P53 Plays a central role in UVA and UVB induced cell damage and apoptosis in Melanoma cells. Cancer Letters 2005; 244: 229-38.

[83] Aguirre R, May JM. Inflammation in the vascular bed: importance of vitamin C. Pharmacol Ther 2008; 119: 96-103.

[84] Beatty S, Boulton M, Henson D, Koh HH, Murray IJ. Macular pigment and age related macular degeneration. Br J Ophthalmol 1999; 83: 867-77.

[85] Broekmans WMR, Berendschot TTJM, *et al.* Macular pigment density in relation to serum and adipose tissue concentrations of lutein and serum concentrations of zeaxanthin. Am J Clin Nutr 2002; 76: 595-603.

[86] Khachik F, Beecher GR, Smith JC. Lutein, lycopene, and their oxidative metabolites in chemoprevention of cancer. J Cell Biochem 1995; 22: 236-46.

[87] Pratt S. Dietary prevention of age-related macular degeneration. (1990) J Am Optom Assoc 1990; 70: 39-47.

[88] Snodderly DM. Evidence for protection against age-related macula degeneration by carotenoids and antioxidant vitamins. Am J Clin Nutr 1995; 62:1448S-1461S.

[89] Jain A, Rieger I, Rohr M, Schrader A. Antioxidant efficacy on human skin *in vivo* investigated by UVA-induced chemiluminescence decay analysis *via* induced chemiluminescence of human skin. Skin Pharmacol Physiol 2010; 23: 266-72.

[90] Roberts CK, Sindhu KK. Oxidative stress and metabolic syndrome. Life Sci 2009; 84: 705-12.

[91] Miyake Y, Sasaki S, Tanaka K, Hirota Y. Consumption of vegetables, fruit, and antioxidants during pregnancy and wheeze and eczema in infants. Allergy 2010; 65:758-65.

[92] Oh SY, Chung J, Kim MK, Kwon SO, Cho BH. Antioxidant nutrient intakes and corresponding biomarkers associated with the risk of atopic dermatitis in young children. Eur J Clin Nutr 2010; 64: 245-52.

[93] Ingram D. Diet and subsequent survival in women with breast cancer. Br J Cancer 1994; 69: 71-80.

[94] Age Related Eye Disease Study Research Group AREDS report no 9. A randomized, placebo controlled clinical trial of high dose supplementation with Vit C and E and ß-carotene for age related cataract and vision loss. Arch Ophthalmol 2001; 119: 1439-52.

[95] Age Related Eye Disease Study Research Group AREDS report no 8. A randomized, placebo controlled clinical trial of high dose supplementation with Vit C and E, ß-carotene and zinc for age related cataract and vision loss. Arch Ophthalmol 2001; 119: 1417-36.

[96] Bone RA, Landrum JT, Cains A. Optical Density Spectra of The Macular Pigment *In Vivo* And *In Vitro*. Vision Res 1992; 32: 105-10.

[97] O'Connor I, O'Brien N. Modulation of UVA light-induced oxidative stress by ß-carotene, lutein and astaxanthin in cultured fibroblasts. J Derm Science 1998; 16: 226-30.

[98] Sujak A, Gabrielska J, Grudzinski W, Borc R, Mazurek P, Gruszecki WI. Lutein and zeaxanthin as protectors of lipid membranes against oxidative damage: the structural aspects. Arch Biochem Biophys 1999; 371: 301-7.

[99] Bone RA, Landrum JT, Fernandez L and Tarsis SL. Analysis of macular pigment by HPLC: retinal pigment and age study. Invest Ophthalmol Vis Sci 1988; 29: 843-9.

[100] Kijlstra A, Tian Y, Kelly ER, Berendschot TT. Lutein: More than just a filter for blue light. Prog Retin Eye Res 2012; 31: 303-15.

[101] Krishnaswamy R, Devaraj SN, Padma VV. Lutein protects HT-29 cells against Deoxynivalenol-induced oxidative stress and apoptosis: prevention of NF-kappaB nuclear localization and down regulation of NF-kappaB and Cyclo-Oxygenase-2 expression. Free Radic Biol Med 2010; 49: 50-60.

[102] Wingerath T, Sies H, Stahl W. Xanthophyll esters in human skin. Arch Biochem Biophys 1998; 355: 271-4.

[103] Astner S, Wu A, Chen J, *et al.* Dietary lutein/zeaxanthin reduces photoaging and photocarcinogenesis in chronically UVB irradiated SKH-1 hairless mice. Skin Pharmacol Physiol 2007; 20: 283-1.

[104] González S, Astner S, An W, Goukassian D, Pathak MA. Dietary lutein/zeaxanthin decreases ultraviolet B-induced epidermal hyperproliferation and acute inflammation in hairless mice. J Invest Dermatol 2003; 121: 399-405.

[105] Evans JA, Johnson EJ. The Role of Phytonutrients in Skin Health. Nutrients 2010; 2: 903-28.

[106] Millen AE, Tucker MA, Hartge P, *et al.* Diet and melanoma in a case-control study. Cancer Epidemiol Biomarkers Prev 2004; 13: 1042-51.

[107] Kozuki Y, Miura Y, Yagasaki K. Inhibitory effects of carotenoids on the invasion of rat ascites hepatoma cells in culture. Cancer Lett 2000; 151: 111-5.

[108] Narisawa T, Fukaura Y, Hasebe M, *et al.* Inhibitory effects of natural carotenoids, ol-carotene, B-carotene, lycopene and lutein, on colonic aberrant crypt foci formation in rats. Cancer Letters 1996; 106: 137-142.

[109] Slattery ML, Benson J, Curtin K, Khe-NI M, Schaeffer D, Potter JD. Carotenoids and colon cancer. Am J Clin Nutr 2000; 71: 575-82.

[110] Satia JA, Littman A, Slatore CG, Galanko JA, White E. Long-term use of beta-carotene, retinol, lycopene, and lutein supplements and lung cancer risk: results from the Vitamins and lifestyle (VITAL) study. Am J Epidemiol 2009; 169: 815-28.

[111] Benavente CA, Jacobson MK, Jacobson EL. NAD in skin: therapeutic approaches for niacin. Current Pharmaceutical Design 2009; 15: 29–38.

[112] Liu H, Knabb JR, Spike BT, Macleod KF. Elevated poly-(ADP-ribose) polymerase activity sensitizes retinoblastoma-deficient cells to DNAdamage-induced necrosis. Mol Cancer Res 2009; 7: 1099-109.

[113] Grange PA, Raingeaud J, Calvez V, Dupin N. Nicotinamide inhibits Propionibacterium acnes-induced IL-8 production in keratinocytes through the NF-kappaB and MAPK pathways. J Dermatol Sci 2009; 56: 106-12.

[114] Lappas M, Riley C, Lim R, Barker G, Rice GE, Menon R, Permezel M. MAPK and AP-1 proteins are increased in term pre-labour fetal membranes overlying the cervix: regulation of enzymes involved in the degradation of fetal membranes. Placenta 2011; 32: 1016-25.

[115] Kamat JP, Devasagayam TP. Methylene blue plus light-induced lipid peroxidation in rat liver microsomes: inhibition by nicotinamide (vitamin B3) and other antioxidants. Chem. Biol. Interact 1996; 99: 1-16.

[116] Bissett DL, Oblong JE, Berge CA. Niacinamide: A B vitamin that improves aging facial skin appearance. Dermatol Surg 2005; 31: 860-5.

[117] Kawada A, Konishi N, Oiso N, Kawara S, Date A. Evaluation of anti-wrinkle effects of a novel cosmetic containing niacinamide. J. Dermatol 2008; 35: 637-42.

[118] Fairfield K, Fletcher R. Vitamins for chronic disease prevention in adults. *JAMA*. 2002; 287: 3116-26.

[119] Cahill M, Stinnett SS, Fekrat S, Meta-analysis of plasma homocysteine, serum folate, serum vitamin B_{12}, and thermolabile MTHFR genotype as risk factors for retinal vascular occlusive disease. Am J Opthal 2003; 136: 1136-50.

[120] Dauchet L, Amouyel P, Hercberg S, Dallongeville J. Fruit and vegetable consumption and risk of coronary heart disease: a meta-analysis of cohort studies. J Nutr 2006; 136: 2588-93

[121] Evans J. Antioxidant supplements to prevent or slow down the progression of AMD: a systematic review and meta-analysis. Eye (Lond). 2008; 22: 751-60.

[122] Frei B. Efficacy of dietary antioxidants to prevent oxidative damage and inhibit chronic disease. J Nutr 2004; 134: 3196S-8S.

[123] Pozzilli P, Browne PD, Kolb H. Meta-analysis of nicotinamide treatment in patients with recent-onset IDDM. The nicotinamide trialists. Diabetes Care. 1996; 19: 1357-63.

Send Orders for Reprints on reprints@benthamscience.net
Frontiers in Clinical Drug Research – Anti Allergy Agents, Vol. 1, **2013, 265-329**

CHAPTER 8

A Novel Therapeutic Anti-allergy Approach: The Nontraditional Signaling Pathways of Adiponectin and Estrogen

Jianli Zhao, Wayne Bond Lau and Yajing Wang*

Department of Anesthesiology, the First Affiliated Hospital and Department of Physiology, Shanxi Medical University, Shanxi, Taiyuan, China and Department of Emergency Medicine, Thomas Jefferson University, Philadelphia, PA, USA

Abstract: Diseases of allergy affecting respiratory and integumentary systems are costly in terms of public health and finance worldwide. Epidemiologic data reveal upwards of 40% of the population in many countries are sensitized to environmental allergens such as grass, tree pollen, dust mite excreta, and animal dander, and exhibit a preponderance of allergic disease. In the face of limited available pharmaceutics, efficacious therapies (particularly those modifying or halting disease progression), are in great need. Despite intense research, a complete understanding of allergic etiology remains elusive. During allergic exacerbation, polarization of T-lymphocyte responses enhances secretion of cytokines involved in regulation of immunoglobulin E, mast cells, basophils, and eosinophils, ultimately provoking inflammation and disease. Traditional pharmacotherapy for allergic disease focuses upon ameliorating the immune response flare to allergen sensitization. A comprehensive understanding of the cellular and molecular mechanisms of allergic disease atop the complex contribution of both genetic and environmental factors will reveal new potential interventions augmenting public health. In 1995, discovery of the novel adipocytokine (a signaling hormone of adipose origin) adiponectin garnered great attention for the protein's potential role in diabetic and metabolic pathophysiology. In the decades since, research has demonstrated the protein's strong potential link with asthma. Beyond its essential role in sex hormone signaling, the estrogen membrane receptor also exerts anti-inflammatory properties. We shall review the most current information regarding adiponectin and estrogen in context to allergic pathology, encompassing asthma, allergic rhinitis, and immune system components pertaining to inflammation. We will discuss anti-inflammatory mechanisms underlying non-traditional pathways of these proteins, including adiponectin's AMPK-independent signaling pathway and estrogen's effects *via* its membrane receptor. Finally, we will provide perspective about the future of research concerning these proteins, and assess their potential therapeutic benefits for allergic disease.

Keywords: Allergic disease, allergy treatment, inflammatory cells, adiponectin, adiponectin receptor, AMPK-independent, estrogen, estrogen receptor, non-genomic effect, oxidative stress.

***Address correspondence to Yajing Wang:** Department of Physiology, Shanxi Medical University, Taiyuan, Shanxi, China; Tel: +8613934154811; Fax: 2155034458; Email: yajingwang@163.com

Atta-ur-Rahman (Ed)

INTRODUCTION

The prevalence of allergic sensitization continually increases in industrialized countries. Despite several environmental factors having been implicated in the development of allergic diseases, none fully explain this phenomenon [1, 2]. However, modern societal lifestyle elements, including diet, alcohol consumption, physical inactivity, and obesity, are the subject of scrutiny [3, 4]. Indeed, a rise in affluence, typical of developed nations, contributes to increased food availability and decreased physical labor, potentially promoting obesity. Asthmatics are heavier than patients without asthma, and obesity is often correlated with poorer disease control [5]. Moreover, increasing weight gain in adults increases the risk for development of allergic disorders later in life. Taken together, epidemiologic data prompts the concern weight gain has certain association with allergic disease.

Many studies report obesity as a risk factor for asthma development, and that obesity precedes asthma development. Patients with allergic rhinitis tend to have greater body mass index (BMI) than normal subjects, and BMI is significantly related to bronchial hyperreactivity [6-9]. Some studies speculate a possible relationship between increased BMI and respiratory allergic diseases such as asthma and rhinitis [9-14]. As both asthma and obesity are characterized by inflammation, a common inflammatory pathway has been proposed as a plausible explanation for the frequent association of the two diseases. Along adiponectin was founded, adipokines conception was extended, the relationship between asthma and obesity get more clarified.

In this chapter, we shall focus upon two proteins, adiponectin and estrogen, with unique anti-allergy therapeutic potential.

Discovered in 1995, the molecule adiponectin belongs to a group of proteins known as adipocytokines (or adipokines), cell signaling proteins of adipose origin [15]. In addition to its numerous metabolic and cardioprotective/vasculoprotective properties, adiponectin also exerts anti-allergic effects, which shall be the focus of our exposition.

Females of all ages experience significantly decreased allergy prevalence and resultant mortality than men [16-24]. Similarly, a gender discrepancy between inherent inflammatory responses (greater in women compared to men) has long been noted. Whereas a heightened inflammatory response is advantageous in response to infection and sepsis, it is unfavorable in immune responses against the self; indeed, the rate of autoimmune disorders is greatly increased in women compared to men [25-27]. Epidemiological and immunological evidence suggests female sex hormones play a role in the etiology and course of allergic inflammatory diseases, given the influential nature of the menstrual cycle, pregnancy, and menopause [28-31]. Estrogen is immuno-modulating, and with complex pro- and anti-inflammatory effects, depending upon several factors (to be discussed later in this chapter).

CURRENT ALLERGIC DISEASE THERAPY STRATEGIES

Increasing in prevalence over the past 30 years, allergic diseases affect nearly 100 million people worldwide. Epidemiological studies have identified several factors associated with increased atopy:

1. Home designs featuring augmented insulation and declined ventilation, thereby increasing exposure to indoor allergens such as dust mites, pet dander, and cockroach antigens [32, 33].

2. Improved hygienic habits and vaccinations, thereby decreasing childhood infections (*e.g.,* measles, hepatitis A, tuberculosis, and lactobacillus) [34-40] .

3. Increased air pollution, particularly diesel exhaust particles potentially serving as adjuvants for allergic inflammation [41, 42].

An exhaustive list of the specific environment factors responsible for increased prevalence (and resultant associated morbidity) of atopic disease remains incomplete. The ability to prevent inherent genetic predisposition for atopic disease remains a therapy of the future. Reliance upon pharmacological management will realistically continue for decades to come. Currently available medications treating allergic disease are sufficiently diverse to adequately manage the majority of patients suffering allergic sequelae. Corticosteroids, which inhibit many aspects of atopic inflammation, are among the most efficacious and widely utilized medications in the treatment of allergic disease. Despite the increased safety of topical preparations, the long-tern toxicity of corticosteroids remains a major problem, and this concern in the context of increased worldwide allergic disease prevalence has prompted intense research in the development of novel and efficacious treatment options [43, 44].

Immunotherapy provides another avenue for the treatment of allergic rhinitis, allergic asthma, and insect venom hypersensitivity. Diagnosis of these specific pathologic entities is made by history and physical examination, and further testing confirming IgE sensitization. Such testing usually involves skin prick or intradermal injection, but *in vitro* tests such as the radio allergosorbent test (RAST) are an alternative when skin testing is contraindicated [45, 46]. For more than a century, allergen immunotherapy has been a therapeutic option, its use supported by multiple placebo-controlled trials. Allergen immunotherapy alters disease course by a series of mixed extract injections composed of clinically relevant allergens [47-52]. While currently there is no "cure" for allergic disease, allergen immunotherapy is the modality available closest to it, but requires long term commitment. The World Health Organization has replaced the term allergen extract with allergen vaccine to reflect that allergen vaccines are used in medicine as immune modifiers [53].

Immunotherapy is also effective for allergies to pollen, mold, animal dander, dust mite, and cockroaches. Patients suffering allergic rhinitis and asthma refractory to allergen avoidance and pharmacotherapy are immunotherapy candidates. Immunotherapy may also be suitable for candidates enduring adverse medication reactions, or those desiring avoidance of long-term pharmacotherapy. Immunotherapy has the added benefit of potentially preventing sensitization to new allergens, or progression of allergic rhinitis to asthma, particularly in children.

A second form of immunotherapy involves the intravenous injection of monoclonal anti-IgE antibodies, which bind to both free and B-cell associated IgE, tagging them for elimination. Such antibodies do not bind to IgE already bound to the Fc receptor upon basophils and mast cells, which would stimulate the allergic inflammatory response. Omalizumab is the first agent of this class. While this immunotherapy type is very effective in treating several atopy types, it is not suitable for treating the majority of food-related allergies. Yet another subtype of immunotherapy is sublingual immunotherapy, which capitalizes upon oral immune tolerance to non-pathogenic antigens, such as foods and resident bacteria. Already well accepted in Europe, sublingual immunotherapy is gaining support in the United States among traditional allergists and physicians [54, 55].

Traditional treatment and allergy management consisted of simply avoiding the instigating allergen or reducing exposure. It is difficult, however, to avoid pollen or similar air-borne allergens. Nonetheless, strict avoidance of allergens is still considered a useful treatment method, and is a mainstay option in managing food allergies. Frontier pharmaceuticals on the allergy front must consider the whole body immune system. The adipocytokine adiponectin has been demonstrated to exert strong anti-inflammatory effect. With its broad anti-inflammatory role, adiponectin has great potential in future allergy therapy treatment strategies (Fig. **1**). Estrogen has modulatory effect upon inflammatory diseases with beneficial impact. Estrogen or estrogen plant substitutes may be valuable in combination anti-allergy therapies.

THE INFLAMMATORY BASIS OF ALLERGIC DISEASE AND ADIPONECTIN'S ROLE

An abundance of data supports the categorization of allergic disease as a subset of inflammatory conditions. Inflammation is a linchpin pathophysiological feature of several medical conditions including allergic asthma, atopic dermatitis, allergic rhinitis, and several ocular allergic diseases. Allergic reactions are generally divided into the early and late phase reactions. While contribution to the development of symptoms from each of the phases varies greatly between diseases, each phase is usually present and provides us a framework for understanding the inflammatory state of allergic disease [56-61]. Both *in vitro* and *in vivo* studies suggest that adiponectin may interference with the two phases of allergic disease through interactions with inflammatory cells including leukocytes, endothelial cells, and adipocytes.

The early phase of the allergic reaction is commonly referred to as the immediate allergic reaction, or the Type I allergic reaction, and occurs within seconds to minutes after allergen exposure. The reaction is caused by the release of histamine and mast cell granule proteins in a process called degranulation, with concomitant mast cell production of leukotrienes, prostaglandins, and cytokines following the cross-linking of allergen specific IgE molecules bound to mast cell FcRI receptors [62]. The release of these mediators affects neurons causing itching [63], smooth muscle cells causing contraction (causing airway narrowing seen in allergic asthma) [62], goblet cells causing mucus production, and endothelial cells causing vasodilatation and edema [62].

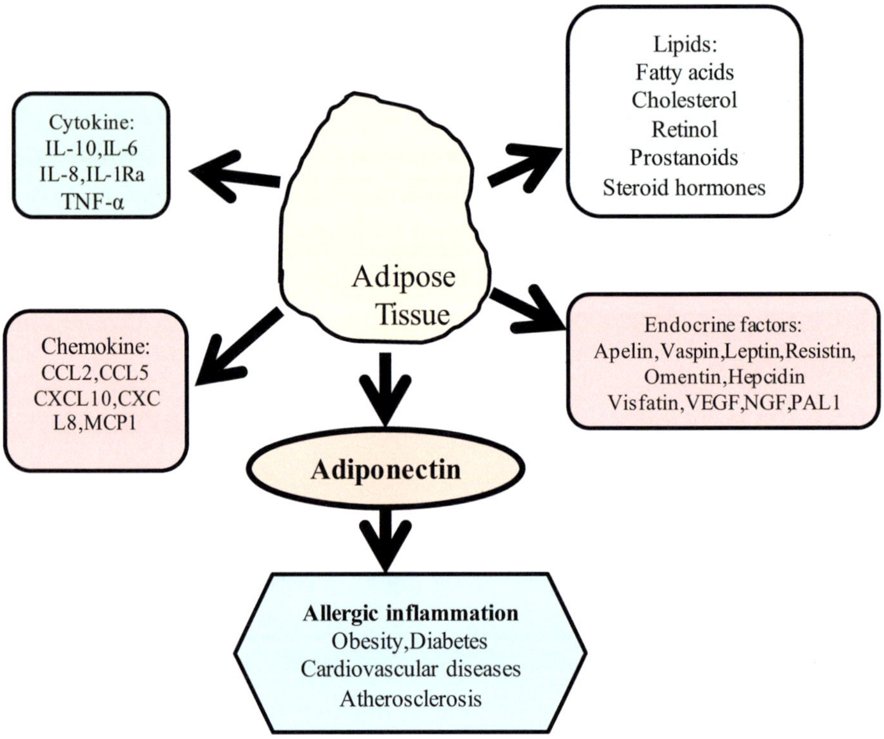

Figure 1: Adiponectin as a kind of adipokines secreted from white adipose tissue involved in against many inflammatory disease. The adipocyte fraction of white adipose tissue secretes adiponectin, leptin, visfatin and resistin as well as pro- and anti-inflammatory cytokines, chemokine, endocrine factors and being in charge of uptake, storage, synthesis of lipids.Adiponectin after secreted from white adipose tissue modulates the inflammatory response and protects against atherosclerosis, cardiovascular dysfunction and diabetes. Inflammatory or immune diseases to which adiponectin mainly contribute by action or omission are depicted in boxes. Adipocyte-derived factors and their downstream signals might constitute therapeutic options for the treatment of these diseases. Abbreviations: CCL, CC-chemokine ligand (CCL); CXCL, CXC-chemokine ligand (CXCL); IL, interleukin; IL1-Ra, interleukin-1-receptor antagonist; NGF, nerve growth factor; PAI1, plasminogen activator inhibitor 1; VEGF, vascular

endothelial growth factor; IL-10, interleukin-10; IL-6, interleukin-6; IL-1β, interleukin-1 beta; TNF-α, tumor necrosis factor alpha; IL-8, interleukin-8; MCP-1, monocyte chemotactic protein-1.

The late phase of a Type 1 reaction (mediated by mast cells, developing 8-12 hours post allergen exposure) [64, 65] should not be confused with delayed hypersensitivity Type IV allergic reaction (mediated by T cells, developing 48-72 hours post allergen exposure). The products of the early phase reaction include chemokines and molecules that act upon endothelial cells, inducing their expression of intercellular adhesion molecules (*e.g.*, vascular cell adhesion molecules and selectins), which recruit and activate circulating leukocytes to the site of the allergic reaction [66, 67]. Typically, the infiltrating cells observed in allergic reactions contain a high proportion of lymphocytes and, particularly, eosinophils. The degranulation of recruited eosinophils releases cytotoxic molecules such as IL-5 [59, 60]. T-cells present are typically of the Th2 (T helper 2 cells) variety, whose production of cytokines further recruits mast cells and eosinophils. The binding of IgE to mast cell FcRI receptors primes the individual for future allergic responses. Understanding these two phases of the allergic reaction has led to development of approaches ameliorating cytotoxic molecule release from inflammatory cells, but results are only fair.

When it was discovered nearly twenty years ago in 1995, adiponectin's potential as an anti-inflammatory molecule was not anticipated. Produced largely by white adipose tissue, adiponectin (also known as GBP28, apM1, Acrp30, or AdipoQ) is a 244-residue protein sharing structural homology with collagens VIII and X, as well as complement factor C1q, and circulates in the blood in relatively large quantities in different oligomers [68, 69]. Clinical data reveals adiponectin levels are elevated in classic chronic inflammatory/autoimmune diseases such as rheumatoid arthritis, systemic lupus erythematosus, inflammatory bowel disease, type 1 diabetes, cystic fibrosis, and some other autoimmune allergic diseases [70-73]. In such conditions, adiponectin levels correlate positively with autoimmune inflammatory markers. However, although adiponectin's role in allergic disorder is complicated, recently, researchers have demonstrated several interesting relationships between allergic disorders and adiponectin:

- Asthmatics weigh consistently more than patients without asthma. The degree of obesity is often positively correlated with poorer asthma control.

- Asthma and obesity are both conditions characterized by inflammation. A common inflammatory pathway could explain the frequent association of the two diseases.

- Another adipokine, serum leptin levels are associated with several clinical and immunological parameters (including BMI, eosinophil, and immunoglobulin E levels).

- Adiponectin exerts both anti-inflammatory and pro-inflammatory effects, depending upon the immunological milieu present.

- Sublingual immunotherapy slightly increases leptin and adiponectin serum levels.

Adiponectin exerts a wide range of effects in diseases harboring immune and inflammatory pathophysiology, such as cardiovascular disease, type 2 diabetes, metabolic syndrome and rheumatoid arthritis. The effects of adiponectin upon innate and adaptive immunity are listed in Table **1**. Interfering with many inflammatory cells, adiponectin inhibits phagocytic activity, and production of IL-6 and TNF. It reduces B-cell lymphopoiesis, decreases T-cell response, and induces the production of important anti-inflammatory factors such as IL-10 and IL-1RA by human monocytes, macrophages, and dendritic cells. In the following sections, detailed information will be provided regarding the characteristics of adiponectin supporting its strong potential as an anti-allergic therapeutic.

Table 1: The effects of adiponectin upon innate and adaptive immunity. HMW, high molecular weight; IFN, interferon; IL, interleukin; NF-kB, nuclear factor kB; TNF, tumor necrosis factor; LPS, lippolysaccharide.

Effect on immunity			
Adaptive Innate			**Reference**
Adiponectin	↓B cell lymphopoiesis	↓ Phagocytosis	[74, 75]
	↓T cell response	↓ Endothelial adhesion molecules	[75, 76]
		↑IL-10, ↑ IL-1RA, ↓IFN-γ	[75]
		↓TNF, ↓NF-κB, ↓IL-6	[76-79]
		↑IL-8(CXCL8) HMW form, LPS	

Adiponectin and the cellular and molecular mechanisms of allergy

Involvement of the Adiponectin Receptor in the Immune Response of Allergic Inflammation

Adiponectin acts *via* two described receptors, one (adiponectin receptor 1, AdipoR1) found predominantly in skeletal muscle and the other (adiponectin 2, AdipoR2) in the liver. These membrane-spanning receptors are structurally and topologically distinct from G-protein coupled receptors, and are predicted to contain seven transmembrane domains. Though predominantly found in their major organs, both receptors are expressed in numerous cell types, including adipocytes and inflammatory cells and by means of that adiponectin could influence function of various organ or tissues (Fig. **2**). Each receptor type exhibits different binding affinity for the globular domain and full length adiponectin isoforms. AdiopR1 has a high affinity for the globular adiponectin and a very low affinity for the full length form, whereas AdipoR2 has intermediate affinity for both the full length and globular forms of adiponectin [80]. Transduction of the adiponectin signal by AdipoR1 and AdipoR2 involves the activation of the protein kinase AMPK (AMP-activated protein kinase), PPAR (peroxisome proliferator-activated receptor) alpha, PPAR gamma, and other signaling molecules [81].

To better elucidate the role of adiponectin in allergic disease, Kim *et al.* investigated the expression and distribution pattern of AdipoR1 and AdipoR2 in healthy, mild, and moderate/severe persistent allergic nasal mucosa. AdipoR1 was expressed in healthy, mild, and moderate/severe persistent allergic nasal mucosa. However, AdipoR2 was not expressed in the nasal mucosa of any allergic severity type. Expression of AdipoR1 was decreased in mild and moderate/severe persistent allergic nasal mucosa compared to healthy nasal mucosa, but not significantly different between mild and moderate/severe persistent allergic nasal mucosa, suggesting that AdipoR1 may play an important role in the pathogenesis of allergic nasal mucosa [82]. Yamauchi *et al.* demonstrated simultaneous disruption of AdipoR1 and AdipoR2 in leptin$^{-/-}$ mice significantly altered oxidative stress (a major pro-inflammatory factor increasing the expression of genes encoding chemokines), decreased the expression of genes encoding molecules reducing oxidative stress,

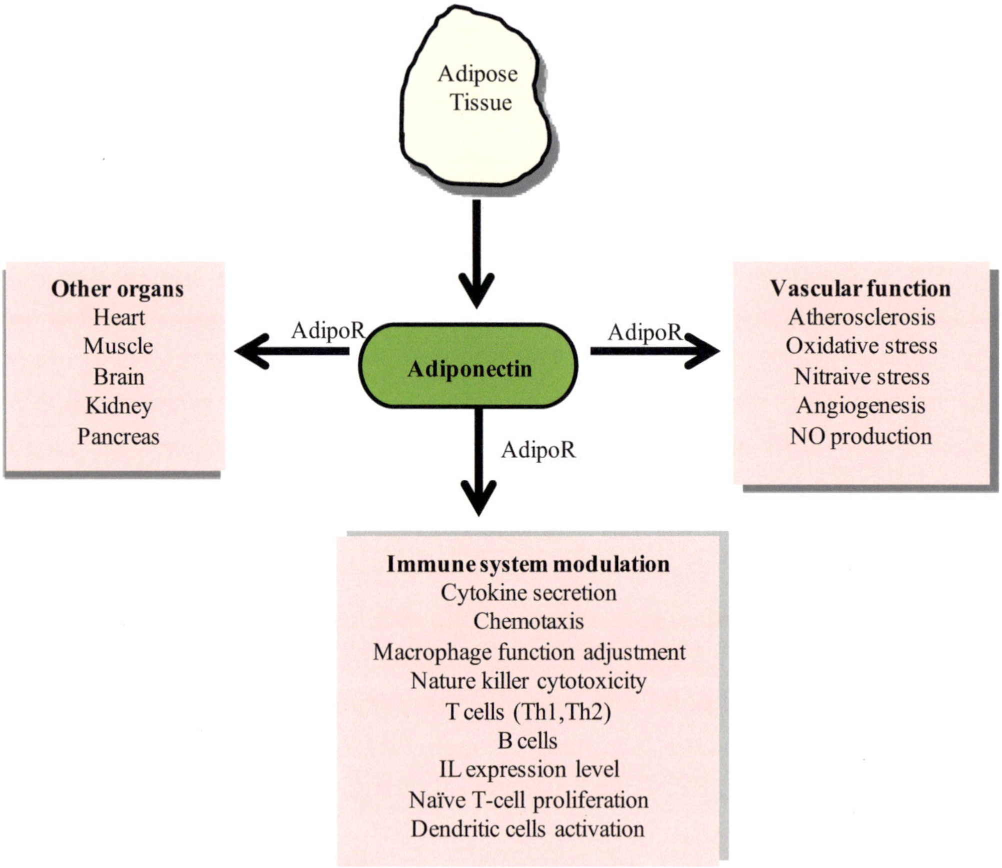

Figure 2: A schematic diagram depicting the pleiotropic nature of adiponectin since the discovery of adiponectin in 1995. Adiponectin have been described as a modulator on key organ/tissue linking metabolism and many aspects of immunity and inflammation through binding with adipoR1/adipoR2. Abbreviations: IL, interleukin; NO, nitric oxide; Th1, T-helper lymphocyte type 1; Th2, T-helper lymphocyte type 2.

and increased the expression of genes augmenting peripheral tissue oxidative stress [80]. Furthermore, adenoviral-mediated overexpression of AdipoR2 reduced both inflammatory and oxidative stress genes, TNF, and chemokine ligand 2, and increased catalase and super-oxide dismutase 1 *via* amplified PPARα (Peroxisome proliferator-activated receptor alpha) expression. Both PPARα and PPARγ can antagonize NF-κB and activator protein 1 pathways, inhibiting pro-inflammatory gene expression [83]. However, AdipoR1 overexpression in these leptin$^{-/-}$ mice increased hepatic AMPK activation by adiponectin, which was not observed during AdipoR2 overexpression [80].

Oxidative Stress/Nitrative Stress in Allergic Disease and Adiponectin AMPK Independent Signaling

Adiponectin is a known activator of AMPK in numerous cell types [80, 84, 85]. Similar to PPARα, AMPK may play a role in the anti-inflammatory effects of adiponectin [86]. Recent studies demonstrate that a chemical activator of AMPK, 5-aminoimidazole-4-carboximide 1-β-D-ribo-furanoside, or expression of constitutively active AMPK [87] disrupts NF-κB-mediated gene expression in several cell types. Furthermore, AMPK regulates the transcriptional activity of NF-κB and CCAAT/enhancer binding protein δ *via* inhibition of their nuclear translocation, and controls NF-κB transcriptional activity by inhibiting LPS-induced I-kappa kinase α/β activity and phosphorylation/degradation of IκBα [84]. The CCAAT/enhancer binding protein is known to regulate the expression of TNF-α, IL-1β, IL-6, inducible nitric oxide synthase (iNOS), IL-8, and IL-12 [88] (Fig. **3**). Together, through upregulation of AMPK and PPARα, disruption of NF-κB transcriptional activity, and mitigation of downstream pro-inflammatory gene expression, adiponectin attenuates inflammation. Although the anti-inflammatory actions of adiponectin are due largely to counteraction of NF-κB and pro-inflammatory cytokine production, Masaie *et al.* demonstrated adiponectin's anti-inflammatory effects may be additionally mediated through chemokine binding with its globular head domain [89]. However, the dose of full-length recombinant adiponectin utilized in Masaie's study did not influence chemokine-receptor interactions.

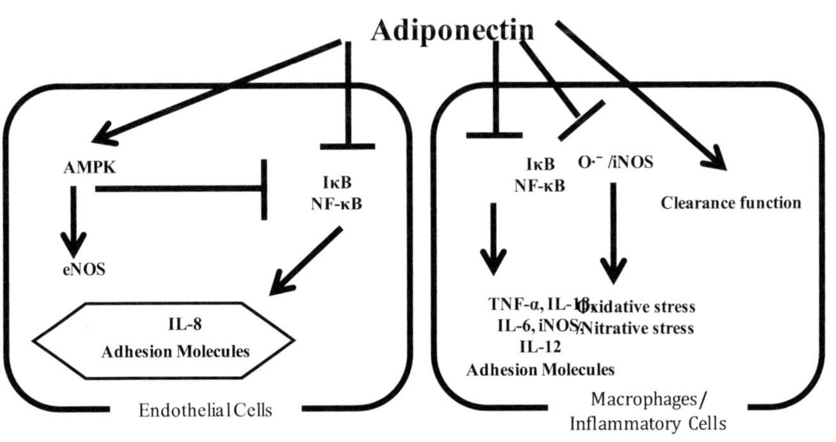

Figure 3: Anti-inflammatory actions of adiponectin. Adiponectin inhibits NF-κB activation in endothelial cells, at least in part, by its ability to activate AMPK (AMPK dependent pathway).

Inhibition of NF-κB by adiponectin results in downregulation of IL-8, and adhesion molecule expression. In macrophages or other inflammatory cells, adiponectin attenuates TNF-α, IL-1β, IL-6, iNOS, IL-12 and adhesion molecules production through its ability to suppress NF-κB activation, and it promotes the clearance of apoptotic cells or fibrosis by macrophages. Adiponectin also can through ameliorate superoxide to further inhibit oxidative stress/nitrative stress.

When the research of adiponectin's AMPK dependent pathway grows vigorously, surprisingly, Wang *et al.* first reported that adiponectin has a partial anti-inflammatory role independent of the AMPK axis, *via* reducing both oxidative and nitrative stress [90]. As mentioned previously, oxidative and nitrative stress are significant sources of inflammatory molecule generation. Many observations support the role of oxidative/nitrative stress in the pathogenesis of allergic disease [91-93]. Despite the difficulty of directly measuring levels of reactive oxygen species in allergic patients, recent studies of exhaled gases from asthmatic patients demonstrate increased hydrogen peroxide [94-96] and nitric oxide levels [97, 98]. Furthermore, increased reactive oxygen species (ROS) production is inversely correlated with FEV1 (forced expiratory volume in 1 second) [99]. Airway inflammatory cells are the likely source of such ROS burst. For instance, airway macrophages from asthmatic patients produce more superoxide than those from control subjects [100], and antigen challenge increases spontaneous reactive oxygen species in airway eosinophils in asthmatics [101-103]. Circulating inflammatory cells might also be a source; activation of peripheral blood monocytes by IgE binding to membrane receptors results in superoxide secretion [104, 105], and eosinophils isolated from asthmatics 24 hours after antigen challenge produce more hydrogen peroxide when antigen-challenged [106, 107]. Blood eosinophils and monocytes produce more reactive oxygen species in allergic patients compared to control subjects [93, 103, 108, 109]. Together, both airway and intravascular inflammatory cells contribute to elevated oxidative stress in allergic disease (Fig. **4**). The direct mechanisms by which reactive oxygen species exacerbate asthma include effects upon both smooth muscle and mucin secretion. Even so, adiponectin has shown good talents on diminishing oxidative stress in well document proofing [110-116], adiponectin could through stimulate increased IFN-γ to blunt this response in allergic patients [104, 117].

The association between inflammation and reactive oxygen species could set up a positive-feedback loop perpetuating both lung and airway tissue injury. Numerous cytokines are found in the lung during inflammation, including TNF-α, epidermal growth factor, fibroblast growth factor, and serotonin, which activate oxidases increasing reactive oxygen species in cell culture [118-122]. Treating allergic disease *via* anti-oxidative therapeutics is a novel method not requiring complete patient isolation from the inciting allergen. The anti-oxidative signaling mechanisms underlying adiponectin's AMPK independent pathways underline the protein's anti-allergic applications. Recently, Wang *et al.* demonstrated caveolin-3 plays an essential role in the anti-oxidative effects of adiponectin [123]. Ceramidase which is presents on the cell membrane, could induce superoxide generation under many circumstance *via* upregulating superoxide dismutase expression [124, 125], adiponectin also diminishes adhesive molecule expression *via* the ceramidase-s1p shifting pathway as well. Increasing evidence demonstrates that nitric oxide is dysregulated in allergic disease as well [126, 127]. Corticosteroids have been demonstrated to suppress exhaled nitric oxide levels [128-132]. Wang *et al.* demonstrated adiponectin ameliorates nitrative stress as well, which provide a good evidence for adiponectin as a high potential drug to against allergic disease [90].

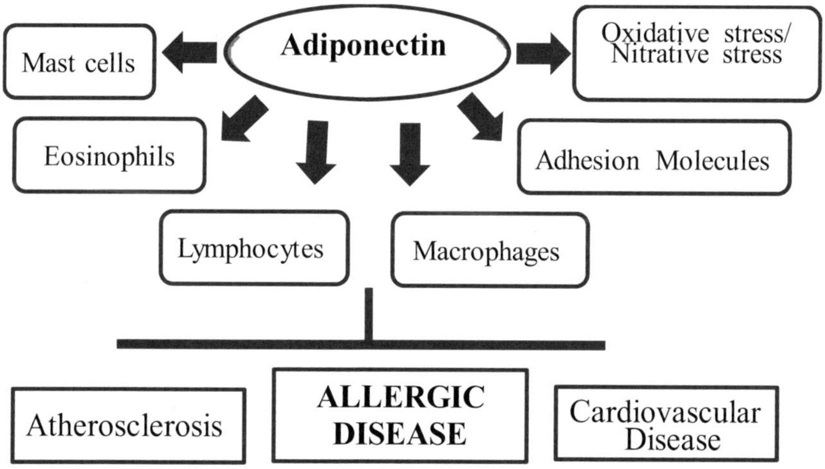

Figure 4: From adiponectin to inflammatory disease. The diagram describes adiponectin associated with inflammatory disease to ameliorating allergic disease and cardiovascular risks. Inflammatory cells activated by allergen is associated with an increased risk of allergic, cardiovascular inflammation. This phenomenon is linked to a series of cellular events and modifications inhibiting generation of reactive oxygen species/nitric oxide, adhesion molecule and inflammatory cytokines. These factors affect local and systemic functions which influences endothelial function and predisposes to the development of allergic inflammation.

As the role of nitric oxide is complicated in ROS generation, it is important to quickly review the three distinct sources of nitric oxide, the nitric oxide synthases (NOSs). NOS I (nNOS, or neuronal NOS) is present at nonadrenergic nerve terminals of smooth muscle and may induce nitric oxide-mediated bronchodilation [133-137]. NOS III (eNOS or endothelial NOS) is found primarily in the endothelium, and mediates vasodilation [138, 139]. NOS II (iNOS or inducible NOS) exists within a variety of inflammatory and epithelial cell types [140-143]. Both nNOS and eNOS are constitutively active. However, in asthma conditions, inducible NOS is primarily responsible for augmented exhaled nitric oxide levels. Lack of significant broncho-relaxation associated with nitric oxide in asthma suggests impaired signaling pathways within bronchial smooth muscle. Increased production of reactive oxygen species during inflammation might be genesis of such impairment. Nitric oxide signaling might not occur to the presence of reactive oxygen species. Nitric oxide rapidly reacts with superoxide to form peroxynitrite [144, 145]. Peroxynitrite formation increases during inflammation, and though toxic to microbes, it can also induce airway hyper-responsiveness [146]. Peroxynitrite formation decreases the amount of nitric oxide available for smooth muscle bronchodilation. Peroxynitrite formation is therefore advantageous at sites of inflammation and infection, but detrimental at sites where nitric oxide-mediated signaling must be preserved, such as the endothelium and respiratory smooth muscle [145, 147, 148]. This explains enhanced vascular vulnerability during allergic exacerbation states.

Preservation of nitric oxide requires two important pathways (1) shifting nitric oxide into a more stable species, such as an S-nitrosoglutathione, or (2) reducing the local concentrations of reactive oxygen species *via* elevated concentrations of antioxidant enzymes in the extracellular space. Recent literature reports S-nitrosoglutathione as a major contributor to smooth muscle airway relaxation in asthma [149, 150]. The superoxide-dismutase (SOD) family of enzymes critically preserves nitric oxide activity. SOD is abundant in the pulmonary vasculature and smooth muscle-laden airways. Although the specific role of SOD in asthma exacerbations remains unsubstantiated, it is nevertheless plausible SOD may preserve nitric-oxide mediated smooth muscle bronchodilation and vasoregulation under normal conditions. During inflammatory allergic flare, however, amplified oxidative or nitrative stress overwhelms ambient SOD, resulting in pathologic bronchospasm and vasodysregulation.

Adiponectin has been demonstrated to not only decrease oxidative stress, but also nitrative stress *via* inhibiting inducible NOS [90, 151, 152], and in this manner has strong potential to be therapeutic against allergic disease.

Adiponectin and Inflammatory Cells

Because of the numerous inflammatory cells involved in allergic inflammation, and the precise role of each cell type is not yet certain, no single inflammatory cell accounts for the complex pathophysiology of allergic disease. However, some cells predominate in allergic inflammation (Fig. **4**).

In allergen immunotherapy, treatment strategy involves shifting a patient's immune response to a particular allergen from a predominantly allergic T-lymphocyte (Th2) response to a "nonallergic" T-lymphocyte (Th1) response. Th2 phenotype lymphocytes typically produce IL-4 and IL-5, cytokines necessary for IgE production and eosinophil survival [153]. However, increased IFN-γ production and decreased production of IL-4 and IL-5 have not been consistently demonstrated post immunotherapy [154, 155]. Increased production of allergen-specific IL-10 has been consistently confirmed [156-158]. IL-10 causes a shift in allergen-specific IgE to allergen-specific IgG, a change possibly coordinated by regulatory T cells downregulating allergic immune responses partly *via* release of IL-10 and T-cell growth factor alpha (TGF-α) [159-161]. During allergen immunotherapy, the seasonal increase in allergen-specific IgE is blunted while protective allergen-specific IgG production is increased. Unfortunately, changes in IgE and IgG may not correlate with clinical efficacy, and periodic skin testing or *in vitro* IgE antibody assays may not be indicative of immunotherapy responsiveness [162-164].

In normal individuals, adiponectin circulates at very high levels (3-30 μg/ml), the most abundant human adipose tissue-specific protein produced [165]. Is the high circulatory adiponectin level associated with an inflammatory state induced by allergic disease? Adiponectin is an anti-inflammatory, anti-proliferative adipokine [165-168], reducing the production and activity of TNF, IgE, IL-6, IL-5 [169,

170], reducing expression of adhesion molecules (*e.g.*, intracellular adhesion molecule 1 and vascular cellular adhesion molecule), and promoting production of IL-10 and IL-1 receptor antagonist (Fig. **4**).

Recent studies have shown that adiponectin may also exert pro-inflammatory effects. Adiponectin levels are positively correlated with inflammatory markers in osteoarthritis and rheumatoid arthritis [171]. It has since been demonstrated that adiponectin may also promote inflammation by upregulating two major proinflamatory mediators, IL-6 and matrix metalloproteinase 1 [172]. Such conflicting data is difficult to reconcile. However, adiponectin may certainly interfere with stages of allergy progression, but under diabetes condition, adiponectin's role will be hurt because considerable literature emphasizes the relationship between adiponectin dearth in conditions of obesity or diabetes. The mechanism underlying adiponectin deficiency in obesity-associated/metabolic inflammatory disorders is likely complex and multifactorial, possibly involving adiponectin resistance and differential oligomeric distribution. So, under this kind of conditions, adiponectin's anti-inflammation roles maybe get influence by its low concentration and activity. Interestingly, adiponectin serum levels are elevated in patients with classic chronic inflammatory/autoimmune diseases that are unrelated to increased adipose tissue, such as systemic lupus erythematosus, inflammatory bowel disease, type 1 diabetes, and cystic fibrosis [70, 173-175]. In such diseases, adiponectin levels correlate with inflammatory markers. Adiponectin may be regulated in a certain fashion and exert beneficial function in classic *vs.* obesity-associated inflammatory disorders. A recent report demonstrated elevated serum adiponectin levels in male patients with pollen-induced allergic rhinitis than normal male subjects outside the pollen season [176, 177]. We next discuss the regulation or influence of adiponectin upon various inflammatory cells in different stages of allergic disease.

Adiponectin, Mast Cells, and Eosinophils

Any discussion of asthma symptomatology must mention mast cells [178], which initiate the acute bronchoconstrictor responses to allergens and likely other indirect stimuli, such as exercise, fog, and hyperventilation (*via* osmolality or thermal changes), and viral infections. Mast cells in airway smooth muscle appear to distinguish asthma from chronic eosinophilic bronchitis, in which patients have chronic cough [179]. Mast cells also induce rhinitis symptoms after allergen exposure (*e.g.,* grass pollen). The number of mast cells within induced-sputum samples from seasonal allergic rhinitis patients is related to the degree of methacholine responsiveness. Treatment of asthmatic patients with prednisone decreases the number of tryptase-positive mast cells [180]. Mast cell tryptase appears to influence airway remodeling, as tryptase stimulates human lung fibroblast proliferation [181, 182]. Mast cells also secrete certain cytokines, such as interleukin (IL)-4 that may be involved in maintaining the allergic inflammatory response and tumor necrosis factor-α (TNF-α) [183]. Adiponectin has been demonstrated to inhibit IL-4 secretion [184]. Adiponectin receptor 1 distribution in nasal mucosa and can be altered in varying stages of persistent allergic nasal mucosa [82]. Both laboratory and clinical investigations demonstrate correlation of adiponectin levels in patients with both allergic and seasonal rhinitis [176, 177, 185, 186].

Clinical use of anti-IgE therapy has applied to mast cells in asthma *via* omalizumab, which significantly reduces asthma exacerbations, and reduces maintenance doses of inhaled or oral corticosteroids [187, 188]. This treatment is also effective in allergic rhinitis. Adiponectin may serve as advantageous adjuvant strategy further decreasing corticosteroid utilization necessity.

Although mast cells are traditionally regarded as mediators of allergic responses, they have been implicated in many diseases including obesity and diabetes. Liu *et al.* demonstrated that mast cells accumulated in obese adipose tissue prior to macrophage appearance [178]. Mast cell depletion resulted in decreased weight gain and reduced adipose tissue macrophage content during obesity, suggesting their involvement in adipose tissue macrophage recruitment [189-192]. Mast cell expression of IL-6 and IFN-γ increased adipose protease expression, which play a key role in angiogenesis by degrading anti-angiogenic molecules [178]. Mast cell-induced angiogenesis may further facilitate leukocyte recruitment to the adipose tissue.

However, available data demonstrates adiponectin deficiency does not affect acute allergic airway inflammation. Medoff *et al.* utilized a mouse model challenged with chicken ovalbumin aerosolized immunization to induce allergic airway inflammation [73]. The authors conclude that adiponectin therapy has better efficacy on chronic treatment or prophylaxis rather than acute exacerbation.

Eosinophilic infiltration is a characteristic feature of allergic inflammation. More accurately, asthma might be described as chronic eosinophilic bronchitis. At the late stage of allergy, allergen inhalation results in markedly increased eosinophilia within bronchoalveolar lavage fluid, with correlation between eosinophil counts in peripheral blood and bronchial lavage [193]. Eosinophils are linked to the development of airway hyperreactivity *via* release of basic proteins and oxygen-derived free radicals [194]. Experimentally activated eosinophils have been shown to induce airway epithelial damage, characteristic of asthmatics [195-197]. Similar nasal epithelial shedding is not observed in patients with allergic rhinitis, indicating differential sensitivity of epithelial cell types to eosinophilic effects. Although no enough evidence to address that adiponectin can directly influence eosinophils themselves, there are adiponectin knockout mice data proving that adiponectin deficiency mice develop increased allergic airway inflammation compared with wild-type mice, with greater accumulation of eosinophils and monocytes in the airways associated with elevated lung chemokine levels [72, 73]. Therefore, these data provide a possible mechanism for the association between obesity and asthma, and suggest a potential novel link with eosinophils between obesity, inflammatory lung disease.

Several mechanisms, including cytokine secretion and adhesive molecule overexpression, are involved in eosinophilic recruitment into the site of allergic inflammation. Eosinophils are derived from bone marrow precursors. After allergen challenge, eosinophils appear during the late response phase, in association with decreased peripheral eosinophil counts, and eosinophil progenitor appearance in the circulation [198, 199]. The signal for increased eosinophil production is presumably derived from the inflamed airway. Eosinophil recruitment initially involves adhesion of eosinophils to vascular endothelial cells in the airway circulation, migration into the submucosa, and subsequent activation. The role of individual adhesion molecules, cytokines, and mediators in coordinating these responses has been extensively investigated. Eosinophilic adhesion involves the expression of specific glycoprotein molecules on the eosinophil surface (integrins) and intercellular adhesion molecule-1 (ICAM-1) upon vascular endothelial cells [200-202]. Pharmaceutics directed at ICAM-1 markedly inhibiting eosinophil accumulation in the airways post allergen exposure also block accompanying hyperresponsiveness [203, 204]. However, since ICAM-1 is not selective for eosinophils and cannot account for the selective recruitment of eosinophils in allergic inflammation. So, although adiponectin has strong adhesive molecules inhibitory effect, it cannot directly draw a conclusion that adiponectin could straightly have inhibitory role on eosinophils's moving. Very Late Antigen-4 (VLA4, expressed upon eosinophils which interacts with VCAM-1) appears to be more selective for eosinophils, and IL-4 increases VCAM-1 expression upon endothelial cells [205, 206]. Adiponectin effectively downregulates eosinophilic VLA-4 expression, and additionally decreases IL-5, prevent chronic hyperesponsiveness [169]. Eosinophil migration may be due to the effects of lipid mediators (*e.g.*, leukotrienes) and cytokines (*e.g.*, GM-CSF and IL-5), which may be crucial for eosinophil survival in the airways, and for 'priming' eosinophils to exhibit enhanced responsiveness. Superoxide generated during allergic flare activates VLA-4 and VCAM-1 as well, further drawing eosinophils to sites of inflammation [205-208]. In summation, adiponectin decreases recruitment of eosinophils to inflammatory sites by decreasing requisite adhesive molecule expression, and attenuates allergic airway inflammation, hypersensitivity, and long term pulmonary vascular remodeling *via* indirect inhibition of selective adhesion molecule and super oxide [73, 107, 169, 209].

To further clarify the role of eosinophils in allergy response, Evans *et al.* demonstrated asthmatic patient eosinophils manifest exaggerated response to some antigens, compared to eosinophils from atopic non-asthmatic individuals, a phenomenon exacerbated by allergen challenge [106], suggesting priming by circulatory cytokine exposure. Several mediators are involved in eosinophil migration from the circulation to the airway surface. The most potent and selective agents are chemokines, such as RANTES, eotaxins 1–3, and MCP-4, expressed in epithelial cells. These chemokines have been shown to upregulate adiponectin receptors in the endometrium; in adiponectin deficient mice, chemokines are responsible for exaggerated airway inflammation [210, 211]. Adiponectin blocks chemokine secretion in epithelial cells. There appears to be a cooperative interaction between IL-5 and chemokines, as both are requisite for eosinophilic response in the airways [212-214]. Once recruited, eosinophils require various growth factors, most importantly GM-CSF and IL-5 [107, 215]. In the absence of growth factors eosinophils may undergo apoptosis, programmed cell death. Given its effect upon chemokines and cytokines, adiponectin has the potential to prevent eosinophil recruitment, promote their dispersal, and initiate their demise- thereby abating acute allergic reactions, or serving as prophylaxis therapy.

Currently, a humanized monoclonal antibody to IL-5 has been administered to asthmatic patients [216]; in animal studies, a profound and prolonged reduction in circulating eosinophils is observed. Despite completely blocked eosinophilic recruitment into the airway post inhaled allergen challenge, there remains limited effect upon clinical response, and no significant reduction in airway hyperresponsiveness. *In vivo* adiponectin deficiency results in significantly increased C-C chemokine, interleukin (IL)-5, exotoxin, tumor necrosis factor-alpha, and IL-10 in an allergic model [72, 73, 107, 217, 218]. However, a clinical study investigating an antibody blocking IL-5 demonstrated a profound reduction in circulating eosinophils, but no improvement in clinical parameters measuring asthma control [219]. Other studies suggest eosinophils are not actually completely depleted from the airways, and may still exert considerable effect [220-222]. Together, these data question the pivotal role of eosinophils in airway hyperresponsiveness and asthma, and shape the approaches requisite for utilizing adiponectin in blocking allergic response to allergen and augment respiratory function during asthma exacerbation.

Adiponectin and Lymphocytes

T lymphocytes coordinate the inflammatory response in asthma *via* release of specific cytokine patterns, recruiting eosinophils, and maintaining mast cells in the airways. T lymphocytes expressing a distinctive cytokine pattern similar to murine T helper-2 (Th2) lymphocytes, which characteristically express IL-4, IL-5, and IL-13, are associated with allergic responses [223, 224]; adiponectin has been demonstrated to downregulate the Th2 phenotype [225, 226]. Evidence supports that children with atopy retain the Th2 phenotype more than non-atopic patients.

The balance between Th1 and Th2 cells is believed to be determined by locally released cytokines such as IL-12 (which favors Th1 cells) or IL-4/IL-13 (which favor Th2 emergence). Corticosteroid treatment may differentially affect the balance between IL-12 and IL-13 expression [227]. Murine asthma models strongly suggest IL-13 is both necessary and sufficient for asthmatic phenotype induction [228-231]. Adiponectin may alter Th1 cell cytokine expression (*via* upregulation of IL-12 and IFN-γ) to inhibit Th2 cells [215]. Adiponectin may additionally aid regulatory T (Treg) cells suppress the immune response *via* secretion of inhibitory cytokines, such as IL-10 and TGF-β, suppressing Th1 and Th2 responses [232, 233]. CD4+CD25+ cells utilize the transcription factor FoxP3 to suppress the immune response [234, 235]. Evidence supports CD4+CD25+ regulatory T cells are defective in patients with allergic rhinitis [236]. Adiponectin has been demonstrated to modulate CD4+CD25+ T cells in a novel immunotherapy mechanism, as well as augment Tregs production of IL-10 [237, 238].

CD8+ cells are not usually prominent in asthmatic airways, but may appear in severe asthmatics, and have been linked to rapid decline in pulmonary function [239]. Termed Tc2 cells, CD8+ cells in asthma may express IL-4, IL-5, and IL-13 [240]. In a murine model, adiponectin has been demonstrated to inhibit an allograft transplantation rejection in a CD8+ mediated fashion [241].

Adiponectin and Macrophages

Macrophages, derived from blood monocytes, are pro-inflammatory cells that traffic into airways during asthma, and may be activated by allergens *via* low affinity IgE receptors [242]. Leukotriene (LT) also stimulates macrophages to release inflammatory products, such as TNF-α and nitric oxide [243]. Macrophages have ability to produce a large variety of cytokines mediating different inflammatory responses. Previous studies have demonstrated adiponectin may have anti-inflammatory effects on macrophages [244-248], but the role of the adiponectin in relation to macrophages has only recently been investigated. Ohashi *et al.* determined adiponectin promotes macrophage polarization to an anti-inflammatory phenotype, and reduces reactive oxygen species levels [246]. Adiponectin suppresses IL-5, and induces IL-6 and IL-10 [249]. In addition, these effects are mediated *via* cAMP, NF-kB signaling, and ERK1/2. Alveolar macrophages normally suppress lymphocyte function, but this may be impaired after allergen exposure. The amplification of macrophage IL-10 production by adiponectin may help mitigate the reduction of IL-10 in alveolar macrophages seen in asthmatics [75, 245, 250, 251]. Macrophages from normal individuals also inhibit the IL-5 secretion from T lymphocytes, probably *via* IL-12 release, but this is defective in allergic asthmatics [252]. However, adiponectin-mediated suppression of IL-5 may promote recovery to normal conditions [107]. Macrophages may prevent allergic inflammation development, but their functions are limited during allergic flares. Adiponectin may help mitigate deficiencies and augment macrophage function during such circumstances.

Finally, macrophages may act as antigen-presenting cells, which process allergen for presentation to T lymphocytes, illustrating a function of macrophages entirely separate from one invoking inflammation response. During allergic conditions, there may exist macrophage subtypes that perform deranged functions. However, no differences in the macrophage populations have been noted between normal and asthmatic sputum samples [253].

Adiponectin and Cellular Adhesion in Allergic Inflammation

Under allergic inflammatory circumstances, both tissue-resident cells (mast cells, macrophages, dendritic cells), as well as peripheral blood leukocytes (eosinophils, T cells, Th cells), play a key role in tissue inflammatory response. Coordinated cellular adhesion events occur between circulating leukocytes and the vascular endothelium, ultimately leading to recruitment of circulating leukocytes to inflammation sites, where a wide range of tissue inflammatory responses associated with allergy commence.

Dependent upon the nature of the inciting stimulus eliciting the inflammatory response (*i.e.,* allergen), one or more of the circulating leukocyte subsets (eosinophils, T cells, Th cells, macrophages, *etc.*) may be recruited [254-259]. Cell adhesion molecules (CAMs) contribute to the selective recruitment of circulating leukocytes to inflammation sites *via* promoting cell–cell and cell–matrix interactions. Based upon different structural features and functions, CAMs have been subdivided into three families: selectins, integrins, and immunoglobulin gene super family (IgSF) members [260-262]. Adhesion molecules belonging to one of these families, with some exceptions, promote a series of leukocyte interactions with endothelial cells within blood vessels. Such interaction may mediate subsequent leukocyte migration across the endothelium, followed by directed leukocyte migration into the tissues where the allergic response is occurring. We shall next focus specifically upon those CAMs associated with allergic inflammation or immunodeficiencies, and how adiponectin may help restore normal function.

When endobronchial allergens increase VCAM-1, epithelial ICAM-1, and E-selectin expression, eosinophil flux occurs. Soluble forms of adhesion molecules have been identified in bronchial alveolar lavage from allergic disease. Airway allergen challenge is associated with modified levels of adhesion molecules expressed by circulating leukocytes. The effect of adiponectin upon VCAM-1 produced by leukocytes during allergic conditions has not been addressed. However, it has been demonstrated that adiponectin deficiency promotes endothelial activation, and greatly exacerbates adhesion molecule expression [263]. Bronchial mucosal biopsies reveal increased endothelial cell E-selectin expression in allergic patients compared to healthy subjects, which is further increased after allergen challenge, coinciding with the recruitment of esoinophils, neutrophils, and lymphocytes into the airway mucosa. Adiponectin effectively decreases E-selectin expression levels [264].

While studies involving allergen challenge in allergic diseases demonstrate increased expression of adhesion molecules, studies of adhesion molecule expression in conditions unrelated to allergen challenge are somewhat contradictory, perhaps due to differences of patient severity and treatments. Several studies have examined adhesion molecule expression in the airways of mild asthmatics [265-268]. Similar levels of endothelial ICAM-1 and E-selectin were found in bronchial mucosal biopsies from subjects with mild allergic asthma and normal subjects, despite an increased number of mucosal eosinophils in mild asthmatic patients [269-271]. Treatment of mild asthmatics with inhaled corticosteroids reduced tissue eosinophilia without altering ICAM-1 or E-selectin expression [272, 273]. Taken together, adiponectin as monotherapy would not be most efficacious in terms of adhesion molecule inhibition in inflammatory cells; combination therapy with another agent would likely be most beneficial.

Possible Avenues for Therapeutic Action and Conclusion

The multiple protective effects of adiponectin serve as the basis for its numerous potential therapeutic applications. A significant body of literature has demonstrated promising associations of adiponectin in relation to anti-inflammatory, anti-allergy effects. We have reviewed here at length the potential applications of adiponectin in different aspects of allergy related pathophysiology, from broad strategy to specific cellular scope. As a novel therapeutic with exciting advantages over current mainstay pharmacotherapy, adiponectin may be pivotal in the treatment of antigen-induced inflammatory diseases in the future.

ESTROGEN, ESTROGEN RECEPTOR, AND ALLERGIC DISEASE

Approximately 50 million people in the United States and 80 million people in Europe suffer from allergic disease, with increasing prevalence over the past 20-30 years [274-278]. Allergy problems are now not restricted to seasons and regions; people note numerous environmental allergens and experience multiple symptoms associated with allergic asthma, allergic rhinitis, food allergies, and dermatological problems such as allergic eczema and urticaria [279-282]. As the prevalence of allergic disorders such as asthma is higher among women than men, the identification of factors influencing asthma disease course among women may shed light upon potential mechanisms capable of reducing morbidity. Evidence suggests that estrogen and progesterone may influence pulmonary function and asthma disease [283-287] (Fig **5**). Therefore, we shall address the potential impact of both endogenous and exogenous estrogen and progesterone upon the allergic disease asthma, critically appraise the strengths and weaknesses of available evidence, and suggest future directions for research and pharmacotherapeutic strategies.

Estrogen is produced in the ovaries and in various target cells from the precursor dehydroepiandrosterone [288, 289]. Estrogen and progesterone are immune modulators [28, 290, 291]. The immune system is arguably the most complex physiologic system in the body. Several cell lines within the immune system produce specific responses in the form of regulatory cytokine release in reaction to various stimuli. Estrogen affects most cytokines in varying manner, even within similar cytokine families [285, 292-294]. It acts upon two estrogen receptors (ER). ER are predominantly localized in the plasma membrane, cytosol, and nucleus of various cells, from many organs of the body, including the uterus, prostate, ovary, brain, lung, bladder, testes, pituitary gland, kidney, epididymis, adrenal gland, bone, neurons of the central and peripheral nervous system, thymus, spleen, and the immune system [295-299]. Activated ER is localized predominantly in the nucleus, whereas ER is mainly located in the cytoplasm [300-302]. Estrogen and other steroids diffuse through the cell membrane to form complexes with cytosolic and/or nuclear receptors, ultimately inducing both genomic and nongenomic effects. Wang *et al.* demonstrated the existence of membrane receptors in endothelial cells (Fig. **6**), and acts as a functional channel for calcium influx to the cytosol [303, 304] (Fig. **7**). *Via* this membrane receptor, estrogen has anti-inflammatory effects, particularly against antigen specific allergens (*e.g.*, nicotine). However, estrogen appears to have opposing effects upon allergic disorders *via* its two traditional receptors. Whereas, estrogen receptor-α (alpha) appears to promote bronchial asthma [300, 301], estrogen receptor-β (beta) may ameliorate the inflammatory response [301] .

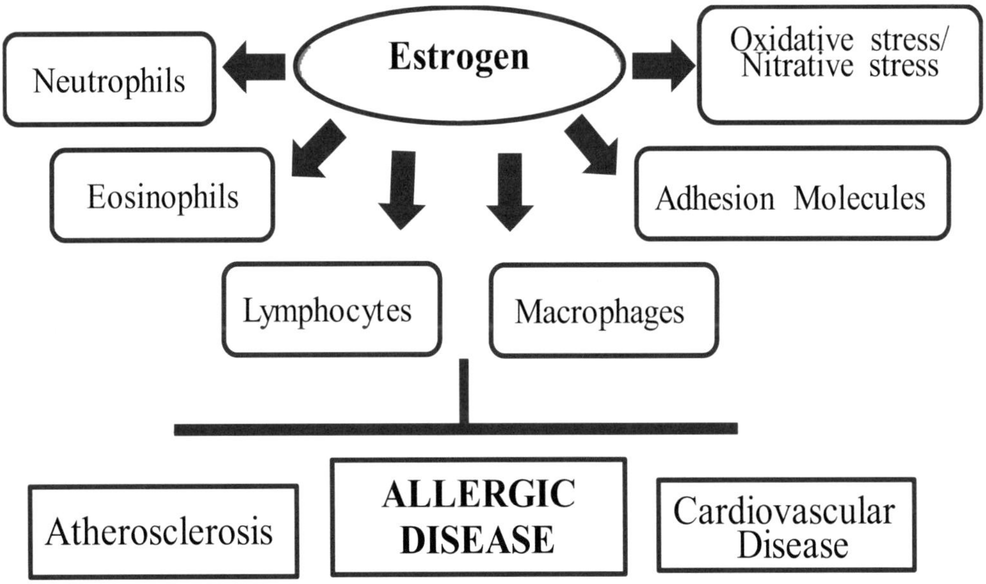

Figure 5: From estrogen to inflammatory disease. The diagram depicts estrogen can through modulate inflammatory cells to further ameliorate allergic disease and cardiovascular risks. Estrogen's influence is linked to a series of cellular actions and modifications decreasing generation of reactive oxygen species/nitrite oxide, adhesion molecules and inflammatory cytokines, which factors affects local and systemic functions and influences endothelial function and predisposes to the development of allergic inflammation.

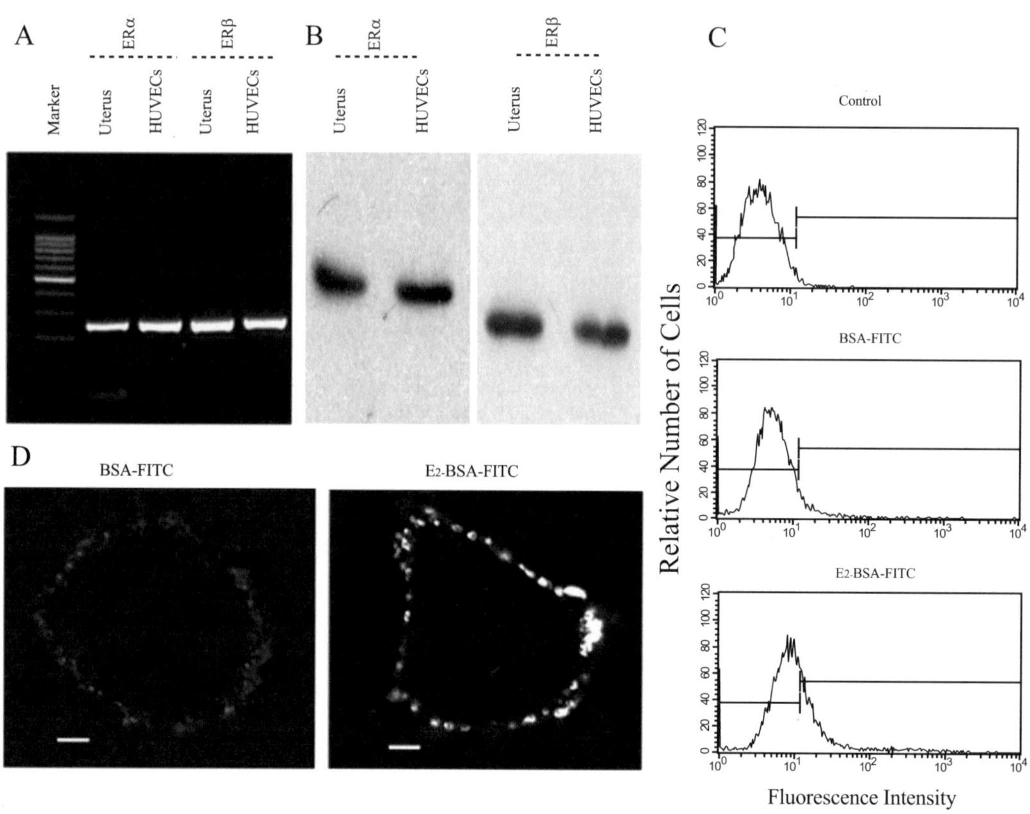

Figure 6: Existence of ER in HUVECs. (A) RT-PCR detecting ERα, ERβ. The predicted bands were revealed in ER mRNA from HUVECs. (B)Western blot showing ERα, ERβ existed in HUVECs. (C) Flow cytometric analysis of intact HUVECs labeled with E2-BSA-FITC and BSA-FITC. (D) Using CLSM, E2-BSA-FITC localized but not BSA-FITC on the surface of HUVECs. Bars represent 10 μm. The positive control was from uterus.

Estrogen and its effects upon allergic inflammation

Animal models demonstrate that estrogen stimulates, whereas progesterone and androgens suppress, the immune system in terms of allergic inflammation. Progesterone promotes T-helper 2 cell development, triggering antibody production, and antagonizing the emergence of T-helper 1 cells and pro-inflammatory cytokines [305-307]. Specifically however, these results were pivotally dependent upon the receptor type expression profile of different diseases. In states of increased estrogen receptor beta expression, augmented anti-inflammatory function was demonstrated in allergic disorders [300, 301, 308, 309]. An analysis of cytokine/chemokine secretion by specific T cells revealed divergently unique estrogen receptor-α and estrogen receptor-β genotype-dependent regulation. Estrogen receptor-α negatively regulated IFN-γ secretion; estrogen receptor-β negatively regulated TNF-α secretion [309]. Although estrogen demonstrates variable influence upon cytokine secretion *via* its two receptors, both estradiol and progesterone significantly inhibit human peripheral monocyte production of IL-1, a strong mediator of inflammation [310]. Estradiol has also been found to exhibit anti-inflammatory properties in leukocyte studies [311, 312]. In general, estrogen has immuno-modulating capability through interaction with its two receptors, and considerable evidence supports estrogen receptor-β as being suppressive of the allergic inflammatory response.

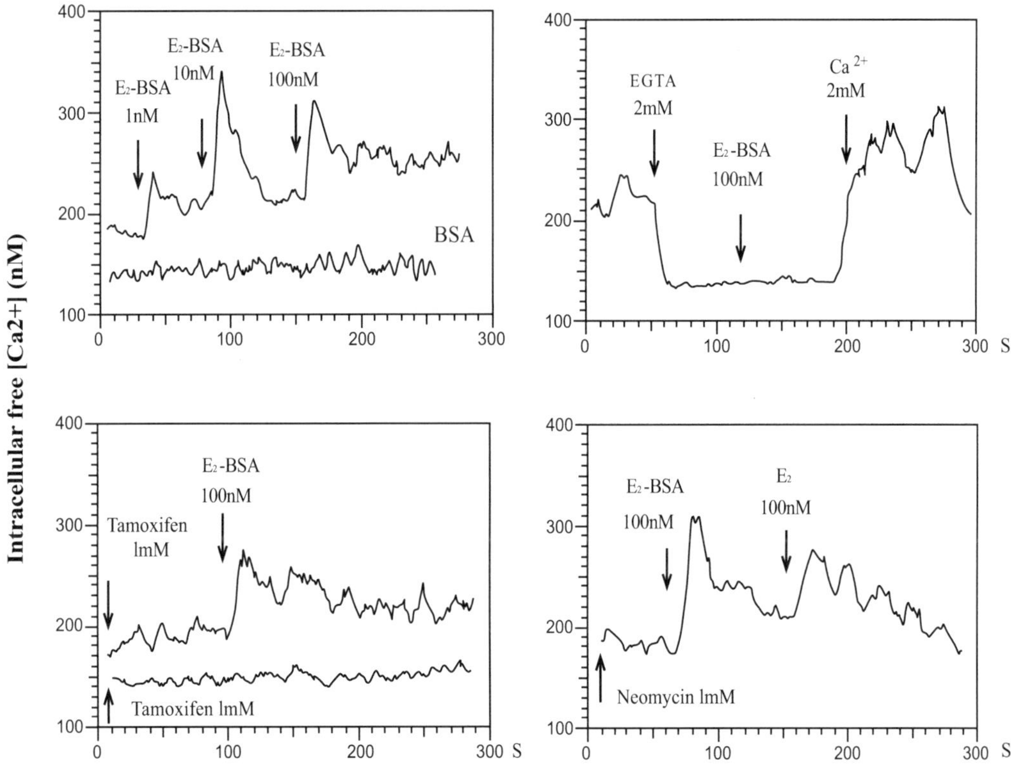

Figure 7: E_2 caused rise in $[Ca^{2+}]$ of HUVECs through estrogen membrane receptor. Cells stimulated with E_2-BSA could triggere an immediate increase in $[Ca^{2+}]$ in inside of cells. If cells preincubated with estrogen receptor inhibitor (tamoxifen) for 1 h before E_2-BSA application, the Ca^{2+} influx could be largely blocked, whereas tamoxifen alone did not affect $[Ca^{2+}]$. If cells were incubated with 2 mM EGTA (an extracellular Ca^{2+} chelator) for 1 min, before the addition of E_2-BSA, E_2-BSA could not make any rise of $[Ca^{2+}]$. Phospholipase C inhibitor neomycin couldnot block E_2-BSA induced the increase of $[Ca^{2+}]$. $[Ca^{2+}]$: calcium concentration inside of cells. The arrows showed the addition of reagents with the indicated concentrations to HUVECs suspensions.

Estrogens and Oxygen Radicals

Reactive oxygen species (ROS) generation is an important pro-inflammatory function evolutionarily conserved to neutralize infection. However, ROS generation is also a feature of allergic inflammatory diseases. We next discuss the effects of estrogen upon ROS generation.

Various studies demonstrate increased ROS production post ovarectomy, whereas supplementation of pregnancy-level estrogen decreased ROS production [313-317]. Cardiac cells expressing ERβ were protected against H_2O_2-induced apoptosis in the presence of estrogen maintained at pregnancy-level. Estradiol increased the expression of glutaredoxin and γ-glutamylcysteine synthase (a rate-limiting enzyme for glutathione synthesis), an effect blocked by estrogen receptor inhibitor ICI 182780 [318]. In primary rat microglia and a microglial cell line (N9), pretreatment with estrogen to pregnancy-levels attenuated phorbol-12-myristate-13-acetate-stimulated superoxide release [319, 320]. Both NADPH oxidase and myeloperoxidase are important for oxygen radical generation. In various cell lines, estrogen at pregnancy-levels decreased the expression of NADPH oxidase [321] and myeloperoxidase [322-324], each significantly decreasing ROS generation.

In conclusion, overwhelming evidence demonstrates estrogen, at proestrus to pregnancy-levels, inhibits ROS formation. Estrogen's inhibition of ROS generation may be blocked depending upon cell type and the microenvironmental conditions leading to catechol estrogen formation [325, 326]. Additionally, ROS formation may still occur in the setting of estrogen below proestrus levels, leading to a pro-inflammatory state post-menopause.

Estrogen's Nongenomic Effects Upon Anti-Allergic Inflammation

Within minutes of interacting with its membrane receptor, estrogen activates mitogen-activated protein kinase (MAPK). Estrogen interaction with its membrane receptor also opens a selective channel permitting calcium influx to the cytosol, with anti-inflammatory effect, by inhibiting calmodulin overexpression [327]. Patch clamp recording techniques demonstrate that the estrogen membrane receptor can trigger a weak positive calcium current with protective effect in human umbilical vein endothelial cells [304]. Such protective effect is not limited to endothelial cells. In macrophages, the estrogen membrane receptor invokes an anti-inflammatory response, reliant upon the p38/ ERK1/2 pathway [328]. In breast cancer cells, the responsible signaling pathway involves c-Src/Shc/Grb/Ras activation [329]; in endothelial cells, the regulatory subunit of phosphatidyl inositol 3 kinase (PI3K) mediates anti-inflammatory effect [330, 331].

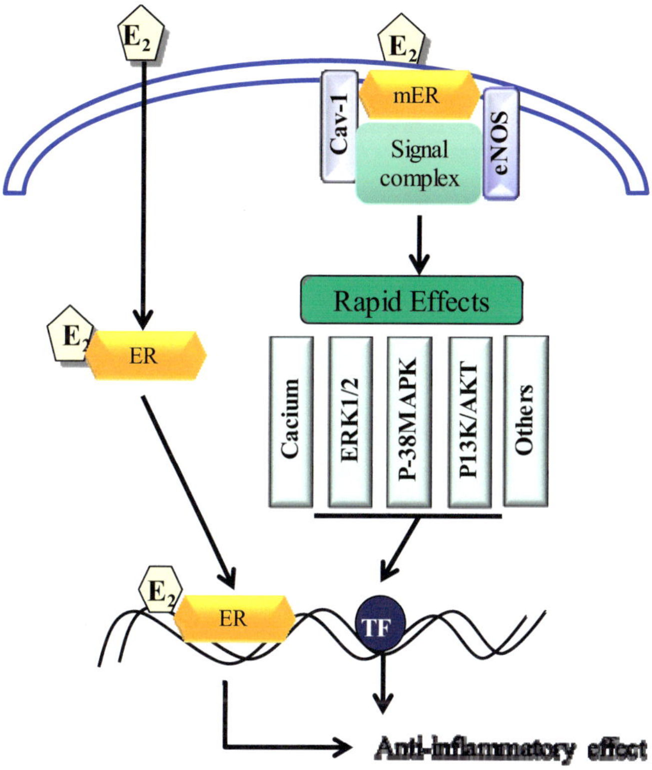

Figure 8: Proposed model of E_2 (estrogen) mechanisms involved in anti-inflammatory effect in inflammatory cells. E_2 action involves nuclear and membrane-associated estrogen receptor (ERα/β) to transfer signaling to the nucleus. The activation of several signaling pathways in response to E_2 regulates inflammatory signaling alteration through influencing interaction behavior of transcription factors (TF). In addition, E_2 can adjust inflammatory gene transcription through the estrogen receptor interaction with the estrogen response element in DNA. Cav-1,Caveolin-1. ER, estrogen receptor.

We mention previously the importance of nitric oxide in allergic disorder pathophysiology. Activation of the estrogen receptor induces long-term vasodilation, dependent upon activation of genes encoding prostacyclin synthase and nitric oxide synthase (NOS) [332, 333]. In pulmonary vascular endothelial cells, estrogen induces PI3K-Akt–dependent activation of endothelial NOS (eNOS or NOS3), increasing production of nitric oxide and causing vessel dilation (optimization of this effect requires active heat shock protein 90) [334, 335]. In pulmonary epithelial cells, estrogen stimulates NO production *via* NOS3 activation [336]; in smooth muscle cells, estrogen increases NO production by phosphorylation of neuronal NOS (nNOS or NOS1) [337]. *Via* estrogen receptor activation, estrogens inhibit smooth muscle cell migration and proliferation [338, 339].

The nontraditional estrogen pathway, *via* the estrogen membrane receptor, therefore carries significant signaling mechanisms influencing inflammation and pathways of allergic response (Fig. **8**).

Estrogen and Inflammatory Cells

Estrogen and Eosinophils

Increased activated eosinophils in the airway epithelium and submucosa are pathognomonic of allergic response [311, 340]. Allergen challenge increases eosinophil count in bronchoalveolar lavage; peripheral blood eosinophil count correlates with bronchial hyperresponsiveness degree in asthmatics [341-343]. Respiratory epithelial cells contain elevated levels of eosinphil granule proteins, such as major basic protein (MBP) [343]. MBP triggers direct degranulation of mast cells and basophils, a key component in allergic disease. Estrogen has been demonstrated to regulate eosinophilic granulocytes *via* MBP modulation [344, 345]. Estrogen receptors are expressed in the eosinophils of patients with vernal keratoconjunctivitis (VKC), an allergic eosinophilic atopic disease, similar to asthma, rhinitis and eczema. Estrogens increase uterine eosinophilic infiltration [346-348], and promote splenic eosinophilic degranulation. However, dietary supplementation of phytoestrogens decreases eosinophil lung infiltration in an animal asthmatic model [349]. Such effect may be due to estrogen effect upon mast cells, which have been demonstrated to contain the estrogen receptor [350]. Genistein, a plant estrogen mimicker, inhibits eosinophilic leukotriene synthesis [351]. Estrogen may control eosinophilia *via* estrogen receptor-α [352]. Together, these experimental data provide multiple avenues for eosinphilic manipulation by estrogen and its receptor.

Estrogen and Neutrophils

Neutrophils are found in both sputum and bronchoalveolar lavage from patients during acute allergic illness [353]. Neutrophils secrete serine proteases, including neutrophil elastase, cathepsin G, and proteinase-3. These enzymes are not only potent mucus stimulants, but may also contribute to alveolar destruction [354, 355]. Airway neutrophil recruitment involves vascular adhesion molecules, and during allergic flare, E-selectin is upregulated in the pulmonary endothelium [356-358]. Neutrophils therefore contribute to the acute stage of allergic inflammatory response. Estrogen exerts cellular immunosuppressive effect upon various chemotactic agents, diminishing phagocytosis, impairing the adhesive potential of immunocytes to vasculature endothelial lining [359-361], and inhibiting oxidative burst [362], which profiles all highly related with neutrophils number in flare locale. Estrogen reduces neutrophil mobilization specifically by interfering with CXCL12, p38, and MAPK families [363-366].

The NOS system is essential in allergic inflammatory processing. In women, circulating estrogen concentrations are associated with neutrophilic expression of NOS protein [367]. Estrogen receptors have been identified in neutrophils from both men and women. Both estrogen and genistein (a natural soy phytoestrogen) upregulate eNOS activity and downregulate iNOS expression in neutrophils [368-372]. However, gender differences exist: neutrophils from premenopausal women express both estrogen receptor-α and -2 subtypes, which both increase following incubation with 17-estradiol *in vitro*, but only estrogen receptor-α expression increases in male neutrophils following *in vitro* incubation with estrogen [373]. Estrogen treatment reduces neutrophilic influx, and inflammation degree in myocardial ischemia [374], skeletal muscle, and ischemic liver disease models [375, 376]. In the lung, estrogen prevents neutrophilic infiltration in pulmonary injury models, an effect involving downregulation of neutrophilic chemoattractant factors and adhesion molecules [377]. Administration of a soy estrogen mimicker in an allergic animal model promisingly decreased oxidative and nitrative stress [369, 370].

Estrogens and Macrophages

Macrophages are activated by antigens (such as cigarette smoke and other inhaled irritants), and drive the inflammatory process in allergic disease. The number of macrophages in the alveolar wall correlates with the extent of parenchymal destruction in emphysema [378-380]. The number of airway macrophages highly correlates with the severity of airway obstruction, the end point of unmitigated allergic response [381, 382]. Estrogens decrease macrophage cytokine production through modulation of CD16 expression *via* estrogen receptor-β [383], decrease macrophage recruitment in the brain *via* estrogen receptor-α [384], and control nuclear factor kappa B (NF-κB) nuclear translocation [385]. Estrogen receptor-β activation increases eNOS activity [313, 386], and decreases TNF-α and IL-1 production in nicotine-treated murine macrophages [303, 304, 387]. Estrogen administered to macrophages prevents CD4+ T cell amplification and suppresses allergic inflammation in experimental allergic encephalomyelitis [388]. In the lung, estrogen enhances macrophage bacteriostatic activity [389, 390]. In summary, estrogen has complex and sometimes opposing actions upon macrophage cytokine secretion and activity. Such divergent effects are likely due to the different estrogen receptors, which facilitate different signal transduction pathways during allergic inflammation.

Estrogens and Lymphocytes

The T helper type 1 (Th1) cell immune response drives cell-mediated immunity, causing tissue damage in chronic inflammatory autoimmune diseases [391]. In contrast, T helper type 2 (Th2) cells invoke the inflammatory reaction in allergic disorders by increasing cytokine (IL-4, IL-5, IL-9, IL-13) release [392-397]. The Th1 and Th2 pathways reciprocally inhibit each other [398, 399]. Cytokines IFN-γ, IL-12, and TNF facilitate the Th1 reactions [397, 400-403], and IL-4, IL-5, and IL-10 enact Th2 responses. Meanwhile, B lymphocyte secretion of immunoglobulin E (IgE) further contributes to allergic inflammation. Estrogens modulate the lymphocytic immunologic response in a variety of manner. Estrogen inhibits B cell development in the bone marrow [404, 405], influences peripheral B-cell development [406], blocks early T-cell development in the thymus [407], and increases the CD4/CD8 ratio. Whether estrogen-induced involution of T-cell development is advantageous in chronic inflammatory states remains unknown, because both auto-aggressive and auto-tolerant T cells may be eliminated. Estrogens also directly elicit a Th2 response, with consequently increased Th2 cytokines [292, 408]. However, the Th1/Th2 ratio has been shown to be increased in pregnancy, a high-estrogen level state; estrogen may therefore exert a balancing effect dependent upon the particular environment [306, 409]. Data also suggests that low concentration estrogen may favorable down-regulate T cell-dependent immunity in allergic disorders [410]. Based on some conflict data saying, if estrogen has higher level or falls to postmenopausal levels (metestrus) before initiation or during the course of an autoimmune disease [411], estrogen shows elevate the sensitivity of immuosystem, which might through alter T helper cell situation to reach out this effect.

Estrogen and Adhesion Molecules

Adhesion molecules are important factors during allergic inflammation, as they enable appropriate migration of inflammatory cells to sites of activity. Essentially, estrogen inhibits expression of adhesion molecules, dependent upon estrogen concentration. *In vitro* human and mice/rat cells studies demonstrate that pregnancy-level estrogen inhibits expression of adhesion molecules, but this effect is lost at low estrogen levels. Cultured human umbilical vein endothelial cells (HUVECs) were pretreated with pregnancy-level estrogen for 48 hours before IL-1 activation. Estrogen strongly inhibited IL-1-induced expression of membrane E-selectin, vascular cell adhesion molecule-1 (VCAM-1), and intercellular adhesion molecule-1 (ICAM-1) [412, 413]. Other studies demonstrate estrogen at pregnancy-levels decreased expression of TNF-α-induced VCAM-1 in HUVECs [314, 414, 415]. Such effects appear to be mediated *via* estrogen receptor-α; in an endothelial cell line overexpressing estrogen receptor-α (ECV-304), estrogen at pregnancy-levels inhibited the effects of TNF-α upon VCAM-1 expression and U937 cell adhesion [416]. In normal human female iliac artery endothelial cells, high-level estrogen decreased IL-1β-stimulated VCAM-1 and ICAM-1 membrane expression [416]. In ECV-304 cells, the E-selectin promoter is down-regulated by estradiol (no effect seen at lowest estradiol concentration 10^{-11} M, increasing effect at increased estradiol concentrations 10^{-10} and 10^{-5} M) [417]. In cultured brain endothelial cells, estrogen at suprapregnancy-levels blocked basal and IL-1β-stimulated expression of ICAM-1 [361, 416, 418]. These studies clearly demonstrate the inhibitory effect of high-level estrogen upon various adhesion molecule expressions. Estrogens at low levels may exert opposing effect. Estrogen at diestrus-levels upregulates L-selectin and α4-integrin dependent adhesion pathways in endothelium and lymphocytes [419]. Postmenopausal women with coronary artery disease exhibit increased serum levels of soluble E-selectin, ICAM-1, and VCAM-1, indicating upregulation of membrane-bound adhesion molecules [420-423].

In conclusion, estrogen has different effect with different dose administration. Higher concentration estrogen (pregnancy-levels) decreases membrane expression of adhesion molecules and cell adhesion to endothelial cells, an effect possibly mediated by estrogen receptor-α. Some studies indicate that lower estrogen concentration (diestrus to ovariectomy/postmenopausal-levels) increases adhesion molecule expression. Even a marginal increase of estrogen to 10^{-10} M under estrogen replacement therapy (ERT) in postmenopausal women reduces soluble forms of adhesion molecules, likely indicative of downregulation of membrane-bound adhesion molecules. Again, a dichotomy of estrogen effects is observed, but related to its dose, and not receptor specificity. Such data gives evidence for the utilization of estrogen supplementation as a feasible therapy for allergic disorder. We next discuss estrogen supplementation regiments.

From Estrogen Replacement Therapy (ERT) and Hormone Replacement Therapy (HRT) to Plant Estrogen Supplementation

ERT ameliorates the impaired immune response observed in postmenopausal women, giving evidence to the role of estrogen in regulating immune function. ERT significantly decreases production of IL-2 and IL-4 [424] and increases serum IFN–γ concentration [425]. Estrogen attenuates endotoxin release of TNF-α in postmenopausal women [426]. If subject to comparable injuries, aged mice are more immunosuppressed than young mice. Immunosuppression in severely injured patients is associated with a Th1-Th2 shift. Clinical observations indicate exacerbation of asthma after menopause, and increased asthma incidence after menopause onset. It remains controversial whether ERT is beneficial to asthma development, as there is evidence supporting ERT increases asthma risk [427] and decreases it [428]. Asthmatic postmenopausal women secrete less estrogen than postmenopausal healthy women. ERT increases estrogen levels, with normalization of asthmatic symptoms [429]. However, accumulating evidence suggests oral contraceptives abrogate or alleviate asthmatic symptoms in premenstrual women [428]. Patients taking oral contraceptives experience attenuated menstrual cycle-mediated airway hyper-responsiveness, as well as reduced diurnal peak expiratory flow rate variability (typically associated with the luteal cycle phase), compared to control [430-432]. It is worthy to note that estradiol was utilized in animal studies, but rarely is a synthetic estradiol derivative administered to women as sole hormonal therapy.

Currently, hormone replacement therapy (HRT) is more widely utilized as therapy than ERT. HRT is a combination therapy of naturally occurring or synthetic estrogens together with progestins or synthetic progestins [433-435]. Therefore, a separate analysis of estrogen and progestin effects is impossible, and observed effects must be attributed to both estrogens and progestins in combination [436]. HRT utilizes different estrogen types, most often employing conjugated equine estrogens (CEE) or synthetic estradiol derivatives. Conjugated equine estrogens may have different effects, pharmacodynamics, and pharmacokinetics compared to estradiol [436-438]. It bears mentioning serum estrogen levels during hormonal therapy only increase to a relatively small extent [439, 440]. Estradiol alone or in combination with progestins demonstrates little or no effect upon pro-inflammatory cytokines [441]. However, estradiol in combination with progestins or CEE with/without progestins decrease serum levels of monocyte chemotactic protein-1 (MCP-1) and other important soluble adhesion molecules, deemed favorable in the treatment of atherosclerosis, and likely other chronic inflammatory diseases [420, 442, 443]. Decreased cell surface soluble adhesion molecules reflect decreased leukocyte migration into sites of tissue inflammation. Estrogen dose and route are important considerations as well, as only oral (not transdermal) therapy increases C-reactive protein [444], demonstrating possibly hepatic conversion of estradiol to downstream estrogens might produce pro-inflammatory metabolites.

We mention many aspects of estrogen favoring inhibition of allergic inflammation. However, there remain questions challenging estrogen side effects. Plant estrogen alternatives have been the subject of intense investigation. Spinach leaves contain active components, such as flavonoids, exhibiting anti-oxidative, anti-proliferative, and anti-inflammatory effects [445]. Appropriate intake of foods with anti-allergic potency may prevent onset of allergic diseases and/or ameliorate allergic symptoms. Flavonoids, particular luteolin, apigenin, fisetin, hesperidin, isoquercitrin, and epigallocatechin-3-gallate, are ubiquitously present in vegetables, fruits, or teas. These compounds exert anti-allergic activities [446-453]. Flavonoids inhibit inflammatory cell release of histamine, synthesis of IL-4 and IL-13, and expression of CD40 ligand [450, 452]. Havsteen *et al.* demonstrated that luteolin, ayanin, apigenin, and fisetin were the strongest inhibitors of IL-4 production [454]. By investigating the mechanism by which flavonoids exert their effect, researchers demonstrate flavonoids inhibit IL-4, IL-5, and IL-13 ligand expression, with subsequent inhibition of T cell nuclear factor activation *via* the AP-1, NF-κB pathway, and MAPK/ERK axis; IL-4 IL-5, and IL-13 are important markers in the allergic response pathway [447-452, 455, 456]. Additionally, as oxidative stress is an exacerbating allergic inflammation, luteolin demonstrates anti-oxidant and anti-inflammatory properties [457, 458]. Flavonoid administration in atopic dermatitis-prone mice conferred preventative and ameliorative effect [446, 457-461]. Recent epidemiological studies report that a significantly decreased incidence of asthma was observed in a population with high flavonoid intake [462]. Such encouraging evidence supports the development of dietary menus including appropriate flavonoids optimized to complement any allergic disease preventative strategy.

INTERVENTIONS FOR THE TREATMENT OF ALLERGIC DISEASES

The current first line therapy for allergic disease symptoms includes over the counter medications available in commercial pharmacies. While self-medication with physician guidance may benefit many patients, those with severe illness, refractory symptoms, and/or highly poly-sensitized require more aggressive treatment options. For patients with persistent and severe symptoms, consultation with a physician, prescription medications, and vigilance provides the best method for controlling allergic disease. Significant allergy treatment advances over recent decades offer treatment options for even the most persistent allergic exacerbations. Table **2** lists the most common forms of allergy treatment, and potential future therapies:

Table 2: Treatment options for allergy treatment, established and anticipated.

Treatment Classification and Description			
Established	Antihistamines (oral)	The gold standard treatment for acute allergic disease (excluding asthma); effective and widely available; prescribed for ~30% of all allergic disorders	[463-466]
	β2-agonists (inhaled)	For acute exercise-induced asthma and wheezing; not recommended for long term use (except long acting formulations)	[467]
	Corticosteroids (oral and inhaled)	For long term use in asthmatics with intermediate and severe asthma; inhaled corticosteroids utilized for daily therapy	[468, 469]
	Anticholinergic drugs (inhaled and oral)	For nocturnal asthma, adjuvant therapy to β2 agonists, useful for situations where side effects of β2-agonists are not acceptable	[469-471]
	Immunotherapy	Administered over three year treatment period; not recommended for severe asthmatics or highly poly-sensitized patients	[472, 473]
	Adrenaline (epinephrine, subcutaneous or intravenous)	Rapid injection for anaphylaxis	[474, 475]
	Others	Anti-IgE for severe allergic asthma; xanthine, cromolyn sodium and sodium nedocromil for asthma treatment (mast cell stabilization)	[476, 477]
Anticipated	Adiponectin	Anti-inflammatory, for late phase adjuvant therapy	
	Plant estrogen	Luteolin, apigenin, fisetin, hesperidin, and isoquercitrin for allergy prophylaxis and long term suppressive therapy	

CONCLUSIONS

Many components are central to the pathogenesis of allergic disease. Successful treatment must derive from an appreciation of the complexity of the interaction of these components, including but not limited to: the instigating immune stimuli itself (foreign antigens or autoantigens), the cellular types involved in response (not limited to immune cells alone), and the target tissues and organs affected.

In this chapter, we have discussed the potential applications of adiponectin and estrogen in anti-allergic role. Adiponectin's anti-inflammatory role has been demonstrated in the cardiovascular system at length, and available evidence presented in this chapter concerning its applicability in allergic medicine therapeutics is promising. Its anti-oxidative and anti-nitrative stress properties are well documented, and would be advantageous during antigen-induced allergic flare recruitment of inflammatory cells to sites of injury. Evidence presented in this chapter concerning estrogen reveals its dichotomous effects, usually attributable to its two different traditional cytosol receptors, estrogen receptor-α and -β. Estrogen's membrane receptor has critical implication in the treatment of allergic disease, as it mediates the anti-inflammatory effects of estrogen. Estrogen inhibits a variety of the immune cell players involved with allergic response at pregnancy-levels, and its suitability as an anti-allergic therapeutic has new promise in plant estrogen supplementations.

Allergic diseases transcend season, region, and socioeconomics, affecting millions worldwide. Industrialization has increased quality of life in developed nations, but unfortunately modern lifestyles expose us to constantly more aggressive allergens. Prevalence will likely continue to climb in the years to come. Fortunately, many allergic diseases can be successfully treated with the right intervention and avoidance strategies, with minimal costs of mortality. However, more can and must be done to alter the outcome of disease and treat morbidity for all patients.

To maximize the best practice for the control and treatment of allergic disease, we must:

1. Recognize allergic diseases as a public health priority.
2. Conduct epidemiological research regarding allergic disease prevalence and trends.
3. Ensure healthcare systems educate the public properly and provide access to professional healthcare and efficacious medications.
4. Establish guidelines for the cost-effective management of allergic therapy.
5. Establish programs developing new medications efficacious for early prophylaxis.
6. Agree each person has responsibility to maintain an allergy-friendly environment for all.

ACKNOWLEDGEMENTS

This work was supported by grants from the National Scientific Foundation of China (NSFC 30900592, 81170199 to Y-J.W, and 81270185 to J-L.Z.) and ADA 1-11-JF56 (to Y-J.W.). We are greatly appreciative to Xin-Liang Ma, MD, PhD for his support and guiding vision.

CONFLICT OF INTEREST

The author(s) confirm that this chapter content has no conflict of interest.

REFERENCES

[1] Dixon A. The treatment of asthma in obesity. Expert Rev Respir Med. 2012; 6: 331-40.
[2] Visness CM, London SJ, Daniels JL, *et al.* Association of obesity with IgE levels and allergy symptoms in children and adolescents: results from the National Health and Nutrition Examination Survey 2005-2006. J Allergy Clin Immunol. 2009; 123: 1163-9, 9 e1-4.
[3] Gil A, Bengmark S. [Advanced glycation and lipoxidation end products--amplifiers of inflammation: the role of food]. Nutr Hosp. 2007; 22: 625-40.
[4] Herz U, Petschow B. Perinatal events affecting the onset of allergic diseases. Curr Drug Targets Inflamm Allergy. 2005; 4: 523-9.
[5] Perez-Padilla R, Rojas R, Torres V, *et al.* Obesity among children residing in Mexico City and its impact on lung function: a comparison with Mexican-Americans. Arch Med Res. 2006; 37: 165-71.
[6] Telenga ED, Tideman SW, Kerstjens HA, *et al.* Obesity in asthma: more neutrophilic inflammation as a possible explanation for a reduced treatment response. Allergy. 2012; 67: 1060-8.
[7] Deesomchok A, Fisher T, Webb KA, *et al.* Effects of obesity on perceptual and mechanical responses to bronchoconstriction in asthma. Am J Respir Crit Care Med. 2010; 181: 125-33.
[8] Machado D, Tavares B, Loureiro G, *et al.* Body mass index and airway hyper-responsiveness in individuals without respiratory disease. Eur Ann Allergy Clin Immunol. 2008; 40: 130-7.
[9] Kusunoki T, Morimoto T, Nishikomori R, *et al.* Obesity and the prevalence of allergic diseases in schoolchildren. Pediatr Allergy Immunol. 2008; 19: 527-34.
[10] Holguin F, Bleecker ER, Busse WW, *et al.* Obesity and asthma: an association modified by age of asthma onset. J Allergy Clin Immunol. 2011; 127: 1486-93 e2.
[11] Farah CS, Kermode JA, Downie SR, *et al.* Obesity is a determinant of asthma control independent of inflammation and lung mechanics. Chest. 2011; 140: 659-66.
[12] Giouleka P, Papatheodorou G, Lyberopoulos P, *et al.* Body mass index is associated with leukotriene inflammation in asthmatics. Eur J Clin Invest. 2011; 41: 30-8.

[13] Mansell AL, Walders N, Wamboldt MZ, *et al.* Effect of body mass index on response to methacholine bronchial provocation in healthy and asthmatic adolescents. Pediatr Pulmonol. 2006; 41: 434-40.

[14] Celedon JC, Palmer LJ, Litonjua AA, *et al.* Body mass index and asthma in adults in families of subjects with asthma in Anqing, China. Am J Respir Crit Care Med. 2001; 164: 1835-40.

[15] Scherer PE, Williams S, Fogliano M, Baldini G, Lodish HF. A novel serum protein similar to C1q, produced exclusively in adipocytes. J Biol Chem. 1995; 270: 26746-9.

[16] Tual S, Godard P, Bousquet J, Annesi-Maesano I. The decrease in asthma-related mortality in France. Rev Mal Respir. 2010; 27: e1-5.

[17] Fuhrman C, Jougla E, Uhry Z, Delmas MC. Deaths with asthma in France, 2000-2005: a multiple-cause analysis. J Asthma. 2009; 46: 402-6.

[18] Moorman JE, Rudd RA, Johnson CA, *et al.* National surveillance for asthma--United States, 1980-2004. MMWR Surveill Summ. 2007; 56: 1-54.

[19] Watson L, Turk F, James P, Holgate ST. Factors associated with mortality after an asthma admission: a national United Kingdom database analysis. Respir Med. 2007; 101: 1659-64.

[20] Santo AH. [Asthma-related mortality, Brazil, 2000: a study using multiple causes of death]. Cad Saude Publica. 2006; 22: 41-52.

[21] de Marco R, Locatelli F, Cazzoletti L, *et al.* Incidence of asthma and mortality in a cohort of young adults: a 7-year prospective study. Respir Res. 2005; 6: 95.

[22] Naberan Tona K, Alberti Jaume J. [Mortality due to asthma in the city of Barcelona (1983-1993)]. Aten Primaria. 2004; 33: 13-9.

[23] Picard E, Barmeir M, Schwartz S, *et al.* Rate and place of death from asthma among different ethnic groups in Israel: national trends 1980 to 1997. Chest. 2002; 122: 1222-7.

[24] Varsano S. Bronchial asthma in Israel. Isr Med Assoc J. 2002; 4: 661-3.

[25] Lockshin MD. Sex differences in autoimmune disease. Lupus. 2006; 15: 753-6.

[26] Mayes MD. Epidemiologic studies of environmental agents and systemic autoimmune diseases. Environ Health Perspect. 1999; 107 Suppl 5: 743-8.

[27] Denman AM. Sex hormones, autoimmune diseases, and immune responses. BMJ. 1991; 303: 2-3.

[28] Hughes GC. Progesterone and autoimmune disease. Autoimmun Rev. 2012; 11: A502-14.

[29] Kasperska-Zajac A, Brzoza Z, Rogala B. Dehydroepiandrosterone and dehydroepiandrosterone sulphate in atopic allergy and chronic urticaria. Inflammation. 2008; 31: 141-5.

[30] Gompel A, Pelissier C, Kuttenn F, Mauvais-Jarvis P. [Hormones and lupus]. Rev Med Interne. 1985; 6: 543-52.

[31] Steinberg AD, Melez KA, Raveche ES, *et al.* Approach to the study of the role of sex hormones in autoimmunity. Arthritis Rheum. 1979; 22: 1170-6.

[32] Bukantz SC, Bagg AS, Lockey RF. Adverse effects and fatalities associated with subcutaneous allergen immunotherapy. Clin Allergy Immunol. 2008; 21: 455-68.

[33] Lockey RF, Nicoara-Kasti GL, Theodoropoulos DS, Bukantz SC. Systemic reactions and fatalities associated with allergen immunotherapy. Ann Allergy Asthma Immunol. 2001; 87: 47-55.

[34] Davies JM, Voskamp A, Dang TD, *et al.* The dominant 55 kDa allergen of the subtropical Bahia grass (Paspalum notatum) pollen is a group 13 pollen allergen, Pas n 13. Mol Immunol. 2011; 48: 931-40.

[35] Piconi S, Trabattoni D, Rainone V, *et al.* Immunological effects of sublingual immunotherapy: clinical efficacy is associated with modulation of programmed cell death ligand 1, IL-10, and IgG4. J Immunol. 2010; 185: 7723-30.
[36] Giannarini L, Maggi E. Decrease of allergen-specific T-cell response induced by local nasal immunotherapy. Clin Exp Allergy. 1998; 28: 404-12.
[37] Semple MG, Taylor-Robinson DC, Lane S, Smyth RL. Household tobacco smoke and admission weight predict severe bronchiolitis in infants independent of deprivation: prospective cohort study. PLoS One. 2011; 6: e22425.
[38] Kusel MM, de Klerk N, Holt PG, Sly PD. Antibiotic use in the first year of life and risk of atopic disease in early childhood. Clin Exp Allergy. 2008; 38: 1921-8.
[39] Eichenfield LF, Thaci D, de Prost Y, Puig L, Paul C. Clinical management of atopic eczema with pimecrolimus cream 1% (Elidel) in paediatric patients. Dermatology. 2007; 215 Suppl 1: 3-17.
[40] Harris JM, Mills P, White C, *et al.* Recorded infections and antibiotics in early life: associations with allergy in UK children and their parents. Thorax. 2007; 62: 631-7.
[41] Zaidi AK, MacGlashan DW. Regulation of Fc epsilon RI expression during murine basophil maturation: the interplay between IgE, cell division, and Fc epsilon RI synthetic rate. J Immunol. 2010; 184: 1463-74.
[42] Pruzansky JJ, Patterson R. Evidence for *in vitro* regulation of IgE receptors on the human basophil membrane by their removal and reexpression: effects of Ca2+, Mg2+, some metabolic inhibitors and fetal calf serum. Int Arch Allergy Appl Immunol. 1988; 85: 368-73.
[43] Bajin MD, Cingi C, Oghan F, Gurbuz MK. Global warming and allergy in Asia Minor. Eur Arch Otorhinolaryngol. 2012.
[44] Peterson B, Saxon A. Global increases in allergic respiratory disease: the possible role of diesel exhaust particles. Ann Allergy Asthma Immunol. 1996; 77: 263-8; quiz 9-70.
[45] Potter PC, Berman D, Toerien A, Malherbe D, Weinberg EG. Clinical significance of aero-allergen identification in the western Cape. S Afr Med J. 1991; 79: 80-4.
[46] Osterhage F, Wippler M, Kalden JR, Deicher H. Determination of specific IgE and IgG serum antibodies during immunotherapy in hay fever patients by RAST. Z Immunitatsforsch Immunobiol. 1977; 153: 189-203.
[47] Abramson MJ, Puy RM, Weiner JM. Injection allergen immunotherapy for asthma. Cochrane Database Syst Rev. 2010: CD001186.
[48] Nelson HS. Multiallergen immunotherapy for allergic rhinitis and asthma. J Allergy Clin Immunol. 2009; 123: 763-9.
[49] Casanovas M, Martin R, Jimenez C, Caballero R, Fernandez-Caldas E. Safety of immunotherapy with therapeutic vaccines containing depigmented and polymerized allergen extracts. Clin Exp Allergy. 2007; 37: 434-40.
[50] Scheiblhofer S, Stoecklinger A, Gruber C, *et al.* Gene gun immunization with clinically relevant allergens aggravates allergen induced pathology and is contraindicated for allergen immunotherapy. Mol Immunol. 2007; 44: 1879-87.
[51] Incorvaia C, Frati F, Puccinelli P, Riario-Sforza GG, Dal Bo S. Dose dependence of efficacy and safety of subcutaneous immunotherapy. Monaldi Arch Chest Dis. 2006; 65: 41-3.
[52] Casanovas M, Martin R, Jimenez C, Caballero R, Fernandez-Caldas E. Safety of an ultra-rush immunotherapy build-up schedule with therapeutic vaccines containing depigmented and polymerized allergen extracts. Int Arch Allergy Immunol. 2006; 139: 153-8.

[53] Bousquet J, Lockey R, Malling HJ. Allergen immunotherapy: therapeutic vaccines for allergic diseases. A WHO position paper. J Allergy Clin Immunol. 1998; 102: 558-62.
[54] Compalati E, Rogkakou A, Villa E, Passalacqua G, Canonica GW. Emerging sublingual immunotherapy drugs. Expert Opin Pharmacother. 2010; 11: 2963-72.
[55] Canonica GW, Bousquet J, Casale T, *et al.* Sub-lingual immunotherapy: World Allergy Organization Position Paper 2009. Allergy. 2009; 64 Suppl 91: 1-59.
[56] Sicherer SH, Leung DY. Advances in allergic skin disease, anaphylaxis, and hypersensitivity reactions to foods, drugs, and insects in 2008. J Allergy Clin Immunol. 2009; 123: 319-27.
[57] von Bubnoff D, Koch S, Bieber T. Dendritic cells and atopic eczema/dermatitis syndrome. Curr Opin Allergy Clin Immunol. 2003; 3: 353-8.
[58] Holtzman MJ, Morton JD, Shornick LP, *et al.* Immunity, inflammation, and remodeling in the airway epithelial barrier: epithelial-viral-allergic paradigm. Physiol Rev. 2002; 82: 19-46.
[59] Karol MH, Macina OT, Cunningham A. Cell and molecular biology of chemical allergy. Ann Allergy Asthma Immunol. 2001; 87: 28-32.
[60] Leung DY. Molecular basis of allergic diseases. Mol Genet Metab. 1998; 63: 157-67.
[61] Kihara Y, Ishii S, Kita Y, *et al.* Dual phase regulation of experimental allergic encephalomyelitis by platelet-activating factor. J Exp Med. 2005; 202: 853-63.
[62] Broide DH. Molecular and cellular mechanisms of allergic disease. J Allergy Clin Immunol. 2001; 108: S65-71.
[63] Lommatzsch M, Braun A, Renz H. Neurotrophins in allergic airway dysfunction: what the mouse model is teaching us. Ann N Y Acad Sci. 2003; 992: 241-9.
[64] Peters-Golden M, Henderson WR, Jr. The role of leukotrienes in allergic rhinitis. Ann Allergy Asthma Immunol. 2005; 94: 609-18; quiz 18-20, 69.
[65] Szabo Z, Szilasi M, Brugos L, *et al.* Differences in the changes of allergen-specific IgE serum levels and the chemiluminescence of peripheral blood phagocytes in patients with allergic rhinoconjunctivitis during the ragweed season. Immunol Lett. 2000; 74: 201-5.
[66] Gelfand EW. Inflammatory mediators in allergic rhinitis. J Allergy Clin Immunol. 2004; 114: S135-8.
[67] Hansen I, Klimek L, Mosges R, Hormann K. Mediators of inflammation in the early and the late phase of allergic rhinitis. Curr Opin Allergy Clin Immunol. 2004; 4: 159-63.
[68] Oh DK, Ciaraldi T, Henry RR. Adiponectin in health and disease. Diabetes Obes Metab. 2007; 9: 282-9.
[69] Kadowaki T, Yamauchi T. Adiponectin and adiponectin receptors. Endocr Rev. 2005; 26: 439-51.
[70] Fantuzzi G. Adiponectin and inflammation: consensus and controversy. J Allergy Clin Immunol. 2008; 121: 326-30.
[71] Williams AS, Kasahara DI, Verbout NG, *et al.* Role of the adiponectin binding protein, T-cadherin (cdh13), in allergic airways responses in mice. PLoS One. 2012; 7: e41088.
[72] Calixto MC, Lintomen L, Schenka A, *et al.* Obesity enhances eosinophilic inflammation in a murine model of allergic asthma. Br J Pharmacol. 2010; 159: 617-25.
[73] Medoff BD, Okamoto Y, Leyton P, *et al.* Adiponectin deficiency increases allergic airway inflammation and pulmonary vascular remodeling. Am J Respir Cell Mol Biol. 2009; 41: 397-406.

[74] Yokota T, Meka CS, Kouro T, *et al.* Adiponectin, a fat cell product, influences the earliest lymphocyte precursors in bone marrow cultures by activation of the cyclooxygenase-prostaglandin pathway in stromal cells. J Immunol. 2003; 171: 5091-9.
[75] Wolf AM, Wolf D, Rumpold H, Enrich B, Tilg H. Adiponectin induces the anti-inflammatory cytokines IL-10 and IL-1RA in human leukocytes. Biochem Biophys Res Commun. 2004; 323: 630-5.
[76] Ouchi N, Kihara S, Arita Y, *et al.* Novel modulator for endothelial adhesion molecules: adipocyte-derived plasma protein adiponectin. Circulation. 1999; 100: 2473-6.
[77] Yokota T, Oritani K, Takahashi I, *et al.* Adiponectin, a new member of the family of soluble defense collagens, negatively regulates the growth of myelomonocytic progenitors and the functions of macrophages. Blood. 2000; 96: 1723-32.
[78] Yamaguchi N, Argueta JG, Masuhiro Y, *et al.* Adiponectin inhibits Toll-like receptor family-induced signaling. FEBS Lett. 2005; 579: 6821-6.
[79] Maeda N, Shimomura I, Kishida K, *et al.* Diet-induced insulin resistance in mice lacking adiponectin/ACRP30. Nat Med. 2002; 8: 731-7.
[80] Yamauchi T, Kamon J, Ito Y, *et al.* Cloning of adiponectin receptors that mediate antidiabetic metabolic effects. Nature. 2003; 423: 762-9.
[81] Tsuchida A, Yamauchi T, Takekawa S, *et al.* Peroxisome proliferator-activated receptor (PPAR)alpha activation increases adiponectin receptors and reduces obesity-related inflammation in adipose tissue: comparison of activation of PPARalpha, PPARgamma, and their combination. Diabetes. 2005; 54: 3358-70.
[82] Kim HK, Kim TH, Kim KH, *et al.* The expression of adiponectin receptor is altered in mild and moderate/severe persistent allergic nasal mucosa. Am J Rhinol Allergy. 2011; 25: 318-22.
[83] Fujii H. [Anti-inflammatory action of PPARs]. Nihon Rinsho. 2005; 63: 609-15.
[84] Giri S, Nath N, Smith B, *et al.* 5-aminoimidazole-4-carboxamide-1-beta-4-ribofuranoside inhibits proinflammatory response in glial cells: a possible role of AMP-activated protein kinase. J Neurosci. 2004; 24: 479-87.
[85] Neumeier M, Weigert J, Schaffler A, *et al.* Different effects of adiponectin isoforms in human monocytic cells. J Leukoc Biol. 2006; 79: 803-8.
[86] Gonon AT, Widegren U, Bulhak A, *et al.* Adiponectin protects against myocardial ischaemia-reperfusion injury *via* AMP-activated protein kinase, Akt, and nitric oxide. Cardiovasc Res. 2008; 78: 116-22.
[87] Ruderman NB, Cacicedo JM, Itani S, *et al.* Malonyl-CoA and AMP-activated protein kinase (AMPK): possible links between insulin resistance in muscle and early endothelial cell damage in diabetes. Biochem Soc Trans. 2003; 31: 202-6.
[88] Poli V. The role of C/EBP isoforms in the control of inflammatory and native immunity functions. J Biol Chem. 1998; 273: 29279-82.
[89] Masaie H, Oritani K, Yokota T, *et al.* Adiponectin binds to chemokines *via* the globular head and modulates interactions between chemokines and heparan sulfates. Exp Hematol. 2007; 35: 947-56.
[90] Wang Y, Tao L, Yuan Y, *et al.* Cardioprotective effect of adiponectin is partially mediated by its AMPK-independent antinitrative action. Am J Physiol Endocrinol Metab. 2009; 297: E384-91.
[91] Brindicci C, Ito K, Barnes PJ, Kharitonov SA. Effect of an inducible nitric oxide synthase inhibitor on differential flow-exhaled nitric oxide in asthmatic patients and healthy volunteers. Chest. 2007; 132: 581-8.

[92] Brindicci C, Ito K, Barnes PJ, Kharitonov SA. Differential flow analysis of exhaled nitric oxide in patients with asthma of differing severity. Chest. 2007; 131: 1353-62.

[93] Reynaert NL, Ckless K, Wouters EF, van der Vliet A, Janssen-Heininger YM. Nitric oxide and redox signaling in allergic airway inflammation. Antioxid Redox Signal. 2005; 7: 129-43.

[94] Emelyanov A, Fedoseev G, Abulimity A, *et al.* Elevated concentrations of exhaled hydrogen peroxide in asthmatic patients. Chest. 2001; 120: 1136-9.

[95] Ichinose M, Sugiura H, Yamagata S, Koarai A, Shirato K. Increase in reactive nitrogen species production in chronic obstructive pulmonary disease airways. Am J Respir Crit Care Med. 2000; 162: 701-6.

[96] Ganas K, Loukides S, Papatheodorou G, Panagou P, Kalogeropoulos N. Total nitrite/nitrate in expired breath condensate of patients with asthma. Respir Med. 2001; 95: 649-54.

[97] Kharitonov SA, O'Connor BJ, Evans DJ, Barnes PJ. Allergen-induced late asthmatic reactions are associated with elevation of exhaled nitric oxide. Am J Respir Crit Care Med. 1995; 151: 1894-9.

[98] Kharitonov SA, Yates D, Springall DR, *et al.* Exhaled nitric oxide is increased in asthma. Chest. 1995; 107: 156S-7S.

[99] Jarjour NN, Calhoun WJ. Enhanced production of oxygen radicals in asthma. J Lab Clin Med. 1994; 123: 131-6.

[100] Calhoun WJ, Reed HE, Moest DR, Stevens CA. Enhanced superoxide production by alveolar macrophages and air-space cells, airway inflammation, and alveolar macrophage density changes after segmental antigen bronchoprovocation in allergic subjects. Am Rev Respir Dis. 1992; 145: 317-25.

[101] Lukan N, Racz O, Paulovicova E, Mocnejova I, Petrovicova J. Determination of immunological stress and oxygen free radical formation in white blood cells during allergen immunotherapy. Med Sci Monit. 2012; 18: PR13-7.

[102] Osakabe N, Takano H, Sanbongi C, *et al.* Anti-inflammatory and anti-allergic effect of rosmarinic acid (RA); inhibition of seasonal allergic rhinoconjunctivitis (SAR) and its mechanism. Biofactors. 2004; 21: 127-31.

[103] Shanmugasundaram KR, Kumar SS, Rajajee S. Excessive free radical generation in the blood of children suffering from asthma. Clin Chim Acta. 2001; 305: 107-14.

[104] Demoly P, Damon M, Michel FB, Godard P. IFN-gamma activates superoxide anion production in blood monocytes from allergic asthmatic patients. Ann Allergy Asthma Immunol. 1995; 75: 162-6.

[105] Demoly P, Vachier I, Pene J, *et al.* IgE produces monocyte superoxide anion release: correlation with CD23 expression. Comparison of patients with asthma, patients with rhinitis, and normal subjects. J Allergy Clin Immunol. 1994; 93: 108-16.

[106] Evans DJ, Lindsay MA, O'Connor BJ, Barnes PJ. Priming of circulating human eosinophils following late response to allergen challenge. Eur Respir J. 1996; 9: 703-8.

[107] Weng M, Baron DM, Bloch KD, *et al.* Eosinophils are necessary for pulmonary arterial remodeling in a mouse model of eosinophilic inflammation-induced pulmonary hypertension. Am J Physiol Lung Cell Mol Physiol. 2011; 301: L927-36.

[108] Bao ZS, Hong L, Guan Y, *et al.* Inhibition of airway inflammation, hyperresponsiveness and remodeling by soy isoflavone in a murine model of allergic asthma. Int Immunopharmacol. 2011; 11: 899-906.

[109] Boyce JA. The pathobiology of eosinophilic inflammation. Allergy Asthma Proc. 1997; 18: 293-300.

[110] Sliman SM, Patel RB, Cruff JP, *et al.* Adiponectin Protects Against Hyperoxic Lung Injury and Vascular Leak. Cell Biochem Biophys. 2011.

[111] Lugogo NL, Bappanad D, Kraft M. Obesity, metabolic dysregulation and oxidative stress in asthma. Biochim Biophys Acta. 2011; 1810: 1120-6.

[112] Islam MS, Nagasaka R, Ohara K, *et al.* Biological abilities of rice bran-derived antioxidant phytochemicals for medical therapy. Curr Top Med Chem. 2011; 11: 1847-53.

[113] Holguin F, Rojas M, Brown LA, Fitzpatrick AM. Airway and plasma leptin and adiponectin in lean and obese asthmatics and controls. J Asthma. 2011; 48: 217-23.

[114] Lugogo NL, Kraft M, Dixon AE. Does obesity produce a distinct asthma phenotype? J Appl Physiol. 2010; 108: 729-34.

[115] Hampton T. Cardiac studies reveal clues into asthma and decreased lung function. JAMA. 2008; 300: 32.

[116] Komakula S, Khatri S, Mermis J, *et al.* Body mass index is associated with reduced exhaled nitric oxide and higher exhaled 8-isoprostanes in asthmatics. Respir Res. 2007; 8: 32.

[117] Yamamoto N, Shichijo M, Kokubo T. Establishment of the superoxide production assay with human monocytic cell line, U937, for the evaluation of Syk kinase inhibitors. J Immunol Methods. 2002; 268: 123-30.

[118] Estrella C, Rocks N, Paulissen G, *et al.* Role of A disintegrin and metalloprotease-12 in neutrophil recruitment induced by airway epithelium. Am J Respir Cell Mol Biol. 2009; 41: 449-58.

[119] Kearley J, Erjefalt JS, Andersson C, *et al.* IL-9 governs allergen-induced mast cell numbers in the lung and chronic remodeling of the airways. Am J Respir Crit Care Med. 2011; 183: 865-75.

[120] Freund V, Frossard N. Expression of nerve growth factor in the airways and its possible role in asthma. Prog Brain Res. 2004; 146: 335-46.

[121] Li XQ, Wang HM, Yang CG, *et al.* Fluoxetine inhibited extracellular matrix of pulmonary artery and inflammation of lungs in monocrotaline-treated rats. Acta Pharmacol Sin. 2011; 32: 217-22.

[122] O'Connor JC, Andre C, Wang Y, *et al.* Interferon-gamma and tumor necrosis factor-alpha mediate the upregulation of indoleamine 2,3-dioxygenase and the induction of depressive-like behavior in mice in response to bacillus Calmette-Guerin. J Neurosci. 2009; 29: 4200-9.

[123] Wang Y, Wang X, Jasmin JF, *et al.* Essential role of caveolin-3 in adiponectin signalsome formation and adiponectin cardioprotection. Arterioscler Thromb Vasc Biol. 2012; 32: 934-42.

[124] Lang F, Ullrich S, Gulbins E. Ceramide formation as a target in beta-cell survival and function. Expert Opin Ther Targets. 2011; 15: 1061-71.

[125] Pahan K, Dobashi K, Ghosh B, Singh I. Induction of the manganese superoxide dismutase gene by sphingomyelinase and ceramide. J Neurochem. 1999; 73: 513-20.

[126] Ojoo JC, Mulrennan SA, Kastelik JA, Morice AH, Redington AE. Exhaled breath condensate pH and exhaled nitric oxide in allergic asthma and in cystic fibrosis. Thorax. 2005; 60: 22-6.

[127] Zimmermann N, King NE, Laporte J, *et al.* Dissection of experimental asthma with DNA microarray analysis identifies arginase in asthma pathogenesis. J Clin Invest. 2003; 111: 1863-74.

[128] Kalpaklioglu AF, Kalkan IK. Comparison of orally exhaled nitric oxide in allergic *vs.* nonallergic rhinitis. Am J Rhinol Allergy. 2012; 26: e50-4.
[129] Banovcin P, Jesenak M, Michnova Z, *et al.* Factors attributable to the level of exhaled nitric oxide in asthmatic children. Eur J Med Res. 2009; 14 Suppl 4: 9-13.
[130] Hon KL, Leung TF, Kam WY, *et al.* Exhaled nitric oxide levels are not correlated with eczema severity in Chinese children with atopic dermatitis. J Asthma. 2006; 43: 417-9.
[131] Payne DN. Nitric oxide in allergic airway inflammation. Curr Opin Allergy Clin Immunol. 2003; 3: 133-7.
[132] Hogman M, Holmkvist T, Wegener T, *et al.* Extended NO analysis applied to patients with COPD, allergic asthma and allergic rhinitis. Respir Med. 2002; 96: 24-30.
[133] Prado CM, Leick-Maldonado EA, Miyamoto L, *et al.* Capsaicin-sensitive nerves and neurokinins modulate non-neuronal nNOS expression in lung. Respir Physiol Neurobiol. 2008; 160: 37-44.
[134] Li Y, Wang Y, Zhang Q. [Expression of cell adhesion molecule and nitric oxide synthase in nasal mucosa in allergic rhinitis]. Lin Chuang Er Bi Yan Hou Ke Za Zhi. 2006; 20: 315-8.
[135] Vallance BA, Dijkstra G, Qiu B, *et al.* Relative contributions of NOS isoforms during experimental colitis: endothelial-derived NOS maintains mucosal integrity. Am J Physiol Gastrointest Liver Physiol. 2004; 287: G865-74.
[136] Chiba Y, Arimoto T, Yoshikawa T, Misawa M. Elevated nitric oxide synthase activity concurrent with antigen-induced airway hyperresponsiveness in rats. Exp Lung Res. 2000; 26: 535-49.
[137] Gradini R, Realacci M, Ginepri A, *et al.* Nitric oxide synthases in normal and benign hyperplastic human prostate: immunohistochemistry and molecular biology. J Pathol. 1999; 189: 224-9.
[138] Kotsantis P, Papadimitropoulos A, Drakopoulos A, Vlachojannis JG, Katsoris P. Albumin upregulates eNOS mRNA through ETRA/B in human proximal tubular epithelial cells. J Nephrol. 2012: 0.
[139] Escribano M, Molero L, Lopez-Farre A, *et al.* Aspirin inhibits endothelial nitric oxide synthase (eNOS) and Flk-1 (vascular endothelial growth factor receptor-2) prior to rat colon tumour development. Clin Sci (Lond). 2004; 106: 83-91.
[140] Beauregard C, Brandt PC, Chiou GC. Induction of nitric oxide synthase and over-production of nitric oxide by interleukin-1beta in cultured lacrimal gland acinar cells. Exp Eye Res. 2003; 77: 109-14.
[141] Schwentker A, Vodovotz Y, Weller R, Billiar TR. Nitric oxide and wound repair: role of cytokines? Nitric Oxide. 2002; 7: 1-10.
[142] Ermert M, Ruppert C, Gunther A, *et al.* Cell-specific nitric oxide synthase-isoenzyme expression and regulation in response to endotoxin in intact rat lungs. Lab Invest. 2002; 82: 425-41.
[143] Mellott JK, Nick HS, Waters MF, *et al.* Cytokine-induced changes in chromatin structure and *in vivo* footprints in the inducible NOS promoter. Am J Physiol Lung Cell Mol Physiol. 2001; 280: L390-9.
[144] Inoue H, Hisamatsu K, Ando K, Ajisaka R, Kumagai N. Determination of nitrotyrosine and related compounds in biological specimens by competitive enzyme immunoassay. Nitric Oxide. 2002; 7: 11-7.
[145] Goldstein BJ, Scalia RG, Ma XL. Protective vascular and myocardial effects of adiponectin. Nat Clin Pract Cardiovasc Med. 2009; 6: 27-35.

[146] Maarsingh H, Zaagsma J, Meurs H. Arginase: a key enzyme in the pathophysiology of allergic asthma opening novel therapeutic perspectives. Br J Pharmacol. 2009; 158: 652-64.
[147] Hu A, Jiao X, Gao E, *et al.* Tonic beta-adrenergic drive provokes proinflammatory and proapoptotic changes in aging mouse heart. Rejuvenation Res. 2008; 11: 215-26.
[148] Lopez BL, Christopher TA, Griswold SK, Ma XL. Bench to bedside: nitric oxide in emergency medicine. Acad Emerg Med. 2000; 7: 285-93.
[149] Foster MW, Yang Z, Potts EN, Michael Foster W, Que LG. S-nitrosoglutathione supplementation to ovalbumin-sensitized and -challenged mice ameliorates methacholine-induced bronchoconstriction. Am J Physiol Lung Cell Mol Physiol. 2011; 301: L739-44.
[150] Olson N, Kasahara DI, Hristova M, *et al.* Modulation of NF-kappaB and hypoxia-inducible factor--1 by S-nitrosoglutathione does not alter allergic airway inflammation in mice. Am J Respir Cell Mol Biol. 2011; 44: 813-23.
[151] Li R, Wang WQ, Zhang H, *et al.* Adiponectin improves endothelial function in hyperlipidemic rats by reducing oxidative/nitrative stress and differential regulation of eNOS/iNOS activity. Am J Physiol Endocrinol Metab. 2007; 293: E1703-8.
[152] Lee S, Zhang H, Chen J, *et al.* Adiponectin abates diabetes-induced endothelial dysfunction by suppressing oxidative stress, adhesion molecules, and inflammation in type 2 diabetic mice. Am J Physiol Heart Circ Physiol. 2012; 303: H106-15.
[153] Tournoy KG, Kips JC, Pauwels RA. The allergen-induced airway hyperresponsiveness in a human-mouse chimera model of asthma is T cell and IL-4 and IL-5 dependent. J Immunol. 2001; 166: 6982-91.
[154] Campbell JD, Buchmann P, Kesting S, *et al.* Allergen-specific T cell responses to immunotherapy monitored by CD154 and intracellular cytokine expression. Clin Exp Allergy. 2010; 40: 1025-35.
[155] Doncarli A, Stasiuk LM, Fournier C, Abehsira-Amar O. Conversion *in vivo* from an early dominant Th0/Th1 response to a Th2 phenotype during the development of collagen-induced arthritis. Eur J Immunol. 1997; 27: 1451-8.
[156] Marcondes Rezende M, Hassing I, Bol-Schoenmakers M, *et al.* CD4(+) CD25(+) T regulatory cells do not transfer oral tolerance to peanut allergens in a mouse model of peanut allergy. Clin Exp Allergy. 2011; 41: 1324-33.
[157] Dubois A, Deruytter N, Adams B, *et al.* Regulation of Th2 responses and allergic inflammation through bystander activation of CD8+ T lymphocytes in early life. J Immunol. 2010; 185: 884-91.
[158] Lent AM, Harbeck R, Strand M, *et al.* Immunologic response to administration of standardized dog allergen extract at differing doses. J Allergy Clin Immunol. 2006; 118: 1249-56.
[159] Rupa P, Mine Y. Oral immunotherapy with immunodominant T-cell epitope peptides alleviates allergic reactions in a Balb/c mouse model of egg allergy. Allergy. 2012; 67: 74-82.
[160] Scadding GW, Shamji MH, Jacobson MR, *et al.* Sublingual grass pollen immunotherapy is associated with increases in sublingual Foxp3-expressing cells and elevated allergen-specific immunoglobulin G4, immunoglobulin A and serum inhibitory activity for immunoglobulin E-facilitated allergen binding to B cells. Clin Exp Allergy. 2010; 40: 598-606.
[161] Ciprandi G, De Amici M, Tosca MA, Pistorio A, Marseglia GL. Sublingual immunotherapy affects specific antibody and TGF-beta serum levels in patients with allergic rhinitis. Int J Immunopathol Pharmacol. 2009; 22: 1089-96.

[162] Tanasa RI, Trad A, Lange H, Grotzinger J, Lemke H. Allergen IgE-isotype-specific suppression by maternally derived monoclonal anti-IgG-idiotype. Allergy. 2010; 65: 16-23.

[163] Kendall M, Mitchell TJ, Costigan G, *et al.* Downregulation of IgE antibody and allergic responses in the lung by epidermal biolistic microparticle delivery. J Allergy Clin Immunol. 2006; 117: 275-82.

[164] Oshiba A, Hamelmann E, Takeda K, *et al.* Passive transfer of immediate hypersensitivity and airway hyperresponsiveness by allergen-specific immunoglobulin (Ig) E and IgG1 in mice. J Clin Invest. 1996; 97: 1398-408.

[165] Okamoto Y, Kihara S, Funahashi T, Matsuzawa Y, Libby P. Adiponectin: a key adipocytokine in metabolic syndrome. Clin Sci (Lond). 2006; 110: 267-78.

[166] Siasos G, Tousoulis D, Kollia C, *et al.* Adiponectin and cardiovascular disease: mechanisms and new therapeutic approaches. Curr Med Chem. 2012; 19: 1193-209.

[167] Matsuzawa Y. Adiponectin: a key player in obesity related disorders. Curr Pharm Des. 2010; 16: 1896-901.

[168] Matsuzawa Y. The metabolic syndrome and adipocytokines. Expert Rev Clin Immunol. 2007; 3: 39-46.

[169] Chen Y, Li D, Tsang JY, *et al.* PPAR-gamma signaling and IL-5 inhibition together prevent chronic rejection of MHC Class II-mismatched cardiac grafts. J Heart Lung Transplant. 2011; 30: 698-706.

[170] Radon K, Schulze A, Schierl R, *et al.* Serum leptin and adiponectin levels and their association with allergic sensitization. Allergy. 2008; 63: 1448-54.

[171] Schaffler A, Ehling A, Neumann E, *et al.* Adipocytokines in synovial fluid. JAMA. 2003; 290: 1709-10.

[172] Ehling A, Schaffler A, Herfarth H, *et al.* The potential of adiponectin in driving arthritis. J Immunol. 2006; 176: 4468-78.

[173] Toussirot E, Binda D, Gueugnon C, Dumoulin G. Adiponectin in autoimmune diseases. Curr Med Chem. 2012.

[174] Barbosa Vde S, Rego J, Antonio da Silva N. Possible role of adipokines in systemic lupus erythematosus and rheumatoid arthritis. Rev Bras Reumatol. 2012; 52: 278-87.

[175] Gomez R, Conde J, Scotece M, *et al.* What's new in our understanding of the role of adipokines in rheumatic diseases? Nat Rev Rheumatol. 2011; 7: 528-36.

[176] Ciprandi G, De Amici M, Tosca M, Marseglia G. Serum adiponectin levels in patients with seasonal allergic rhinitis. Int Immunopharmacol. 2010; 10: 635-8.

[177] Ciprandi G, Murdaca G, Marseglia G, *et al.* Serum adiponectin levels in patients with pollen-induced allergic rhinitis. Int Immunopharmacol. 2008; 8: 945-9.

[178] Liu J, Divoux A, Sun J, *et al.* Genetic deficiency and pharmacological stabilization of mast cells reduce diet-induced obesity and diabetes in mice. Nat Med. 2009; 15: 940-5.

[179] Brightling CE, Bradding P, Symon FA, *et al.* Mast-cell infiltration of airway smooth muscle in asthma. N Engl J Med. 2002; 346: 1699-705.

[180] Bentley AM, Hamid Q, Robinson DS, *et al.* Prednisolone treatment in asthma. Reduction in the numbers of eosinophils, T cells, tryptase-only positive mast cells, and modulation of IL-4, IL-5, and interferon-gamma cytokine gene expression within the bronchial mucosa. Am J Respir Crit Care Med. 1996; 153: 551-6.

[181] D'Agostino B, Roviezzo F, De Palma R, *et al.* Activation of protease-activated receptor-2 reduces airways inflammation in experimental allergic asthma. Clin Exp Allergy. 2007; 37: 1436-43.

[182] Reed CE, Kita H. The role of protease activation of inflammation in allergic respiratory diseases. J Allergy Clin Immunol. 2004; 114: 997-1008; quiz 9.
[183] Galli SJ, Kalesnikoff J, Grimbaldeston MA, *et al.* Mast cells as "tunable" effector and immunoregulatory cells: recent advances. Annu Rev Immunol. 2005; 23: 749-86.
[184] Ionescu LI, Alphonse RS, Arizmendi N, *et al.* Airway delivery of soluble factors from plastic-adherent bone marrow cells prevents murine asthma. Am J Respir Cell Mol Biol. 2012; 46: 207-16.
[185] Hsueh KC, Lin YJ, Lin HC, Lin CY. Serum leptin and adiponectin levels correlate with severity of allergic rhinitis. Pediatr Allergy Immunol. 2010; 21: e155-9.
[186] Ciprandi G, De Amici M, Marseglia G. Serum adipsin levels in patients with seasonal allergic rhinitis: preliminary data. Int Immunopharmacol. 2009; 9: 1460-3.
[187] Sandstrom T. Omalizumab in the management of patients with allergic (IgE-mediated) asthma. J Asthma Allergy. 2009; 2: 49-62.
[188] Busse W, Corren J, Lanier BQ, *et al.* Omalizumab, anti-IgE recombinant humanized monoclonal antibody, for the treatment of severe allergic asthma. J Allergy Clin Immunol. 2001; 108: 184-90.
[189] Divoux A, Moutel S, Poitou C, *et al.* Mast Cells in Human Adipose Tissue: Link with Morbid Obesity, Inflammatory Status, and Diabetes. J Clin Endocrinol Metab. 2012.
[190] Zhang J, Shi GP. Mast cells and metabolic syndrome. Biochim Biophys Acta. 2012; 1822: 14-20.
[191] Altintas MM, Azad A, Nayer B, *et al.* Mast cells, macrophages, and crown-like structures distinguish subcutaneous from visceral fat in mice. J Lipid Res. 2011; 52: 480-8.
[192] Anderson EK, Gutierrez DA, Hasty AH. Adipose tissue recruitment of leukocytes. Curr Opin Lipidol. 2010; 21: 172-7.
[193] Hirota R, Akimaru K, Nakamura H. *In vitro* toxicity evaluation of diesel exhaust particles on human eosinophilic cell. Toxicol *In Vitro*. 2008; 22: 988-94.
[194] Rothenberg ME, Hogan SP. The eosinophil. Annu Rev Immunol. 2006; 24: 147-74.
[195] Yukawa T, Read RC, Kroegel C, *et al.* The effects of activated eosinophils and neutrophils on guinea pig airway epithelium *in vitro*. Am J Respir Cell Mol Biol. 1990; 2: 341-53.
[196] Kikuchi I, Kikuchi S, Kobayashi T, *et al.* Theophylline attenuates the neutrophil-dependent augmentation of eosinophil *trans*-basement membrane migration. Int Arch Allergy Immunol. 2007; 143 Suppl 1: 44-9.
[197] Visnovsky P, Suchankova J, Styrandova M. [Oxygen radicals in the mechanism of lung injury caused by air pollutants]. Bratisl Lek Listy. 1997; 98: 523-6.
[198] Saito H, Howie K, Wattie J, *et al.* Allergen-induced murine upper airway inflammation: local and systemic changes in murine experimental allergic rhinitis. Immunology. 2001; 104: 226-34.
[199] Denburg JA, Woolley MJ, Ellis R, Dahlback M, O'Byrne PM. Allergen-induced changes in bone marrow progenitors and airway responsiveness in dogs. Int Arch Allergy Immunol. 1995; 107: 239-41.
[200] Borish L, Steinke JW. Interleukin-33 in asthma: how big of a role does it play? Curr Allergy Asthma Rep. 2011; 11: 7-11.
[201] Kikuchi M, Tachimoto H, Nutku E, Hudson SA, Bochner BS. Phorbol esters alter alpha4 and alphad integrin usage during eosinophil adhesion to VCAM-1. Cell Commun Adhes. 2003; 10: 119-28.

[202] Yamamoto H, Sedgwick JB, Vrtis RF, Busse WW. The effect of transendothelial migration on eosinophil function. Am J Respir Cell Mol Biol. 2000; 23: 379-88.

[203] Gong JH, Shin D, Han SY, Kim JL, Kang YH. Kaempferol suppresses eosionphil infiltration and airway inflammation in airway epithelial cells and in mice with allergic asthma. J Nutr. 2012; 142: 47-56.

[204] Weinberger M. Respiratory infections and asthma: current treatment strategies. Drug Discov Today. 2004; 9: 831-7.

[205] Okigami H, Takeshita K, Tajimi M, *et al.* Inhibition of eosinophilia *in vivo* by a small molecule inhibitor of very late antigen (VLA)-4. Eur J Pharmacol. 2007; 559: 202-9.

[206] Macchiarulo A, Costantino G, Meniconi M, *et al.* Insights into phenylalanine derivatives recognition of VLA-4 integrin: from a pharmacophoric study to 3D-QSAR and molecular docking analyses. J Chem Inf Comput Sci. 2004; 44: 1829-39.

[207] Soler D, Chapman T, Yang LL, *et al.* The binding specificity and selective antagonism of vedolizumab, an anti-alpha4beta7 integrin therapeutic antibody in development for inflammatory bowel diseases. J Pharmacol Exp Ther. 2009; 330: 864-75.

[208] Chuang KP, Tsai WS, Wang YJ, Shieh CC. Superoxide activates very late antigen-4 on an eosinophil cell line and increases cellular binding to vascular cell adhesion molecule-1. Eur J Immunol. 2003; 33: 645-55.

[209] Hirota R, Ngatu NR, Miyamura M, Nakamura H, Suganuma N. Goishi tea consumption inhibits airway hyperresponsiveness in BALB/c mice. BMC Immunol. 2011; 12: 45.

[210] Miller M, Cho JY, Pham A, Ramsdell J, Broide DH. Adiponectin and functional adiponectin receptor 1 are expressed by airway epithelial cells in chronic obstructive pulmonary disease. J Immunol. 2009; 182: 684-91.

[211] Takemura Y, Osuga Y, Yamauchi T, *et al.* Expression of adiponectin receptors and its possible implication in the human endometrium. Endocrinology. 2006; 147: 3203-10.

[212] Penido C, Costa KA, Costa MF, *et al.* Inhibition of allergen-induced eosinophil recruitment by natural tetranortriterpenoids is mediated by the suppression of IL-5, CCL11/eotaxin and NFkappaB activation. Int Immunopharmacol. 2006; 6: 109-21.

[213] Iino Y, Kakizaki K, Katano H, Saigusa H, Kanegasaki S. Eosinophil chemoattractants in the middle ear of patients with eosinophilic otitis media. Clin Exp Allergy. 2005; 35: 1370-6.

[214] Collins PD, Marleau S, Griffiths-Johnson DA, Jose PJ, Williams TJ. Cooperation between interleukin-5 and the chemokine eotaxin to induce eosinophil accumulation *in vivo*. J Exp Med. 1995; 182: 1169-74.

[215] Dixon AE, Johnson SE, Griffes LV, *et al.* Relationship of adipokines with immune response and lung function in obese asthmatic and non-asthmatic women. J Asthma. 2011; 48: 811-7.

[216] Leckie MJ, ten Brinke A, Khan J, *et al.* Effects of an interleukin-5 blocking monoclonal antibody on eosinophils, airway hyper-responsiveness, and the late asthmatic response. Lancet. 2000; 356: 2144-8.

[217] Fenton JI, Nunez NP, Yakar S, *et al.* Diet-induced adiposity alters the serum profile of inflammation in C57BL/6N mice as measured by antibody array. Diabetes Obes Metab. 2009; 11: 343-54.

[218] Huber J, Kiefer FW, Zeyda M, *et al.* CC chemokine and CC chemokine receptor profiles in visceral and subcutaneous adipose tissue are altered in human obesity. J Clin Endocrinol Metab. 2008; 93: 3215-21.

[219] Kips JC, O'Connor BJ, Langley SJ, *et al.* Effect of SCH55700, a humanized anti-human interleukin-5 antibody, in severe persistent asthma: a pilot study. Am J Respir Crit Care Med. 2003; 167: 1655-9.

[220] Kay AB, Menzies-Gow A. Eosinophils and interleukin-5: the debate continues. Am J Respir Crit Care Med. 2003; 167: 1586-7.

[221] Menzies-Gow A, Flood-Page P, Sehmi R, *et al.* Anti-IL-5 (mepolizumab) therapy induces bone marrow eosinophil maturational arrest and decreases eosinophil progenitors in the bronchial mucosa of atopic asthmatics. J Allergy Clin Immunol. 2003; 111: 714-9.

[222] Flood-Page PT, Menzies-Gow AN, Kay AB, Robinson DS. Eosinophil's role remains uncertain as anti-interleukin-5 only partially depletes numbers in asthmatic airway. Am J Respir Crit Care Med. 2003; 167: 199-204.

[223] Chuang YH, Suen JL, Chiang BL. Fas-ligand-expressing adenovirus-transfected dendritic cells decrease allergen-specific T cells and airway inflammation in a murine model of asthma. J Mol Med (Berl). 2006; 84: 595-603.

[224] Romagnani S. Cytokines and chemoattractants in allergic inflammation. Mol Immunol. 2002; 38: 881-5.

[225] Surendar J, Mohan V, Rao MM, Babu S, Aravindhan V. Increased levels of both Th1 and Th2 cytokines in subjects with metabolic syndrome (CURES-103). Diabetes Technol Ther. 2011; 13: 477-82.

[226] Kay AB. The role of T lymphocytes in asthma. Chem Immunol Allergy. 2006; 91: 59-75.

[227] Musabak U, Demirkaya S, Genc G, Ilikci RS, Odabasi Z. Serum adiponectin, TNF-alpha, IL-12p70, and IL-13 levels in multiple sclerosis and the effects of different therapy regimens. Neuroimmunomodulation. 2011; 18: 57-66.

[228] Hacha J, Tomlinson K, Maertens L, *et al.* Nebulized Anti-IL-13 Monoclonal Antibody Fab' Fragment Reduces Allergen-Induced Asthma. Am J Respir Cell Mol Biol. 2012.

[229] Newcomb DC, Boswell MG, Zhou W, *et al.* Human TH17 cells express a functional IL-13 receptor and IL-13 attenuates IL-17A production. J Allergy Clin Immunol. 2011; 127: 1006-13 e1-4.

[230] Chiba Y, Onoda S, Todoroki M, Nishida Y, Misawa M. Upregulation of interleukin-13 receptor chains in bronchial smooth muscle tissues of mouse experimental asthma. J Smooth Muscle Res. 2010; 46: 49-55.

[231] Vladich FD, Brazille SM, Stern D, *et al.* IL-13 R130Q, a common variant associated with allergy and asthma, enhances effector mechanisms essential for human allergic inflammation. J Clin Invest. 2005; 115: 747-54.

[232] Hersoug LG, Linneberg A. The link between the epidemics of obesity and allergic diseases: does obesity induce decreased immune tolerance? Allergy. 2007; 62: 1205-13.

[233] Delgado J, Barranco P, Quirce S. Obesity and asthma. J Investig Allergol Clin Immunol. 2008; 18: 420-5.

[234] Macaubas C, DeKruyff RH, Umetsu DT. Respiratory tolerance in the protection against asthma. Curr Drug Targets Inflamm Allergy. 2003; 2: 175-86.

[235] Umetsu DT, Akbari O, Dekruyff RH. Regulatory T cells control the development of allergic disease and asthma. J Allergy Clin Immunol. 2003; 112: 480-7; quiz 8.

[236] Ling EM, Smith T, Nguyen XD, *et al.* Relation of CD4+CD25+ regulatory T-cell suppression of allergen-driven T-cell activation to atopic status and expression of allergic disease. Lancet. 2004; 363: 608-15.

[237] Domagala-Kulawik J, Hoser G, Dabrowska M, Safianowska A, Chazan R. CD4+/CD25+ cells in systemic inflammation in COPD. Scand J Immunol. 2011; 73: 59-65.

[238] Tsang JY, Li D, Ho D, *et al.* Novel immunomodulatory effects of adiponectin on dendritic cell functions. Int Immunopharmacol. 2011; 11: 604-9.

[239] van Rensen EL, Sont JK, Evertse CE, *et al.* Bronchial CD8 cell infiltrate and lung function decline in asthma. Am J Respir Crit Care Med. 2005; 172: 837-41.

[240] Cho SH, Stanciu LA, Holgate ST, Johnston SL. Increased interleukin-4, interleukin-5, and interferon-gamma in airway CD4+ and CD8+ T cells in atopic asthma. Am J Respir Crit Care Med. 2005; 171: 224-30.

[241] Okamoto Y, Christen T, Shimizu K, *et al.* Adiponectin inhibits allograft rejection in murine cardiac transplantation. Transplantation. 2009; 88: 879-83.

[242] Peters-Golden M. The alveolar macrophage: the forgotten cell in asthma. Am J Respir Cell Mol Biol. 2004; 31: 3-7.

[243] Menard G, Bissonnette EY. Priming of alveolar macrophages by leukotriene D(4): potentiation of inflammation. Am J Respir Cell Mol Biol. 2000; 23: 572-7.

[244] Ouchi N, Kihara S, Arita Y, *et al.* Adipocyte-derived plasma protein, adiponectin, suppresses lipid accumulation and class A scavenger receptor expression in human monocyte-derived macrophages. Circulation. 2001; 103: 1057-63.

[245] Kumada M, Kihara S, Ouchi N, *et al.* Adiponectin specifically increased tissue inhibitor of metalloproteinase-1 through interleukin-10 expression in human macrophages. Circulation. 2004; 109: 2046-9.

[246] Ohashi K, Parker JL, Ouchi N, *et al.* Adiponectin promotes macrophage polarization toward an anti-inflammatory phenotype. J Biol Chem. 2010; 285: 6153-60.

[247] Odegaard JI, Chawla A. Mechanisms of macrophage activation in obesity-induced insulin resistance. Nat Clin Pract Endocrinol Metab. 2008; 4: 619-26.

[248] Odegaard JI, Ricardo-Gonzalez RR, Red Eagle A, *et al.* Alternative M2 activation of Kupffer cells by PPARdelta ameliorates obesity-induced insulin resistance. Cell Metab. 2008; 7: 496-507.

[249] Kyriazi E, Tsiotra PC, Boutati E, *et al.* Effects of adiponectin in TNF-alpha, IL-6, and IL-10 cytokine production from coronary artery disease macrophages. Horm Metab Res. 2011; 43: 537-44.

[250] Wulster-Radcliffe MC, Ajuwon KM, Wang J, Christian JA, Spurlock ME. Adiponectin differentially regulates cytokines in porcine macrophages. Biochem Biophys Res Commun. 2004; 316: 924-9.

[251] Park PH, Huang H, McMullen MR, Bryan K, Nagy LE. Activation of cyclic-AMP response element binding protein contributes to adiponectin-stimulated interleukin-10 expression in RAW 264.7 macrophages. J Leukoc Biol. 2008; 83: 1258-66.

[252] Tang C, Ward C, Reid D, *et al.* Normally suppressing CD40 coregulatory signals delivered by airway macrophages to TH2 lymphocytes are defective in patients with atopic asthma. J Allergy Clin Immunol. 2001; 107: 863-70.

[253] Zeibecoglou K, Ying S, Meng Q, *et al.* Macrophage subpopulations and macrophage-derived cytokines in sputum of atopic and nonatopic asthmatic subjects and atopic and normal control subjects. J Allergy Clin Immunol. 2000; 106: 697-704.

[254] Bogaert P, Naessens T, De Koker S, *et al.* Inflammatory signatures for eosinophilic *vs.* neutrophilic allergic pulmonary inflammation reveal critical regulatory checkpoints. Am J Physiol Lung Cell Mol Physiol. 2011; 300: L679-90.

[255] Ozdemir C, Akdis M, Akdis CA. Nature of regulatory T cells in the context of allergic disease. Allergy Asthma Clin Immunol. 2008; 4: 106-10.

[256] Bloemen K, Verstraelen S, Van Den Heuvel R, *et al.* The allergic cascade: review of the most important molecules in the asthmatic lung. Immunol Lett. 2007; 113: 6-18.

[257] August A, Mueller C, Weaver V, *et al.* Nutrients, nuclear receptors, inflammation, immunity lipids, PPAR, and allergic asthma. J Nutr. 2006; 136: 695-9.

[258] Trujillo-Vargas CM, Mayer KD, Bickert T, *et al.* Vaccinations with T-helper type 1 directing adjuvants have different suppressive effects on the development of allergen-induced T-helper type 2 responses. Clin Exp Allergy. 2005; 35: 1003-13.

[259] Marshall GD, Jr. Pathophysiology of bronchial inflammation: chemoreceptors as therapeutic targets. Allergy Asthma Proc. 2000; 21: 309-13.

[260] Pucci S, Incorvaia C. Allergy as an organ and a systemic disease. Clin Exp Immunol. 2008; 153 Suppl 1: 1-2.

[261] Fang C, Corrigan CJ, Ying S. The treatment targets of asthma: from laboratory to clinic. Inflamm Allergy Drug Targets. 2008; 7: 119-28.

[262] Bacon AS, McGill JI, Anderson DF, *et al.* Adhesion molecules and relationship to leukocyte levels in allergic eye disease. Invest Ophthalmol Vis Sci. 1998; 39: 322-30.

[263] Teoh H, Quan A, Bang KW, *et al.* Adiponectin deficiency promotes endothelial activation and profoundly exacerbates sepsis-related mortality. Am J Physiol Endocrinol Metab. 2008; 295: E658-64.

[264] Kantartzis K, Rittig K, Balletshofer B, *et al.* The relationships of plasma adiponectin with a favorable lipid profile, decreased inflammation, and less ectopic fat accumulation depend on adiposity. Clin Chem. 2006; 52: 1934-42.

[265] Gorska-Ciebiada M, Ciebiada M, Gorska MM, Gorski P, Grzelewska-Rzymowska I. Intercellular adhesion molecule 1 and tumor necrosis factor alpha in asthma and persistent allergic rhinitis: relationship with disease severity. Ann Allergy Asthma Immunol. 2006; 97: 66-72.

[266] Frew AJ, St-Pierre J, Teran LM, *et al.* Cellular and mediator responses twenty-four hours after local endobronchial allergen challenge of asthmatic airways. J Allergy Clin Immunol. 1996; 98: 133-43.

[267] Hakansson L, Bjornsson E, Janson C, Schmekel B. Increased adhesion to vascular cell adhesion molecule-1 and intercellular adhesion molecule-1 of eosinophils from patients with asthma. J Allergy Clin Immunol. 1995; 96: 941-50.

[268] Raeburn D, Webber SE. Proinflammatory potential of the airway epithelium in bronchial asthma. Eur Respir J. 1994; 7: 2226-33.

[269] Montefort S, Lai CK, Kapahi P, *et al.* Circulating adhesion molecules in asthma. Am J Respir Crit Care Med. 1994; 149: 1149-52.

[270] Montefort S, Gratziou C, Goulding D, *et al.* Bronchial biopsy evidence for leukocyte infiltration and upregulation of leukocyte-endothelial cell adhesion molecules 6 hours after local allergen challenge of sensitized asthmatic airways. J Clin Invest. 1994; 93: 1411-21.

[271] Roche WR, Montefort S, Baker J, Holgate ST. Cell adhesion molecules and the bronchial epithelium. Am Rev Respir Dis. 1993; 148: S79-82.

[272] Williamson PA, Short PM, Vaidyanathan S, Lipworth BJ. Inhaled and Systemic Corticosteroid Response in Severe Asthma Assessed by Alveolar Nitric Oxide: a randomised crossover pilot study of add-on therapy. Br J Clin Pharmacol. 2012.

[273] Wolkerstorfer A, Savelkoul HF, de Waard van der Spek FB, *et al.* Soluble E-selectin and soluble ICAM-1 levels as markers of the activity of atopic dermatitis in children. Pediatr Allergy Immunol. 2003; 14: 302-6.
[274] Gaeta TJ, Clark S, Pelletier AJ, Camargo CA. National study of US emergency department visits for acute allergic reactions, 1993 to 2004. Ann Allergy Asthma Immunol. 2007; 98: 360-5.
[275] Harlan WR, Murt HA, Thomas JW, *et al.* Incidence, utilization, and costs associated with acute respiratory conditions, United States, 1980. Natl Med Care Util Expend Surv C. 1986: 1-63.
[276] Anandan C, Gupta R, Simpson CR, Fischbacher C, Sheikh A. Epidemiology and disease burden from allergic disease in Scotland: analyses of national databases. J R Soc Med. 2009; 102: 431-42.
[277] Canonica GW, Poulsen PB, Vestenbaek U. Cost-effectiveness of GRAZAX for prevention of grass pollen induced rhinoconjunctivitis in Southern Europe. Respir Med. 2007; 101: 1885-94.
[278] McDonald JC, Beck MH, Chen Y, Cherry NM. Incidence by occupation and industry of work-related skin diseases in the United Kingdom, 1996-2001. Occup Med (Lond). 2006; 56: 398-405.
[279] Fokkens WJ, Lund VJ, Mullol J, *et al.* EPOS 2012: European position paper on rhinosinusitis and nasal polyps 2012. A summary for otorhinolaryngologists. Rhinology. 2012; 50: 1-12.
[280] Sicherer SH, Leung DY. Advances in allergic skin disease, anaphylaxis, and hypersensitivity reactions to foods, drugs, and insects in 2011. J Allergy Clin Immunol. 2012; 129: 76-85.
[281] Suskovic S, Keser D. Chronic obstructive pulmonary disease status 2011: long walk home. Respir Med. 2011; 105 Suppl 1: S4-6.
[282] Eaton DK, Kann L, Kinchen S, *et al.* Youth risk behavior surveillance - United States, 2011. MMWR Surveill Summ. 2012; 61: 1-162.
[283] Tam A, Morrish D, Wadsworth S, *et al.* The role of female hormones on lung function in chronic lung diseases. BMC Womens Health. 2011; 11: 24.
[284] Pasaoglu G, Mungan D, Abadoglu O, Misirligil Z. Leukotriene receptor antagonists: a good choice in the treatment of premenstrual asthma? J Asthma. 2008; 45: 95-9.
[285] de Oliveira AP, Domingos HV, Cavriani G, *et al.* Cellular recruitment and cytokine generation in a rat model of allergic lung inflammation are differentially modulated by progesterone and estradiol. Am J Physiol Cell Physiol. 2007; 293: C1120-8.
[286] Gluck JC. The change of asthma course during pregnancy. Clin Rev Allergy Immunol. 2004; 26: 171-80.
[287] Barr RG, Camargo CA, Jr. Hormone replacement therapy and obstructive airway diseases. Treat Respir Med. 2004; 3: 1-7.
[288] Billich A, Bilban M, Meisner NC, *et al.* Confocal fluorescence detection expanded to UV excitation: the first continuous fluorimetric assay of human steroid sulfatase in nanoliter volume. Assay Drug Dev Technol. 2004; 2: 21-30.
[289] Moran FM, Lohstroh P, VandeVoort CA, *et al.* Exogenous steroid substrate modifies the effect of 2,3,7,8-tetrachlorodibenzo-p-dioxin on estradiol production of human luteinized granulosa cells *in vitro*. Biol Reprod. 2003; 68: 244-51.

[290] Clark JA, Alves S, Gundlah C, *et al.* Selective estrogen receptor-beta (SERM-beta) compounds modulate raphe nuclei tryptophan hydroxylase-1 (TPH-1) mRNA expression and cause antidepressant-like effects in the forced swim test. Neuropharmacology. 2012; 63: 1051-63.

[291] Oertelt-Prigione S. The influence of sex and gender on the immune response. Autoimmun Rev. 2012; 11: A479-85.

[292] Cai Y, Zhou J, Webb DC. Estrogen stimulates Th2 cytokine production and regulates the compartmentalisation of eosinophils during allergen challenge in a mouse model of asthma. Int Arch Allergy Immunol. 2012; 158: 252-60.

[293] Dimitropoulou C, Drakopanagiotakis F, Chatterjee A, Snead C, Catravas JD. Estrogen replacement therapy prevents airway dysfunction in a murine model of allergen-induced asthma. Lung. 2009; 187: 116-27.

[294] Matsubara S, Swasey CH, Loader JE, *et al.* Estrogen determines sex differences in airway responsiveness after allergen exposure. Am J Respir Cell Mol Biol. 2008; 38: 501-8.

[295] Younes M, Honma N. Estrogen receptor beta. Arch Pathol Lab Med. 2011; 135: 63-6.

[296] Wu F, Xu R, Kim K, Martin J, Safe S. *In vivo* profiling of estrogen receptor/specificity protein-dependent transactivation. Endocrinology. 2008; 149: 5696-705.

[297] Somponpun SJ, Johnson AK, Beltz T, Sladek CD. Estrogen receptor-alpha expression in osmosensitive elements of the lamina terminalis: regulation by hypertonicity. Am J Physiol Regul Integr Comp Physiol. 2004; 287: R661-9.

[298] Pearce ST, Jordan VC. The biological role of estrogen receptors alpha and beta in cancer. Crit Rev Oncol Hematol. 2004; 50: 3-22.

[299] Menuet A, Anglade I, Flouriot G, Pakdel F, Kah O. Tissue-specific expression of two structurally different estrogen receptor alpha isoforms along the female reproductive axis of an oviparous species, the rainbow trout. Biol Reprod. 2001; 65: 1548-57.

[300] Shah SP, Gohil PV, Shah GB. Role of estrogen receptor- alpha in an experimental model of bronchial asthma. Iran Biomed J. 2010; 14: 41-8.

[301] Catley MC, Birrell MA, Hardaker EL, *et al.* Estrogen receptor beta: expression profile and possible anti-inflammatory role in disease. J Pharmacol Exp Ther. 2008; 326: 83-8.

[302] Riffo-Vasquez Y, Ligeiro de Oliveira AP, Page CP, Spina D, Tavares-de-Lima W. Role of sex hormones in allergic inflammation in mice. Clin Exp Allergy. 2007; 37: 459-70.

[303] Wang Y, Wang Z, Wang L, *et al.* Estrogen down-regulates nicotine-induced adhesion molecule expression *via* nongenomic signal pathway in endothelial cells. Int Immunopharmacol. 2006; 6: 892-902.

[304] Wang LL, Zhao JL, Lau WB, *et al.* Estradiol pretreatment attenuated nicotine-induced endothelial cell apoptosis *via* estradiol functional membrane receptor. Int Immunopharmacol. 2011; 11: 675-82.

[305] Kidd P. Th1/Th2 balance: the hypothesis, its limitations, and implications for health and disease. Altern Med Rev. 2003; 8: 223-46.

[306] Yoneyama Y, Suzuki S, Sawa R, *et al.* The T-helper 1/T-helper 2 balance in peripheral blood of women with hyperemesis gravidarum. Am J Obstet Gynecol. 2002; 187: 1631-5.

[307] Piccinni MP, Maggi E, Romagnani S. Role of hormone-controlled T-cell cytokines in the maintenance of pregnancy. Biochem Soc Trans. 2000; 28: 212-5.

[308] Carey MA, Card JW, Bradbury JA, *et al.* Spontaneous airway hyperresponsiveness in estrogen receptor-alpha-deficient mice. Am J Respir Crit Care Med. 2007; 175: 126-35.

[309] Polanczyk M, Yellayi S, Zamora A, *et al.* Estrogen receptor-1 (Esr1) and -2 (Esr2) regulate the severity of clinical experimental allergic encephalomyelitis in male mice. Am J Pathol. 2004; 164: 1915-24.
[310] Smith SM, Baskin GB, Marx PA. Estrogen protects against vaginal transmission of simian immunodeficiency virus. J Infect Dis. 2000; 182: 708-15.
[311] Bousquet J, Chanez P, Lacoste JY, *et al.* Eosinophilic inflammation in asthma. N Engl J Med. 1990; 323: 1033-9.
[312] Huang CH, Kuo PL, Hsu YL, *et al.* The natural flavonoid apigenin suppresses Th1- and Th2-related chemokine production by human monocyte THP-1 cells through mitogen-activated protein kinase pathways. J Med Food. 2010; 13: 391-8.
[313] Kakui K, Itoh H, Sagawa N, *et al.* Augmented endothelial nitric oxide synthase (eNOS) protein expression in human pregnant myometrium: possible involvement of eNOS promoter activation by estrogen *via* both estrogen receptor (ER)alpha and ERbeta. Mol Hum Reprod. 2004; 10: 115-22.
[314] Mukherjee TK, Nathan L, Dinh H, Reddy ST, Chaudhuri G. 17-epiestriol, an estrogen metabolite, is more potent than estradiol in inhibiting vascular cell adhesion molecule 1 (VCAM-1) mRNA expression. J Biol Chem. 2003; 278: 11746-52.
[315] Barbacanne MA, Rami J, Michel JB, *et al.* Estradiol increases rat aorta endothelium-derived relaxing factor (EDRF) activity without changes in endothelial NO synthase gene expression: possible role of decreased endothelium-derived superoxide anion production. Cardiovasc Res. 1999; 41: 672-81.
[316] Kleinert H, Wallerath T, Euchenhofer C, *et al.* Estrogens increase transcription of the human endothelial NO synthase gene: analysis of the transcription factors involved. Hypertension. 1998; 31: 582-8.
[317] Arnal JF, Clamens S, Pechet C, *et al.* Ethinylestradiol does not enhance the expression of nitric oxide synthase in bovine endothelial cells but increases the release of bioactive nitric oxide by inhibiting superoxide anion production. Proc Natl Acad Sci U S A. 1996; 93: 4108-13.
[318] Dimitrova KR, DeGroot KW, Suyderhoud JP, *et al.* 17-beta estradiol preserves endothelial cell viability in an *in vitro* model of homocysteine-induced oxidative stress. J Cardiovasc Pharmacol. 2002; 39: 347-53.
[319] Marotta F, Mao GS, Liu T, *et al.* Anti-inflammatory and neuroprotective effect of a phytoestrogen compound on rat microglia. Ann N Y Acad Sci. 2006; 1089: 276-81.
[320] Baker AE, Brautigam VM, Watters JJ. Estrogen modulates microglial inflammatory mediator production *via* interactions with estrogen receptor beta. Endocrinology. 2004; 145: 5021-32.
[321] Wagner AH, Schroeter MR, Hecker M. 17beta-estradiol inhibition of NADPH oxidase expression in human endothelial cells. FASEB J. 2001; 15: 2121-30.
[322] Zinnuroglu M, Dincel AS, Kosova F, Sepici V, Karatas GK. Prospective evaluation of free radicals and antioxidant activity following 6-month risedronate treatment in patients with postmenopausal osteoporosis. Rheumatol Int. 2012; 32: 875-80.
[323] Oh PS, Lim KT. Blocking of intracellular ROS production by phytoglycoprotein (30 kDa) causes anti-proliferation in bisphenol A-stimulated Chang liver cells. J Appl Toxicol. 2008; 28: 749-58.
[324] Huang Q, Weber WJ, Jr. Transformation and removal of bisphenol A from aqueous phase *via* peroxidase mediated oxidative coupling reactions: efficacy, products, and pathways. Environ Sci Technol. 2005; 39: 6029-36.

[325] Chen ZH, Na HK, Hurh YJ, Surh YJ. 4-Hydroxyestradiol induces oxidative stress and apoptosis in human mammary epithelial cells: possible protection by NF-kappaB and ERK/MAPK. Toxicol Appl Pharmacol. 2005; 208: 46-56.

[326] Hurh YJ, Chen ZH, Na HK, Han SY, Surh YJ. 2-Hydroxyestradiol induces oxidative DNA damage and apoptosis in human mammary epithelial cells. J Toxicol Environ Health A. 2004; 67: 1939-53.

[327] Russell KS, Haynes MP, Sinha D, Clerisme E, Bender JR. Human vascular endothelial cells contain membrane binding sites for estradiol, which mediate rapid intracellular signaling. Proc Natl Acad Sci U S A. 2000; 97: 5930-5.

[328] Guo Z, Krucken J, Benten WP, Wunderlich F. Estradiol-induced nongenomic calcium signaling regulates genotropic signaling in macrophages. J Biol Chem. 2002; 277: 7044-50.

[329] Migliaccio A, Di Domenico M, Castoria G, *et al.* Tyrosine kinase/p21ras/MAP-kinase pathway activation by estradiol-receptor complex in MCF-7 cells. EMBO J. 1996; 15: 1292-300.

[330] Fehrenbacher JC, Loverme J, Clarke W, *et al.* Rapid pain modulation with nuclear receptor ligands. Brain Res Rev. 2009; 60: 114-24.

[331] Haynes MP, Li L, Sinha D, *et al.* Src kinase mediates phosphatidylinositol 3-kinase/Akt-dependent rapid endothelial nitric-oxide synthase activation by estrogen. J Biol Chem. 2003; 278: 2118-23.

[332] Binko J, Murphy TV, Majewski H. 17Beta-oestradiol enhances nitric oxide synthase activity in endothelium-denuded rat aorta. Clin Exp Pharmacol Physiol. 1998; 25: 120-7.

[333] Bentrari F, Arnould L, Jackson AP, Jeannin JF, Pance A. Progesterone enhances cytokine-stimulated nitric oxide synthase II expression and cell death in human breast cancer cells. Lab Invest. 2005; 85: 624-32.

[334] Hisamoto K, Ohmichi M, Kurachi H, *et al.* Estrogen induces the Akt-dependent activation of endothelial nitric-oxide synthase in vascular endothelial cells. J Biol Chem. 2001; 276: 3459-67.

[335] Haynes MP, Sinha D, Russell KS, *et al.* Membrane estrogen receptor engagement activates endothelial nitric oxide synthase *via* the PI3-kinase-Akt pathway in human endothelial cells. Circ Res. 2000; 87: 677-82.

[336] Sud N, Wiseman DA, Black SM. Caveolin 1 is required for the activation of endothelial nitric oxide synthase in response to 17beta-estradiol. Mol Endocrinol. 2010; 24: 1637-49.

[337] Dimitropoulou C, White RE, Ownby DR, Catravas JD. Estrogen reduces carbachol-induced constriction of asthmatic airways by stimulating large-conductance voltage and calcium-dependent potassium channels. Am J Respir Cell Mol Biol. 2005; 32: 239-47.

[338] Chandrasekar B, Sirois MG, Geoffroy P, *et al.* Local delivery of 17beta-estradiol improves reendothelialization and decreases inflammation after coronary stenting in a porcine model. Thromb Haemost. 2005; 94: 1042-7.

[339] Chandrasekar B, Tanguay JF. Local delivery of 17-beta-estradiol decreases neointimal hyperplasia after coronary angioplasty in a porcine model. J Am Coll Cardiol. 2000; 36: 1972-8.

[340] Romagnoli M, Vachier I, Tarodo de la Fuente P, *et al.* Eosinophilic inflammation in sputum of poorly controlled asthmatics. Eur Respir J. 2002; 20: 1370-7.

[341] Spina D, Page CP. Asthma -- a need for a rethink? Trends Pharmacol Sci. 2002; 23: 311-5.

[342] Leong KP, Huston DP. Understanding the pathogenesis of allergic asthma using mouse models. Ann Allergy Asthma Immunol. 2001; 87: 96-109; quiz 10.

[343] Gleich GJ. The eosinophil and bronchial asthma: current understanding. J Allergy Clin Immunol. 1990; 85: 422-36.
[344] Schubert AK. [Effects of progesterone antagonists on the eosinophilic granulocytes in the rat uterus]. Ann Anat. 1998; 180: 401-8.
[345] Dembele-Duchesne MJ, Badia E, Etienne-Julan M, Capony JP. Identification and tissue localization of an eosinophil 17 kDa protein accumulating in rat uterus upon estradiol treatment. J Steroid Biochem Mol Biol. 1991; 38: 321-30.
[346] Luque EH, Munoz de Toro MM, Ramos JG, Rodriguez HA, Sherwood OD. Role of relaxin and estrogen in the control of eosinophilic invasion and collagen remodeling in rat cervical tissue at term. Biol Reprod. 1998; 59: 795-800.
[347] Corbeil LB, Campero CM, Rhyan JC, *et al.* Uterine mast cells and immunoglobulin-E antibody responses during clearance of Tritrichomonas foetus. Vet Pathol. 2005; 42: 282-90.
[348] Robertson SA, Mau VJ, Young IG, Matthaei KI. Uterine eosinophils and reproductive performance in interleukin 5-deficient mice. J Reprod Fertil. 2000; 120: 423-32.
[349] Regal JF, Fraser DG, Weeks CE, Greenberg NA. Dietary phytoestrogens have anti-inflammatory activity in a guinea pig model of asthma. Proc Soc Exp Biol Med. 2000; 223: 372-8.
[350] Zhao XJ, McKerr G, Dong Z, *et al.* Expression of oestrogen and progesterone receptors by mast cells alone, but not lymphocytes, macrophages or other immune cells in human upper airways. Thorax. 2001; 56: 205-11.
[351] Kalhan R, Smith LJ, Nlend MC, *et al.* A mechanism of benefit of soy genistein in asthma: inhibition of eosinophil p38-dependent leukotriene synthesis. Clin Exp Allergy. 2008; 38: 103-12.
[352] Douin-Echinard V, Calippe B, Billon-Gales A, *et al.* Estradiol administration controls eosinophilia through estrogen receptor-alpha activation during acute peritoneal inflammation. J Leukoc Biol. 2011; 90: 145-54.
[353] Lacoste JY, Bousquet J, Chanez P, *et al.* Eosinophilic and neutrophilic inflammation in asthma, chronic bronchitis, and chronic obstructive pulmonary disease. J Allergy Clin Immunol. 1993; 92: 537-48.
[354] Nadel JA. Role of mast cell and neutrophil proteases in airway secretion. Am Rev Respir Dis. 1991; 144: S48-51.
[355] Sommerhoff CP, Nadel JA, Basbaum CB, Caughey GH. Neutrophil elastase and cathepsin G stimulate secretion from cultured bovine airway gland serous cells. J Clin Invest. 1990; 85: 682-9.
[356] Bosson J, Blomberg A, Pourazar J, *et al.* Early suppression of NFkappaB and IL-8 in bronchial epithelium after ozone exposure in healthy human subjects. Inhal Toxicol. 2009; 21: 913-9.
[357] Grzelewska-Rzymowska I, Pietrzkowicz M. [Role of intra cellular adhesion molecule-1 (ICAM-1) and its soluble form (sICAM) in chronic airway inflammation]. Pol Merkur Lekarski. 2004; 16: 179-82.
[358] Stenfors N, Nordenhall C, Salvi SS, *et al.* Different airway inflammatory responses in asthmatic and healthy humans exposed to diesel. Eur Respir J. 2004; 23: 82-6.
[359] Xing D, Feng W, Miller AP, *et al.* Estrogen modulates TNF-alpha-induced inflammatory responses in rat aortic smooth muscle cells through estrogen receptor-beta activation. Am J Physiol Heart Circ Physiol. 2007; 292: H2607-12.

[360] Miller AP, Xing D, Feng W, *et al.* Aged rats lose vasoprotective and anti-inflammatory actions of estrogen in injured arteries. Menopause. 2007; 14: 251-60.

[361] Miller AP, Feng W, Xing D, *et al.* Estrogen modulates inflammatory mediator expression and neutrophil chemotaxis in injured arteries. Circulation. 2004; 110: 1664-9.

[362] Abrahams VM, Collins JE, Wira CR, Fanger MW, Yeaman GR. Inhibition of human polymorphonuclear cell oxidative burst by 17-beta-estradiol and 2,3,7,8-tetrachlorodibenzo-p-dioxin. Am J Reprod Immunol. 2003; 50: 463-72.

[363] Epstein RJ. The CXCL12-CXCR4 chemotactic pathway as a target of adjuvant breast cancer therapies. Nat Rev Cancer. 2004; 4: 901-9.

[364] Yu HP, Hwang TL, Hsieh PW, Lau YT. Role of estrogen receptor-dependent upregulation of P38 MAPK/heme oxygenase 1 in resveratrol-mediated attenuation of intestinal injury after trauma-hemorrhage. Shock. 2011; 35: 517-23.

[365] Hsu JT, Kan WH, Hsieh CH, *et al.* Mechanism of estrogen-mediated intestinal protection following trauma-hemorrhage: p38 MAPK-dependent upregulation of HO-1. Am J Physiol Regul Integr Comp Physiol. 2008; 294: R1825-31.

[366] Kan WH, Hsu JT, Ba ZF, *et al.* p38 MAPK-dependent eNOS upregulation is critical for 17beta-estradiol-mediated cardioprotection following trauma-hemorrhage. Am J Physiol Heart Circ Physiol. 2008; 294: H2627-36.

[367] Mandhane PJ, Hanna SE, Inman MD, *et al.* Changes in exhaled nitric oxide related to estrogen and progesterone during the menstrual cycle. Chest. 2009; 136: 1301-7.

[368] Intapad S, Dimitropoulou C, Snead C, Piyachaturawat P, Catravas JD. Regulation of asthmatic airway relaxation by estrogen and heat shock protein 90. J Cell Physiol. 2012; 227: 3036-43.

[369] Valsecchi AE, Franchi S, Panerai AE, *et al.* The soy isoflavone genistein reverses oxidative and inflammatory state, neuropathic pain, neurotrophic and vasculature deficits in diabetes mouse model. Eur J Pharmacol. 2011; 650: 694-702.

[370] Valsecchi AE, Franchi S, Panerai AE, *et al.* Genistein, a natural phytoestrogen from soy, relieves neuropathic pain following chronic constriction sciatic nerve injury in mice: anti-inflammatory and antioxidant activity. J Neurochem. 2008; 107: 230-40.

[371] Sakazaki F, Ueno H, Nakamuro K. 17beta-Estradiol enhances expression of inflammatory cytokines and inducible nitric oxide synthase in mouse contact hypersensitivity. Int Immunopharmacol. 2008; 8: 654-60.

[372] Sakazaki F, Ueno H, Nakamuro K. 17beta-estradiol enhances contact hypersensitivity and IFN-gamma expression in inflamed skin of BALB/c mice. Toxicol Lett. 2006; 166: 60-6.

[373] Molero L, Garcia-Duran M, Diaz-Recasens J, *et al.* Expression of estrogen receptor subtypes and neuronal nitric oxide synthase in neutrophils from women and men: regulation by estrogen. Cardiovasc Res. 2002; 56: 43-51.

[374] Booth EA, Marchesi M, Kilbourne EJ, Lucchesi BR. 17Beta-estradiol as a receptor-mediated cardioprotective agent. J Pharmacol Exp Ther. 2003; 307: 395-401.

[375] Tiidus PM. Can oestrogen influence skeletal muscle damage, inflammation, and repair? Br J Sports Med. 2005; 39: 251-3.

[376] Tiidus PM. Influence of estrogen on skeletal muscle damage, inflammation, and repair. Exerc Sport Sci Rev. 2003; 31: 40-4.

[377] Cuzzocrea S, Mazzon E, Sautebin L, *et al.* The protective role of endogenous estrogens in carrageenan-induced lung injury in the rat. Mol Med. 2001; 7: 478-87.

[378] Finkelstein R, Fraser RS, Ghezzo H, Cosio MG. Alveolar inflammation and its relation to emphysema in smokers. Am J Respir Crit Care Med. 1995; 152: 1666-72.
[379] Wang Y, Wang Z, Zhou Y, *et al.* Nicotine stimulates adhesion molecular expression *via* calcium influx and mitogen-activated protein kinases in human endothelial cells. Int J Biochem Cell Biol. 2006; 38: 170-82.
[380] Wang Y, Wang L, Ai X, *et al.* Nicotine could augment adhesion molecule expression in human endothelial cells through macrophages secreting TNF-alpha, IL-1beta. Int Immunopharmacol. 2004; 4: 1675-86.
[381] Di Stefano A, Capelli A, Lusuardi M, *et al.* Decreased T lymphocyte infiltration in bronchial biopsies of subjects with severe chronic obstructive pulmonary disease. Clin Exp Allergy. 2001; 31: 893-902.
[382] Di Stefano A, Capelli A, Lusuardi M, *et al.* Severity of airflow limitation is associated with severity of airway inflammation in smokers. Am J Respir Crit Care Med. 1998; 158: 1277-85.
[383] Kramer PR, Kramer SF, Guan G. 17 beta-estradiol regulates cytokine release through modulation of CD16 expression in monocytes and monocyte-derived macrophages. Arthritis Rheum. 2004; 50: 1967-75.
[384] Vegeto E, Belcredito S, Etteri S, *et al.* Estrogen receptor-alpha mediates the brain antiinflammatory activity of estradiol. Proc Natl Acad Sci U S A. 2003; 100: 9614-9.
[385] Ghisletti S, Meda C, Maggi A, Vegeto E. 17beta-estradiol inhibits inflammatory gene expression by controlling NF-kappaB intracellular localization. Mol Cell Biol. 2005; 25: 2957-68.
[386] Nanni S, Benvenuti V, Grasselli A, *et al.* Endothelial NOS, estrogen receptor beta, and HIFs cooperate in the activation of a prognostic transcriptional pattern in aggressive human prostate cancer. J Clin Invest. 2009; 119: 1093-108.
[387] Wang Y, Wang L, Zhao J, Qiao Z. Estrogen, but not testosterone, down-regulates cytokine production in nicotine-induced murine macrophage. Methods Find Exp Clin Pharmacol. 2005; 27: 311-6.
[388] Pettersson A, Ciumas C, Chirsky V, *et al.* Dendritic cells exposed to estrogen *in vitro* exhibit therapeutic effects in ongoing experimental allergic encephalomyelitis. J Neuroimmunol. 2004; 156: 58-65.
[389] Curran EM, Judy BM, Newton LG, *et al.* Dietary soy phytoestrogens and ERalpha signalling modulate interferon gamma production in response to bacterial infection. Clin Exp Immunol. 2004; 135: 219-25.
[390] Tsuyuguchi K, Suzuki K, Matsumoto H, *et al.* Effect of oestrogen on Mycobacterium avium complex pulmonary infection in mice. Clin Exp Immunol. 2001; 123: 428-34.
[391] Mosmann TR, Cherwinski H, Bond MW, Giedlin MA, Coffman RL. Two types of murine helper T cell clone. I. Definition according to profiles of lymphokine activities and secreted proteins. 1986. J Immunol. 2005; 175: 5-14.
[392] Li Z, Zhang Y, Sun B. Current understanding of Th2 cell differentiation and function. Protein Cell. 2011; 2: 604-11.
[393] Wills-Karp M. Interleukin-13 in asthma pathogenesis. Immunol Rev. 2004; 202: 175-90.
[394] Jarnicki AG, Fallon PG. T helper type-2 cytokine responses: potential therapeutic targets. Curr Opin Pharmacol. 2003; 3: 449-55.
[395] Jenmalm MC, Van Snick J, Cormont F, Salman B. Allergen-induced Th1 and Th2 cytokine secretion in relation to specific allergen sensitization and atopic symptoms in children. Clin Exp Allergy. 2001; 31: 1528-35.

[396] McKenzie AN. Regulation of T helper type 2 cell immunity by interleukin-4 and interleukin-13. Pharmacol Ther. 2000; 88: 143-51.
[397] Bellanti JA. Cytokines and allergic diseases: clinical aspects. Allergy Asthma Proc. 1998; 19: 337-41.
[398] Inoue H, Fukuyama S, Matsumoto K, Kubo M, Yoshimura A. Role of endogenous inhibitors of cytokine signaling in allergic asthma. Curr Med Chem. 2007; 14: 181-9.
[399] Kubo M, Inoue H. Suppressor of cytokine signaling 3 (SOCS3) in Th2 cells evokes Th2 cytokines, IgE, and eosinophilia. Curr Allergy Asthma Rep. 2006; 6: 32-9.
[400] Peric A, Vojvodic D, Radulovic V, *et al.* Proinflammatory cytokine levels in nasal fluid as indicators of severity of nasal polyposis. Acta Clin Croat. 2010; 49: 395-403.
[401] Erin EM, Zacharasiewicz AS, Nicholson GC, *et al.* Topical corticosteroid inhibits interleukin-4, -5 and -13 in nasal secretions following allergen challenge. Clin Exp Allergy. 2005; 35: 1608-14.
[402] Renkl AC, Wussler J, Ahrens T, *et al.* Osteopontin functionally activates dendritic cells and induces their differentiation toward a Th1-polarizing phenotype. Blood. 2005; 106: 946-55.
[403] Wynn TA, Jankovic D, Hieny S, Cheever AW, Sher A. IL-12 enhances vaccine-induced immunity to Schistosoma mansoni in mice and decreases T helper 2 cytokine expression, IgE production, and tissue eosinophilia. J Immunol. 1995; 154: 4701-9.
[404] Medina KL, Kincade PW. Pregnancy-related steroids are potential negative regulators of B lymphopoiesis. Proc Natl Acad Sci U S A. 1994; 91: 5382-6.
[405] Kincade PW, Medina KL, Smithson G. Sex hormones as negative regulators of lymphopoiesis. Immunol Rev. 1994; 137: 119-34.
[406] Grimaldi CM, Michael DJ, Diamond B. Cutting edge: expansion and activation of a population of autoreactive marginal zone B cells in a model of estrogen-induced lupus. J Immunol. 2001; 167: 1886-90.
[407] Rijhsinghani AG, Thompson K, Bhatia SK, Waldschmidt TJ. Estrogen blocks early T cell development in the thymus. Am J Reprod Immunol. 1996; 36: 269-77.
[408] Park J, Kim SH, Cho D, Kim TS. Formononetin, a phyto-oestrogen, and its metabolites up-regulate interleukin-4 production in activated T cells *via* increased AP-1 DNA binding activity. Immunology. 2005; 116: 71-81.
[409] Kiyokawa Y, Yoneyama Y. Relationship between adenosine and T-helper 1/T-helper 2 balance in hyperemesis gravidarum. Clin Chim Acta. 2006; 370: 137-42.
[410] Jansson L, Olsson T, Holmdahl R. Estrogen induces a potent suppression of experimental autoimmune encephalomyelitis and collagen-induced arthritis in mice. J Neuroimmunol. 1994; 53: 203-7.
[411] d'Elia HF, Carlsten H. The impact of hormone replacement therapy on humoral and cell-mediated immune responses *in vivo* in post-menopausal women with rheumatoid arthritis. Scand J Immunol. 2008; 68: 661-7.
[412] Thor D, Zhang R, Anderson L, *et al.* Effects of 17 beta-estradiol on lipopolysacharride-induced intracellular adhesion molecule-1 mRNA expression and Ca(2)+ homeostasis alteration in human endothelial cells. Vascul Pharmacol. 2010; 53: 230-8.
[413] Caulin-Glaser T, Watson CA, Pardi R, Bender JR. Effects of 17beta-estradiol on cytokine-induced endothelial cell adhesion molecule expression. J Clin Invest. 1996; 98: 36-42.
[414] Rodriguez E, Lopez R, Paez A, Masso F, Montano LF. 17Beta-estradiol inhibits the adhesion of leukocytes in TNF-alpha stimulated human endothelial cells by blocking IL-8 and MCP-1 secretion, but not its transcription. Life Sci. 2002; 71: 2181-93.

[415] Mori M, Tsukahara F, Yoshioka T, Irie K, Ohta H. Suppression by 17beta-estradiol of monocyte adhesion to vascular endothelial cells is mediated by estrogen receptors. Life Sci. 2004; 75: 599-609.
[416] Piercy KT, Donnell RL, Kirkpatrick SS, *et al.* Effects of estrogen, progesterone, and combination exposure on interleukin-1 beta-induced expression of VCAM-1, ICAM-1, PECAM, and E-selectin by human female iliac artery endothelial cells. J Surg Res. 2002; 105: 215-9.
[417] Tyree CM, Zou A, Allegretto EA. 17beta-Estradiol inhibits cytokine induction of the human E-selectin promoter. J Steroid Biochem Mol Biol. 2002; 80: 291-7.
[418] Marfella R, Di Filippo C, Portoghese M, *et al.* Proteasome activity as a target of hormone replacement therapy-dependent plaque stabilization in postmenopausal women. Hypertension. 2008; 51: 1135-41.
[419] Chantakru S, Wang WC, van den Heuvel M, *et al.* Coordinate regulation of lymphocyte-endothelial interactions by pregnancy-associated hormones. J Immunol. 2003; 171: 4011-9.
[420] Yasui T, Saijo A, Uemura H, *et al.* Effects of oral and transdermal estrogen therapies on circulating cytokines and chemokines in postmenopausal women with hysterectomy. Eur J Endocrinol. 2009; 161: 267-73.
[421] Yeboah J, Klein K, Brosnihan B, Reboussin D, Herrington DM. Effects of hormone therapy on soluble cell adhesion molecules in postmenopausal women with coronary artery disease. Menopause. 2008; 15: 1060-4.
[422] Song Y, Manson JE, Tinker L, *et al.* Circulating levels of endothelial adhesion molecules and risk of diabetes in an ethnically diverse cohort of women. Diabetes. 2007; 56: 1898-904.
[423] Oger E, Alhenc-Gelas M, Plu-Bureau G, *et al.* Association of circulating cellular adhesion molecules with menopausal status and hormone replacement therapy. Time-dependent change in transdermal, but not oral estrogen users. Thromb Res. 2001; 101: 35-43.
[424] Kamada M, Irahara M, Maegawa M, *et al.* Transient increase in the levels of T-helper 1 cytokines in postmenopausal women and the effects of hormone replacement therapy. Gynecol Obstet Invest. 2001; 52: 82-8.
[425] Kumru S, Godekmerdan A, Yilmaz B. Immune effects of surgical menopause and estrogen replacement therapy in peri-menopausal women. J Reprod Immunol. 2004; 63: 31-8.
[426] Puder JJ, Freda PU, Goland RS, Wardlaw SL. Estrogen modulates the hypothalamic-pituitary-adrenal and inflammatory cytokine responses to endotoxin in women. J Clin Endocrinol Metab. 2001; 86: 2403-8.
[427] Troisi RJ, Speizer FE, Willett WC, Trichopoulos D, Rosner B. Menopause, postmenopausal estrogen preparations, and the risk of adult-onset asthma. A prospective cohort study. Am J Respir Crit Care Med. 1995; 152: 1183-8.
[428] Matsuo N, Shimoda T, Matsuse H, Kohno S. A case of menstruation-associated asthma: treatment with oral contraceptives. Chest. 1999; 116: 252-3.
[429] Kos-Kudla B, Ostrowska Z, Marek B, *et al.* Hormone replacement therapy in postmenopausal asthmatic women. J Clin Pharm Ther. 2000; 25: 461-6.
[430] Tan KS, McFarlane LC, Lipworth BJ. Modulation of airway reactivity and peak flow variability in asthmatics receiving the oral contraceptive pill. Am J Respir Crit Care Med. 1997; 155: 1273-7.
[431] Degano B, Prevost MC, Berger P, *et al.* Estradiol decreases the acetylcholine-elicited airway reactivity in ovariectomized rats through an increase in epithelial acetylcholinesterase activity. Am J Respir Crit Care Med. 2001; 164: 1849-54.

[432] Weinmann GG, Zacur H, Fish JE. Absence of changes in airway responsiveness during the menstrual cycle. J Allergy Clin Immunol. 1987; 79: 634-8.
[433] de Lignieres B. Endometrial hyperplasia. Risks, recognition and the search for a safe hormone replacement regimen. J Reprod Med. 1999; 44: 191-6.
[434] Lupulescu A. Estrogen use and cancer risk: a review. Exp Clin Endocrinol. 1993; 101: 204-14.
[435] Ponte CD, Swinker ML, Madhavan S. Estrogen replacement therapy: a pilot survey of primary care physicians in West Virginia. DICP. 1989; 23: 977-9.
[436] Dubey RK, Imthurn B, Barton M, Jackson EK. Vascular consequences of menopause and hormone therapy: importance of timing of treatment and type of estrogen. Cardiovasc Res. 2005; 66: 295-306.
[437] Yilmazer M, Fenkci V, Fenkci S, *et al.* Hormone replacement therapy, C-reactive protein, and fibrinogen in healthy postmenopausal women. Maturitas. 2003; 46: 245-53.
[438] Burger H. Hormone replacement therapy in the post-Women's Health Initiative era. Report a a meeting held in Funchal, Madeira, February 24-25, 2003. Climacteric. 2003; 6 Suppl 1: 11-36.
[439] Lacroix-Fralish ML, Tawfik VL, Nutile-McMenemy N, DeLeo JA. Progesterone mediates gonadal hormone differences in tactile and thermal hypersensitivity following L5 nerve root ligation in female rats. Neuroscience. 2006; 138: 601-8.
[440] Kos-Kudla B, Ostrowska Z, Marek B, *et al.* Effects of hormone replacement therapy on endocrine and spirometric parameters in asthmatic postmenopausal women. Gynecol Endocrinol. 2001; 15: 304-11.
[441] Hudic I, Szekeres-Bartho J, Fatusic Z, *et al.* Dydrogesterone supplementation in women with threatened preterm delivery--the impact on cytokine profile, hormone profile, and progesterone-induced blocking factor. J Reprod Immunol. 2011; 92: 103-7.
[442] Eilertsen AL, Sandvik L, Steinsvik B, Sandset PM. Differential impact of conventional-dose and low-dose postmenopausal hormone therapy, tibolone and raloxifene on C-reactive protein and other inflammatory markers. J Thromb Haemost. 2008; 6: 928-34.
[443] Sumino H, Ichikawa S, Ohyama Y, *et al.* Effect of transdermal hormone replacement therapy on the monocyte chemoattractant protein-1 concentrations and other vascular inflammatory markers and on endothelial function in postmenopausal women. Am J Cardiol. 2005; 96: 148-53.
[444] Jenkins DJ, Kendall CW, Connelly PW, *et al.* Effects of high- and low-isoflavone (phytoestrogen) soy foods on inflammatory biomarkers and proinflammatory cytokines in middle-aged men and women. Metabolism. 2002; 51: 919-24.
[445] Lomnitski L, Bergman M, Nyska A, Ben-Shaul V, Grossman S. Composition, efficacy, and safety of spinach extracts. Nutr Cancer. 2003; 46: 222-31.
[446] Kawai M, Hirano T, Higa S, *et al.* Flavonoids and related compounds as anti-allergic substances. Allergol Int. 2007; 56: 113-23.
[447] Goh FY, Upton N, Guan S, *et al.* Fisetin, a bioactive flavonol, attenuates allergic airway inflammation through negative regulation of NF-kappaB. Eur J Pharmacol. 2012; 679: 109-16.
[448] Wu MY, Hung SK, Fu SL. Immunosuppressive effects of fisetin in ovalbumin-induced asthma through inhibition of NF-kappaB activity. J Agric Food Chem. 2011; 59: 10496-504.

[449] Wei D, Ci X, Chu X, *et al.* Hesperidin suppresses ovalbumin-induced airway inflammation in a mouse allergic asthma model. Inflammation. 2012; 35: 114-21.
[450] Jin M, Yang JH, Lee E, *et al.* Antiasthmatic activity of luteolin-7-O-glucoside from Ailanthus altissima through the downregulation of T helper 2 cytokine expression and inhibition of prostaglandin E2 production in an ovalbumin-induced asthma model. Biol Pharm Bull. 2009; 32: 1500-3.
[451] Kawai M, Hirano T, Arimitsu J, *et al.* Effect of enzymatically modified isoquercitrin, a flavonoid, on symptoms of Japanese cedar pollinosis: a randomized double-blind placebo-controlled trial. Int Arch Allergy Immunol. 2009; 149: 359-68.
[452] Higa S, Hirano T, Kotani M, *et al.* Fisetin, a flavonol, inhibits TH2-type cytokine production by activated human basophils. J Allergy Clin Immunol. 2003; 111: 1299-306.
[453] Noh SU, Cho EA, Kim HO, Park YM. Epigallocatechin-3-gallate improves Dermatophagoides pteronissinus extract-induced atopic dermatitis-like skin lesions in NC/Nga mice by suppressing macrophage migration inhibitory factor. Int Immunopharmacol. 2008; 8: 1172-82.
[454] Havsteen B. Flavonoids, a class of natural products of high pharmacological potency. Biochem Pharmacol. 1983; 32: 1141-8.
[455] Lorentz A, Wilke M, Sellge G, *et al.* IL-4-induced priming of human intestinal mast cells for enhanced survival and Th2 cytokine generation is reversible and associated with increased activity of ERK1/2 and c-Fos. J Immunol. 2005; 174: 6751-6.
[456] Dumont FJ, Staruch MJ, Fischer P, DaSilva C, Camacho R. Inhibition of T cell activation by pharmacologic disruption of the MEK1/ERK MAP kinase or calcineurin signaling pathways results in differential modulation of cytokine production. J Immunol. 1998; 160: 2579-89.
[457] Seelinger G, Merfort I, Schempp CM. Anti-oxidant, anti-inflammatory and anti-allergic activities of luteolin. Planta Med. 2008; 74: 1667-77.
[458] Martinez-Florez S, Gonzalez-Gallego J, Culebras JM, Tunon MJ. [Flavonoids: properties and anti-oxidizing action]. Nutr Hosp. 2002; 17: 271-8.
[459] Gonzalez-Gallego J, Sanchez-Campos S, Tunon MJ. Anti-inflammatory properties of dietary flavonoids. Nutr Hosp. 2007; 22: 287-93.
[460] Theoharides TC, Bielory L. Mast cells and mast cell mediators as targets of dietary supplements. Ann Allergy Asthma Immunol. 2004; 93: S24-34.
[461] Matsumoto M, Kotani M, Fujita A, *et al.* Oral administration of persimmon leaf extract ameliorates skin symptoms and transepidermal water loss in atopic dermatitis model mice, NC/Nga. Br J Dermatol. 2002; 146: 221-7.
[462] Devereux G. Session 1: Allergic disease: Nutrition as a potential determinant of asthma. Proc Nutr Soc. 2010; 69: 1-10.
[463] Endre L. [Occupational rhinitis]. Orv Hetil. 2010; 151: 941-5.
[464] Niggemann B, Wahn U. [Allergic rhinoconjunctivitis--past and present aspects]. Monatsschr Kinderheilkd. 1992; 140: 156-61.
[465] Valero A, Chivato T, Justicia JL, Navarro AM. Diagnosis and treatment of grass pollen-induced allergic rhinitis in specialized current clinical practice in Spain. Allergy Asthma Proc. 2011; 32: 384-9.
[466] Valovirta E, Scadding G. Parental attitudes toward new dosage forms of desloratadine in an online survey: results from four European countries. Curr Med Res Opin. 2009; 25: 2061-7.

[467] Chavasse R, Seddon P, Bara A, McKean M. Short acting beta agonists for recurrent wheeze in children under 2 years of age. Cochrane Database Syst Rev. 2002: CD002873.
[468] Toogood JH. Complications of topical steroid therapy for asthma. Am Rev Respir Dis. 1990; 141: S89-96.
[469] Vianna EO, Martin RJ. Bronchodilators and corticosteroids in the treatment of asthma. Drugs Today (Barc). 1998; 34: 203-23.
[470] Blaiss M. Current concepts and therapeutic strategies for allergic rhinitis in school-age children. Clin Ther. 2004; 26: 1876-89.
[471] Hughes DT. The use of anticholinergic drugs in nocturnal asthma. Postgrad Med J. 1987; 63 Suppl 1: 47-51.
[472] Ridolo E, Albertini R, Borghi L, *et al.* Acute polyradiculoneuropathy occurring after hymenoptera stings: a clinical case study. Int J Immunopathol Pharmacol. 2005; 18: 385-90.
[473] Pajno GB, Barberio G, De Luca F, Morabito L, Parmiani S. Prevention of new sensitizations in asthmatic children monosensitized to house dust mite by specific immunotherapy. A six-year follow-up study. Clin Exp Allergy. 2001; 31: 1392-7.
[474] Sicherer SH, Simons FE. Self-injectable epinephrine for first-aid management of anaphylaxis. Pediatrics. 2007; 119: 638-46.
[475] Sharkey P, Portnoy J. Rush immunotherapy: experience with a one-day schedule. Ann Allergy Asthma Immunol. 1996; 76: 175-80.
[476] Kennedy JL, Heymann PW, Platts-Mills TA. The role of allergy in severe asthma. Clin Exp Allergy. 2012; 42: 659-69.
[477] Nelson HS. Advances in upper airway diseases and allergen immunotherapy. J Allergy Clin Immunol. 2007; 119: 872-80.

Send Orders for Reprints on reprints@benthamscience.net

CHAPTER 9

Indications for Adrenaline: Use by Patients and Emergency Departments

Miguel A. Tejedor-Alonso*, Maria V. Mugica-Garcia and Mar Moro-Moro

Allergy Unit of University Hospital Fundacion Alcorcon, Spain

Abstract: Experts agree that prompt use of intramuscular adrenaline is beneficial for patients experiencing anaphylaxis. Adrenaline is administered using autoinjectors, which are indicated in patients with a high risk of anaphylaxis, namely, those who have already experienced anaphylactic reactions and have comorbid persistent asthma, those who have reacted to trace amounts of allergen, those who have experienced mild reactions to peanut or tree nut, those with mastocytosis and finally adolescents.

However, the frequency of administration of adrenaline by patients and physicians in clinical settings is low. Autoinjectors are prescribed in less than 50% of cases; availability and use by patients can be less than 75%. Administration of adrenaline in emergency departments is also uncommon, in many cases less than 50%, although many series show increased use of adrenaline when anaphylaxis is severe.

Our main objectives are to conduct a comprehensive review and update of the use of epinephrine in anaphylaxis episodes (the first and recurrences) both by patients and by the emergency services, after synthesizing the most accepted indications of epinephrine use in anaphylaxis. All this information remains dispersed in the literature on anaphylaxis.

Keywords: Adrenaline, auto-injectors, indications, emergency, prescription, availability, administration, adherence, low.

INTRODUCTION

Anaphylaxis is an acute, life-threatening reaction that is mediated by immunologic and nonimmunologic mechanisms and results in sudden systemic release of mast-cell and basophil mediators [1].

Adrenaline (also known as epinephrine in the USA) was first isolated at the turn

***Address correspondence to Miguel A. Tejedor-Alonso:** Allergy Unit, Hospital Universitario Fundacion Alcorcón, Madrid, Avda Budapest 1, 28922 Alcorcón (Madrid), Spain; Tel: +34916219711; +34629864381; Fax: +34916219704; E-mails: m914674227@telefonica.net; matejedor@fhalcorcon.es

Atta-ur-Rahman (Ed)

of the twentieth century [2]. Since then, it has maintained a role in emergency department care and has become the medication of choice for emergency treatment of anaphylaxis. No randomized controlled trials meet sufficiently high standards to draw firm conclusions on the medication used to treat acute anaphylaxis; however, evidence of the effectiveness of adrenaline injection in patients with anaphylaxis is stronger than that of H_1-antihistamines, H_2-antihistamines, and corticosteroids [3, 4]. Randomization to non–adrenaline-based treatment would be unethical, as most findings indicate that immediate treatment with adrenaline is essential for survival [5-7]. Recommendations for prompt injection of adrenaline are based on a century of clinical use and on fatality studies [7, 8], epidemiologic studies [9, 10], and prospective studies [11-13].

In pharmacological terms, adrenaline acts directly in several organs through a sympathomimetic effect (*e.g.*, increased vasoconstriction, decreased mucosal edema, increased inotropy/chronotropy, and bronchodilation). Adrenaline also downregulates further release of histamine, tryptase, and other mediators by mast cells [11, 14].

Prompt administration of adrenaline has been associated with a better outcome [15]. Delayed injection of adrenaline is associated with fatal anaphylaxis [5-8, 16-18], poor outcome [14, 19-21] and biphasic anaphylaxis [14, 19-21].

Adrenaline is currently used by health professionals to treat anaphylaxis in the emergency department and by patients or their caretakers (autoinjectors) in the community. This chapter analyzes the current indications for adrenaline in clinical settings where health care is available and indications for adrenaline autoinjectors when anaphylaxis occurs outside the care setting. We also determine the real use of adrenaline in the emergency department and present data on the prescription and use of adrenaline autoinjectors.

INDICATIONS FOR ADRENALINE IN CLINICAL PRACTICE

No definitive trials examine the indications for adrenaline, and guidelines are consensus-based [22]. Adrenaline is the first-choice agent for patients with acute anaphylaxis, as confirmed internationally by most anaphylaxis consensus guidelines published in English and in other languages over the past 30 years [1, 14, 23-29]. Experts differ on the clinical thresholds by which they define and treat anaphylaxis. However, they all agree that an appropriate dose of intramuscular adrenaline should be administered rapidly once that threshold is reached [30].

INDICATIONS FOR ADRENALINE AUTOINJECTORS

Evidenced-based approaches to the use of adrenaline autoinjectors in a community setting suggest that prescriptions for self-injectable adrenaline should be given to patients who experience a severe systemic reaction (respiratory difficulty or hypotension) to an allergen or to patients who are at high risk, namely, those with asthma or mastocytosis, reactions to trace amount of allergen, a risk of repeated exposure with lack of access to emergency care, and comorbidity increasing the risk of a severe reaction [29, 31].

Although these recommendations seem straightforward, application to individual patients often requires clinical judgment [29, 30]. In the medical literature, benefits and risks are the subject of debate, with some authorities expressing [32] caution about the assumption that it is always good practice to prescribe adrenaline autoinjectors [33, 34]. Some authors claim autoinjectors improve quality of life by relieving concerns over dying from a reaction. However, other authors feel that such reassurance is false, as self-treatment can fail, and provision of adrenaline self-treatment may have an adverse effect on the quality of life [34]. One death has been imputed to the fact that some patients take extra risks because of this reassurance [7].

First Decision: Which Patients Require Prescription of Self-Injectable Adrenaline?

In the review of indications for adrenaline autoinjectors, we follow the methodology of Sicherer and Simons [29].

Previous Life-Threatening Reaction

The severity of the initial reaction should be taken into account when prescribing an autoinjector [6, 32, 35], as evidence indicates that the severity of the initial reaction provides some prediction of the nature of a subsequent reaction. Hourihane *et al.* reported over 600 allergic reactions to peanuts in adults and children. Of the patients whose first reaction was severe (wheeze, cyanosis, collapse, or fainting), the last reaction was also severe in 78% of cases, whilst in those cases with a mild reaction the last one was severe in 32% of cases [36].

Fortunately, death from anaphylaxis appears to be rare, and a potentially high risk of death has a >99.9% chance of being unjustifiable [37]. The ability of autoinjectors to prevent the morbidity of anaphylaxis, however, can be analyzed statistically in terms of medical interventions (*e.g.*, hospital resuscitation and admission) and sequelae [38]. One retrospective review of 68 South Australian children with anaphylaxis suggests that autoinjectors may be associated with decreased morbidity [39]: children who received adrenaline were significantly less likely to be admitted to hospital.

Patients with no history of severe anaphylaxis or only cutaneous symptoms are at risk of experiencing a more severe recurrence. Also important in terms of prescription is the possibility that a physician might identify a patient who has not yet experienced anaphylaxis but who may be at risk of anaphylaxis and thus require self-injectable adrenaline [3]. For instance, children with generalized symptoms limited to the skin after insect sting have a lower risk of anaphylaxis (approximately 10%), yet prescription of self-injectable adrenaline is recommended [40]. The future risk of anaphylaxis is not clear for foods [17, 41-43]. Van der Leek *et al.* [42] showed that of 24 young children with peanut allergy whose first reaction was restricted to the skin after ingestion or contact, 18 (75%) experienced symptoms beyond the skin in a subsequent reaction. In other series, 3 out of every 4 patients dying from food anaphylaxis only had minor reactions in the past [37]; therefore, if prescribed adrenaline, they have very little incentive to carry it or even to use their prescription to obtain an autoinjector [44]. On the other hand, most fatal allergic reactions to food occurred in persons with a history of mild reactions and concomitant uncontrolled asthma [5, 6, 37]. Nearly 2% of patients with pollen-food syndrome might at some time experience anaphylaxis from the same triggers [45, 46]; in the series of Ortolani *et al.* on fruit and vegetable anaphylaxis, this finding was surprisingly common [46].

Therefore, severity of a previous reaction is a poor guide to symptoms during a future reaction.

Reaction to Trace Allergen

The amount of food allergen that triggers a severe reaction is important [35]. Thus, a child who develops mild generalized urticaria following ingestion of half an egg will be at less risk than a child who experiences a respiratory reaction following exposure to a small amount of egg protein in a cake. The EAACI anaphylaxis task force recommends using adrenaline autoinjectors in any reaction to small amounts of food [30, 47].

Subtypes of Anaphylaxis

The risk of recurrence must be borne in mind in the decision to prescribe self-injectable adrenaline. Recurrence of anaphylaxis affects 30-40% of patients in most series, although the risk of recurrence differs with the type of anaphylaxis (*e.g.*, drugs and food) [15, 48, 49]. Atopic patients are predisposed to certain subtypes of anaphylaxis (*e.g.*, food, latex, and idiopathic), as described in the literature [15, 48-52]. Mullins [48] found that idiopathic anaphylaxis and exercise anaphylaxis caused by wheat had higher recurrence rates. Cianferoni *et al.* [49] reported that food anaphylaxis recurred 4.5 times more than the remaining subtypes (*e.g.*, exercise, idiopathic, and drugs). Gold and Sainsbury [15] found that children with food anaphylaxis were 4 times more likely to experience a recurrence than children with hymenoptera anaphylaxis.

Atopic patients are more likely to experience recurrence than nonatopic patients, probably because of their higher predisposition to become sensitized to new allergens or cross-reactivity between different food allergens or between food allergens and latex. However, people with idiopathic anaphylaxis can expect to have almost 3 recurrent episodes each year, whilst for food and insect venom anaphylaxis, 1 recurrent episode could occur every 2 and 7.5 years, respectively [33].

An autoinjector is not usually necessary for patients who have experienced drug-induced anaphylaxis, unless it is difficult to avoid the drug [53].

Specific Triggers Associated with Severe Reaction

Of the 32 deaths due to food anaphylaxis recorded in a registry of the Food Allergy & Anaphylaxis Network [6], all but 1 of the individuals had a known allergy to the food, and peanut or tree nut caused 94% of the reactions (milk and fish caused the others). Most deaths are associated with nut, and, in particular, peanut. Combining mortality results from the USA, UK, and Sweden showed that 34/46 deaths were associated with peanut or tree-nut reactions [6, 54, 55]. In the UK, walnut and Brazil nut cause more severe reactions and deaths than peanut [56]. Deaths from reaction to egg and cow's milk are much less common, even though these foods commonly cause allergy [55].

Therefore, knowledge of the type of food to which a patient is allergic cannot provide an absolute guarantee against severe or fatal anaphylaxis, because fatalities have been reported for foods not usually considered to cause severe reactions, such as cow's milk, soy, and fruit.

Patients with Mastocytosis

Anaphylactic reactions occur in 49 % of adults with mastocytosis, of which 27% are due to hymenoptera allergy [57]. The clinical symptomatology of anaphylaxis of patients with anaphylaxis has been reported to be more severe in allergic patients with mastocytosis or increased tryptase [58, 59]. For example, these patients may suffer from severe anaphylactic shock after hymenoptera stings or during the course of insect venom hyposensitization [58]. Fatal anaphylaxis has been described following hymenoptera stings [17], in the perioperative period [60], and of unknown cause in children and adults with mastocytosis.

Patients with anaphylaxis and mastocytosis have an increased risk to develop repeated anaphylactic reactions (50% of patients >1 episode) [57], and should be provided with emergency medication.

According to conclusions of a prospective study [57], children and adults with mastocytosis differed markedly with regard to anaphylaxis. In children, it was strictly limited to those with severe disease and high tryptase levels, whereas in adults, all patients may be affected. Still it seems justified to recommend adrenaline autoinjectors to children with severe cutaneous disease and/or previous anaphylaxis and adults with mastocytosis.

Age Over 5 Years

Most deaths from anaphylaxis occur in children aged 5 years and older and adults. A cumulative 14 years' observation of 46 fatal reactions in 3 countries revealed that only 3 reactions (7%) occurred in children aged less than 5 years [6, 54, 55]. In contrast, food-induced immediate hypersensitivity reactions most commonly occurred to milk, egg, and peanuts in preschool children; the reactions were frequent for egg and milk and less common for peanut. In the case of egg and milk, reactions often resolve by 5 years of age.

If the UK figures are extrapolated to the Australian pediatric population, Kemp [33] estimated that there would be 1 death in 30 years in children aged under 5 years and 2 deaths in 10 years in the entire pediatric population. In the case of vaccine-preventable meningococcal infection, there would be 1.2 deaths in 10 years. In other words, a food-allergic child aged under 5 years could be 4 times more likely to die from a preventable meningococcal infection than from food anaphylaxis. Therefore, adrenaline should not be indicated in this group based only on the presence of food allergy.

Asthma

The presence of asthma increases the risk of death or severe reactions [5, 6, 37, 54]. Almost all fatal cases of anaphylaxis occur in patients with asthma. This observation has led to the recommendation that patients with both asthma and food allergy should be prescribed an autoinjector. In pediatric patients, it seems reasonable to prescribe an autoinjector to those children with asthma of sufficient severity to require preventive medication [33, 35, 41, 42].

Although asthma is a relatively sensitive marker, the fact that approximately one-third of food-allergic individuals has asthma means that it is not particularly specific; in addition, children without asthma experience life-threatening anaphylaxis. In summary, a history of previous anaphylactic reactions or coexistent asthma can indicate subgroups of food-allergic children at higher risk of anaphylaxis, although it is impossible to identify groups with a very low risk [30].

Use of Nonselective β-Blockers, ACE-Inhibitors and other Substances

Patients receiving nonselective β-blockers and ACE-inhibitors are more likely to experience severe reactions than patients who are not [29]. Other patients might be at increased risk because of defects in mediator degradation pathways or excessive consumption of alcohol or other harmful substances [22].

Persons with Difficulties to Provide Self-Care or to Find Help From Caregivers or Sanitary Professionals

This group includes patients supervised by caregivers with no health care training or experience, patients who are members of dysfunctional families, infants or young children, patients with skin disease (*e.g.*, eczema) or coloring that makes it difficult to detect erythema, patients who are unable to recognize or describe their symptoms accurately (*e.g.*, infants, children, and persons with learning disabilities or language barriers) [29] and finally persons with barriers to prompt treatment by professionals (people living alone, people living in a remote area, people without reliable transportation, and people without a telephone) [12, 61-64].

We should stress the importance to indicate autoinjectors in age groups with an increased risk of death (*e.g.*, teenagers, young adults, and the elderly), who might take more risks in their diet and be reluctant to use self-injectable adrenaline, as well as in patients with learning disabilities and patients who have previously had trouble recognizing or assessing their own symptoms [29].

In addition, physicians cannot assume that patients and caregivers recognize and report all symptoms, because anaphylaxis can even go undetected by trained health care professionals [29]. Therefore, a high index of suspicion is needed to identify those who have had anaphylaxis and require adrenaline [14].

Second Decision: Instructions to the Patient for Use of Self-Injectable Adrenaline

The recommendations for administration of adrenaline to treat anaphylaxis range between two extremes [65]: some physicians advise against injecting adrenaline unless progressive respiratory symptoms, cardiovascular symptoms, or both are present [29]; others such as allergists recommend administration of adrenaline as early as possible after onset of the least severe or minor symptoms, especially if the allergen is administered parenterally or after exposure to a known allergen in the absence of symptoms. In our opinion, neither of these extreme positions is appropriate.

Data from challenge studies (insect stings and foods) in allergy departments indicate that the decision to administer adrenaline to patients with mild symptoms or symptoms affecting the skin only should be taken by trained health professionals [29].

The major themes in several reports on death from food anaphylaxis are concurrent asthma and delay in treatment with adrenaline and identification of particular risks for teens. Most deaths from anaphylaxis occur outside a medical center and usually result from delayed administration of adrenaline. In a retrospective review of 6 fatal and 7 nonfatal episodes of food-induced anaphylaxis in children and adolescents, Sampson *et al.* [5] reported on 6 children with fatal reactions, all of whom had asthma, previous severe reactions to foods, and delay in treatment with adrenaline. None of the children received adrenaline before the onset of severe respiratory symptoms, whereas 7 children with near-fatal food-induced anaphylaxis evaluated during the same period received adrenaline before or within 5 minutes of severe respiratory symptoms. Analysis of data from a national case registry of fatal food-induced anaphylaxis in the USA indicated that very few individuals (7/63) had autoinjectors available at the time of the fatal reaction [6, 8]. Similarly, Pumphrey [17] found that, although adrenaline was administered in 62% of fatal anaphylactic reactions in the UK, it was given before cardiac arrest in only 14% of cases. In a follow-up analysis of 48 cases of fatal food anaphylaxis from 1999 to 2006, Pumphrey and Gowland [7] reported that, although 19 (40%) patients had received epinephrine autoinjectors, more than half of the fatalities occurred in patients whose previous clinical reactions had been too mild to require prescription of an autoinjector.

Although generalized acute urticaria is not life-threatening, patients exposed to an allergen that previously triggered anaphylaxis should receive adrenaline if the exposure occurs outside a medical setting [29, 66]. Adrenaline is not contraindicated in a patient experiencing an anaphylactic reaction. In fact, it is prudent to administer adrenaline in uncertain cases where the patient does not yet fulfill the diagnostic criteria, for example, a person with a history of seafood allergy and anaphylaxis who has inadvertently ingested shrimp and is beginning to experience facial flushing or urticaria [65, 67]

Although trained health professionals can consider postponing adrenaline when symptoms are mild or restricted to the skin, a patient or caregiver might not recognize the symptoms of anaphylaxis or their severity and might fail to inject the adrenaline as instructed. Recommendations for treatment in the real world should therefore be more prudent than they are for situations supervised by trained health professionals. Consequently, the best recommendation is for patients or caregivers to inject adrenaline promptly when symptoms occur after exposure to an allergen that previously caused a significant reaction [29, 65 67, 68].

Reaching peak plasma and tissue adrenaline levels can increase survival, and retrospective studies correlate delayed administration with poor outcome [5, 17]. However, administration during anaphylaxis is not always effective, and patients can still die [5-8, 17, 69]. The reasons for this observation include delayed administration, inadequate doses, inappropriate route of administration, use of adrenaline that has passed its expiry date, or presence of an underlying disease (*e.g.*, poorly controlled asthma, cardiovascular disease, mastocytosis, and other serious systemic disorders) [12, 70]. In their canine study, Bautista *et al.* [71] also demonstrated that reaching peak plasma adrenaline levels and hemodynamic recovery are not as effective when administration is delayed until hypotension has developed.

Although deaths have been attributed to delay in administration of adrenaline, it is impossible to predict how a reaction will develop. In addition, symptoms can worsen quickly or slowly. Furthermore, patient uncertainty over when to use the autoinjector is compounded by the fact that they often do not receive clear instructions from their doctor, most probably because the doctors themselves do not know the best time to use the device [72, 73]. For instance, in patients who report recurrent mild reactions with nausea or itching in the mouth or throat, adrenaline can worsen the panic and generate the sensation of difficulty breathing and hyperventilation. In addition, some cases, patients who injected their adrenaline early died [74].

Therefore, it is not possible to provide simple recommendations for all patients. The evidence that early self-injection reduces the need for hospital care following a reaction [15] indicates that patients often make the right decision. In fact, patients commonly report that they knew a reaction was going to be bad before the worst of the symptoms started: this point seems to be the right time to self-inject.

Third Decision: Dosing for First-Aid Treatment

The recommendation for dosing in children with anaphylaxis, which is based primarily on anecdotal evidence, is to inject 0.01 mg/kg up to 0.30 mg [12, 14]. Adrenaline autoinjectors are currently available in 2 fixed doses: 0.15 and 0.30 mg. Twinject® (0.3 mg or 0.15 mg of adrenaline) (Verus, San Diego, California, USA) allows for administration of a follow-up dose using the same device for persistent or worsening allergic symptoms [29, 75].

A risk for overdosage exists in infants receiving 0.15 mg and small children receiving 0.3 mg and for underdosage in many adolescents receiving 0.15 mg [12, 14].

Therefore, physicians face a dilemma when prescribing adrenaline for infants and children who weigh less than 15 kg [14, 64]. One option may be to prescribe an adrenaline ampule/syringe/needle and instruct caregivers on preparation and administration. However, as parents have many concerns about successfully preparing and administering a dose, this approach should only be used when autoinjectors are not available [65].

In a survey of 29 pediatricians [76], 80% responded that they would prescribe the 0.15-mg autoinjector dose for a child weighing 10 kg, 100% responded that they would prescribe it for a child weighing 15 kg, and 70% responded that they would prescribe it for a child weighing 20 kg. In a study of adrenaline dispensing patterns [10], 72% of prescriptions for infants younger than 6 months (weight <7 kg) were for a 0.15-mg autoinjector and 20% were for an ampule/syringe/needle;

95% of prescriptions for infants aged 6 to 12 months (weight up to 10 kg) were for a 0.15-mg autoinjector.

According to Sicherer and Simons [14], in the absence of strong evidence and a large selection of premeasured autoinjector doses and in light of studies showing elevated plasma concentrations and relatively modest adverse effects in children weighing approximately 25 kg injected with a 1.2-fold overdose of intramuscular adrenaline, it seems appropriate to switch most children from the 0.15-mg dose to the 0.30-mg dose at approximately 25 kg. For children who have asthma or other additional risk factors for fatality from anaphylaxis, switching to the higher dose at a lower weight might be considered [12]. At present, no data support specific recommendations for children weighing less than 15 kg [14]. It is not known whether the adverse effects from a previously studied 1.2-fold overdose are similar in infants and very small young children to those reported in children weighing approximately 25 kg. Considering the ease of use of self-injectable adrenaline compared with the ampule/syringe/needle technique and the preferences of pediatricians [10, 76] and parents [10], it seems reasonable to consider autoinjectors containing 0.15 mg of adrenaline for otherwise healthy infants/young children weighing 10 to 25 kg. Clearly, specific clinical circumstances must be taken into consideration when making this decision. For infants weighing less than 10 kg, dosing with 0.15-mg autoinjectors would exceed the 1.5-fold overdose. Many pediatricians choose this option because of the certainty of an autoinjector dose compared with the uncertainty over having prepared the ideal dose with the adrenaline ampule/syringe/needle technique [12, 14, 68, 77].

Lack of availability of autoinjectors [78] in developing countries often means that the less costly adrenaline ampule/syringe/needle technique is prescribed, despite the fact that it requires additional training, is error prone, and may lead to a delay in injection [79].

The recommendation of a second dose if the first was not effective within 5 to 10 minutes raises the question of how many autoinjectors should be carried by each patient. Given the possible need for a second dose and the fact that 1 or more pens are commonly misused when treating a reaction, the argument in favor of carrying 3 or more pens could be valid [67, 68 74].

Multiple doses are needed by patients with severe or protracted anaphylaxis symptoms that are not relieved by the initial dose and by those with biphasic or multiphasic anaphylaxis [80]. The number of patients reported to require more than 1 dose of adrenaline differs from study to study. In 2 prospective studies in which all or most patients with anaphylaxis after allergen immunotherapy injections received adrenaline injections promptly [14, 20], biphasic reactions occurred in 23% and 10% of the patients, respectively. Community and emergency department data [47, 81-83] suggest that 20% of patients suffering from an anaphylactic event who used a self-injectable adrenaline device received a second dose, and case-series data demonstrate that a single self-injectable adrenaline device may be insufficient to prevent death in some patients [17, 29].

Other reasons to considerer prescribing 2 autoinjectors include the possibility of misfiring [84], remote location without rapid access to medical support, a large child (*e.g.*, >45 kg), or concern over the failure to respond to the first dose.

Finally, self-injectable adrenaline should always be prescribed in the context of an individualized emergency action plan that lists potential anaphylaxis symptoms and covers the indications for self-injectable adrenaline, administration technique, the need to take the patient to an emergency department after the injection, identification of triggers of anaphylaxis, instructions on avoidance (*e.g.*, foods and insects), and medical identification (*e.g.*, bracelet, wallet card) [64]. Finally, the emergency action plan and training on the use of self-injectable adrenaline should be reviewed with the patient on a regular basis.

More outcome studies are needed to create comprehensive evidence-based guidelines for self-management of anaphylaxis in the community.

Contraindications

Given that children do not usually suffer from significant comorbidities, such as coronary heart disease or cardiac arrhythmias, no absolute contraindications exist for the use of adrenaline in this population. However, advice to families may need to be modified in specific situations, for example, a food allergic child at higher risk of tachyarrhythmia because of hypertrophic obstructive cardiomyopathy. In such a case, the pediatrician must weigh up the risks and benefits, remembering that adrenaline can save the patient's life [30].

In middle-aged or elderly patients who might have subclinical or diagnosed coronary artery disease or peripheral vascular disease, the potential cardiac effects of adrenaline should be weighed against the cardiac risks of untreated anaphylaxis. Therefore, it is important to remember that the β-$_2$-adrenergic action of adrenaline usually enhances blood flow in the coronary arteries, thus leading to increased myocardial contractility and increased duration of diastole compared with systole [11, 61].

Patients with untreated hyperthyroidism are also particularly vulnerable to the effects of adrenaline, because the increased number of β-adrenergic receptors in the vasculature of these individuals renders the myocardium more sensitive to β-adrenergic effects of adrenaline [31].

The risk of adverse events from drug interactions might also increase [24, 31, 64], as a result of decreased effectiveness of endogenous catecholamine stores or exogenously administered adrenaline (β-adrenergic blockers), interference with intrinsic compensatory responses to hypotension (angiotensin-converting enzyme inhibitors and possibly angiotensin II receptor blockers), or blockage of adrenaline metabolism that leads to increased plasma and tissue concentrations (tricyclic antidepressants and monoamine oxidase inhibitors). Likewise, β-adrenergic antagonists and α-adrenergic antagonists can exaggerate the pharmacologic effects of adrenaline by permitting unopposed α-adrenergic effects (vasoconstrictor) and β-adrenergic effects (vasodilator), respectively. Cocaine and amphetamines sensitize the myocardium to the effects of adrenaline, thus increasing the risk of toxicity [65].

In short, according to all the information it can be concluded that there is no absolute contraindications to the use of epinephrine in patients with anaphylaxis [22].

PRESCRIPTION, AVAILABILITY, AND USE OF AUTOINJECTORS

Prescription of Autoinjectors

Most studies agree that adrenaline autoinjectors are rarely prescribed [15, 48, 49, 75, 85-89], mainly due to poor availability in many countries (especially for children) [12, 78] and the difficulty in establishing accurate indications and simple algorithms to help patients know when to use their devices.

Availability of Autoinjectors in the World

In a 2007 updated survey sponsored by the WAO, Simons [12] reported that autoinjectors of adrenaline with 0.15 mg and 0.30 mg were available in 59% of countries, although autoinjectors for children under 15 kg had not been marketed at the time of publication. Therefore, the availability of 0.3-mg adrenaline autoinjectors improved slightly compared with the 2003 survey [78], particularly in Europe, although it remained more limited in Asia, South America, and Africa. In countries where 0.30-mg devices were introduced, 0.15-mg autoinjectors were fully available.

Prescription of Adrenaline in Clinical Settings

Prescription of autoinjectors is infrequent in allergy outpatient clinics [15, 48, 49, 85-88] and in the emergency department [75, 90], although in some studies, autoinjectors were prescribed to 100% of patients attended [15, 48, 49].

Several authors have studied the prescription of adrenaline in allergy outpatient clinics. Sicherer *et al.* [86] used a survey to ascertain changes in the prevalence of allergy to peanut and walnut over 5 years (1997-2002) in the general population of the USA. These authors observed that adrenaline autoinjectors were prescribed for 46% of the children and 23% of the adults after hypersensitivity reactions with respiratory or multisystemic involvement in the first episode. The authors also found that 2% of patients presented 5 or more reactions. In 2002, Sicherer *et al.* performed a similar study [85] to determine the prevalence of allergy to fish and shellfish in the general population of the USA. Adrenaline autoinjectors were prescribed to 8.6% of patients, despite the extreme severity and use of adrenaline in the emergency department in 16% of reactions.

Asero *et al.* [87] carried out an observational study in Italy in 2007 to analyze whether adrenaline prescribed to patients with IgE-mediated food allergy attended in the allergy outpatient clinic was administered following clinical guidelines or according to the risk associated with sensitization to specific foods. The drug was prescribed to only 13% of patients.

Other authors report prescription of adrenaline to all patients with anaphylaxis. Mullins [48] reported, in a mail and telephone survey on anaphylaxis conducted from 1995 to 2000 among 432 patients weighing more than 15 kg, that adrenaline autoinjectors were prescribed to all patients. Similarly, Cianferoni *et al.* [49] reported prescription of autoinjectors to 76 children with anaphylaxis attended from 1994 to 1996 and interviewed by phone 7 years later. Finally, between 1996 and 1998, Gold and Sainsbury [15] prescribed anaphylaxis to 86 children (>15 kg) weighing more than 15 kg who had experienced generalized allergic reactions with respiratory and circulatory involvement.

Prescription of autoinjectors in the emergency department has also been examined. In a 1999 North American series on the management of food anaphylaxis in the emergency department, Clark *et al.* [75] reported 22% prescription of autoinjectors of patients with anaphylaxis. In a hospital study performed between 1990 and 2000, Campbell *et al.* [90] observed that adrenaline was prescribed to 36.6% of patients who attended the emergency department.

Despite the existence of clinical guidelines published by the European Academy of Allergy and Clinical Immunology [30] and the American Academy of Allergy and Immunology [24], considerable variability is observed in the prescription of adrenaline autoinjectors by different clinical subspecialists, even for the agreed indications for these devices [24].

In the United Kingdom, Johnson *et al.* [44] surveyed general practitioners and pediatric allergists between 2009 and 2010 to know which clinical guidelines had been followed, the factors that warrant prescription of autoinjectors, and the number of prescriptions made for specific clinical cases. The respondents did not agree on the type of patients for whom autoinjectors were indicated and prescribed according to clinical guidelines in most but not all cases. The authors showed that, although most physicians had read the relevant clinical guidelines on the management of anaphylaxis, the guidelines did not influence their clinical decision. They concluded that implementation of clinical guidelines among pediatricians should be improved.

Asero *et al.* [87] observed that Italian allergists prescribed adrenaline autoinjectors according to the severity of the anaphylaxis episode, an approach that is consistent with clinical guidelines; however, they also observed an emerging trend toward prescription according to the risk of severity associated with specific food allergens.

Prescriptions of Autoinjectors According to Demographic and Clinical Characteristics

Few studies assess differences in prescription of adrenaline autoinjectors between males and females or between different age groups. Mugica [88] found that women had fewer prescriptions than men (10.62% *vs.* 18.88%, $p=0.001$) and that age did not affect prescription habits.

Furthermore, few studies assess prescription of adrenaline according to clinical characteristics. Múgica [88] found that patients with hymenoptera anaphylaxis and exercise anaphylaxis had the highest percentage of prescriptions (>60% in both cases), followed by patients with idiopathic anaphylaxis (30%) and latex and food anaphylaxis (>20%). Patients with drug anaphylaxis and Anisakis anaphylaxis had the lowest percentages of prescriptions (<7.5%) ($p<0.0001$).

In their analysis of anaphylaxis episodes in an emergency department, Campbell *et al.* [90] noted that adrenaline autoinjectors were prescribed more frequently to patients with hymenoptera anaphylaxis.

Several studies have analyzed the association between prescription of autoinjectors and severity and found that the frequency of prescription is low, even in the most severe cases. Sicherer *et al.* [85, 86] in their studies of the prevalence of peanut and seafood allergy in North America, found a low frequency of prescription despite the severity of episodes. Finally, Gold and Sainsbury [15] analyzed generalized allergic reactions in a pediatric population and reported that adrenaline autoinjectors were prescribed more frequently in patients with circulatory and respiratory involvement.

Availability of Adrenaline Autoinjectors

Despite the availability of adrenaline autoinjectors, most studies show that very few patients carry an autoinjector [15, 48, 49, 76, 88, 91].

Mullins [48] analyzed risk factors for recurrence of anaphylaxis and found that 73% of patients carried their devices. In a survey of patients with anaphylaxis 7 years previously, Cianferoni *et al.* [49] observed that only 39% of children had adrenaline autoinjectors at home. In a survey of pediatric patients with immediate-type generalized reactions, Gold and Sainsbury [15] noted that 69% had adrenaline autoinjectors. However, Webb and Lieberman [91] (601 patients collected from 1978 to 2003 in a postal survey) found that 92% of patients carried their autoinjectors. Finally, using outpatient data, Sicherer *et al.* [76] investigated the use of devices by the parents of children with food allergy and found that 71% of families always carried the autoinjector.

The association between availability of autoinjectors and time since prescription has only been studied by 2 authors: Mullins [48] observed that the probability of carrying an autoinjector was inversely correlated with the time since the first assessment in the allergy outpatient clinic. Múgica [88] did not confirm this correlation.

In many cases, patients carry autoinjectors that are out of date. Mullins [48] observed that 65% of patients carried out-of-date autoinjectors. In their study of parents and children with food allergy, Sicherer *et al.* [76] found that only 55% of patients had an autoinjector that was not out of date.

Differences in the availability of autoinjectors in different patient groups are rarely reported. Múgica [88] found that the percentages for purchase of autoinjectors were similar for both genders (69% female and 64% male). However, Mullins [48] observed that males carried adrenaline autoinjectors more frequently than females [72% *vs.* 66%, $p<0.05$). Finally, Múgica [88] noted that the percentage of autoinjectors was bigger ($p=0.01$) in hymenoptera, food, and idiopathic anaphylaxis (>70%) than in exercise, drug, and Anisakis anaphylaxis (<50%).

Use of Adrenaline Autoinjectors

Even though patients have a prescription for an adrenaline autoinjector, purchase the device, and carry it, studies show that many patients do not use the autoinjector when necessary [15, 48, 88, 91].

Mullins [48] reported that, only 8% of patients used their device during a recurrence. In the study by Webb and Lieberman [91], only 36.8% of patients used their autoinjector during a recurrence. Simons *et al.* [92] carried out a mail survey on 1885 patients who had survived an anaphylaxis episode and noted that only 27% of those who answered had self-administered adrenaline or received adrenaline from another person. Only Gold and Sainsbury [15] reported significantly higher figures: 71% of children received adrenaline during a new episode. Múgica [88] found that age was not a predictor of the use of autoinjectors.

Use of Adrenaline Autoinjectors According to Clinical Characteristics

Several authors have published differences in the use of autoinjectors according to the cause of anaphylaxis [15, 88, 92]. Patients with hymenoptera anaphylaxis used their autoinjectors more than patients with other types of anaphylaxis. Gold and Sainsbury [15] noted that patients with hymenoptera anaphylaxis used autoinjectors more often than patients with food or idiopathic anaphylaxis. In the study by Simons *et al.* [92], patients with anaphylaxis due to peanuts, fish, and insect bites used their autoinjector more than other groups.

These and other findings enable us to conclude that use of an autoinjector is associated with the severity of anaphylaxis [88, 92]. Múgica [88] showed that patients with several recurrences involving or almost always involving circulatory symptoms more frequently used adrenaline autoinjectors than patients whose new episodes of anaphylaxis never or almost never involved circulatory symptoms. Múgica [88] also showed that the severity of the first episode affected self-administration. Simons *et al.* [92] found that, among patients who had survived a previous episode, those who used adrenaline autoinjectors more often had respiratory symptoms than those who did not.

Knowledge of Use of Adrenaline Autoinjector by Patients and Caregivers

Studies on children and their parents show that many patients use their adrenaline autoinjectors incorrectly [76, 93].

Sicherer *et al.* [76] analyzed children with food allergy who had been prescribed an adrenaline autoinjector and found that only 21% of families knew how to use the device properly. Huang [93] analyzed patients and parents of children in order to assess their knowledge of how to use an autoinjector. Only 37% of patients knew how to use the autoinjector correctly.

According to some studies, autoinjectors could be used incorrectly because the prescriber does not provide adequate training to patients, training is not reinforced at each visit, or the prescriber's knowledge of the device is poor [76, 94 -97].

In a survey of pediatricians, Sicherer *et al.* [19] noted that only 24% gave written instructions to their patients and only 18% were able to use the device correctly themselves (21% for EpiPen®).

Kim *et al.* [94] sent a questionnaire to the parents of children with food allergy who were prescribed an autoinjector to determine whether poor use of the device was associated with a feeling of unease due to lack of knowledge about correct administration and the lack of continuous training at visits to the physician. The authors found that only 8% of parents had administered adrenaline to their children and that the factors associated with feeling comfortable using the device were previous administration of adrenaline ($p=0.009$), previous training with the device ($p=0.005$), and reinforcement of device use at subsequent visits ($p<0.0005$). However, the presence of a previous episode of anaphylaxis, knowledge of anaphylaxis symptoms, or indications for autoinjectors were not associated with higher percentages of feeling comfortable with administration. The authors highlighted the importance of continuous training in the use of the devices at each visit.

Pouessel *et al.* [95] also used questionnaires to assess autoinjector use (Anapen®) in the families of children with food allergy. The investigators analyzed training in device management and found that the devices were used by 97% of families, training was with placebo devices in 76% of cases, written instructions were provided in 49% of cases, and families received a new demonstration in 19% of cases.

Grouhi *et al.* [96] performed a survey among medical specialists (emergency physicians, family physicians, and pediatricians) to analyze knowledge of adrenaline autoinjectors and training provided to patients. They observed that most physicians (81%) did not have a placebo autoinjector and that only 25% knew the 3 steps for proper administration of autoinjectors.

Table 1: Prescription and use of adrenaline auto-injectors. NA, not applicable.

	POPULATION	**PRESCRIPTION**		**AVAILABILITY**	**USE**
		Allergy Outpatient Clinic	**Emergency Department**		
MÚGICA (Spain 2011)	Adults and children	14.09%	NA	67.15%	49.15%
SICHERER (USA 2003)	Adults and children	46% adults 23% children	NA	NA	NA
SICHERER (USA 2004)	Adults	8.6%	NA	NA	NA
ASERO (Italy 2010)	Adults	13%	NA	NA	NA
MULLINS (Australia 2003)	Adults	100%	NA	73%	8%
CIANFERONI (Italy 2004)	Children	100%	NA	39%	NA
GOLD (Australia 2000)	Children	100%	NA	69%	71%
CLARK (USA 2004)	Adults and children	NA	22%	NA	NA
CAMPBELL (USA 2008)	Adults and children	NA	36.6%	NA	NA
SICHERER (USA 2000)	Children	NA	NA	71%	NA
WEBB (USA 2006)	Adults and children	NA	NA	NA	36.8%
SIMONS (USA-CANADA 2009)	Adults and children	NA	NA	NA	27%

Mehr *et al.* [97] also reported that 49% of physicians who prescribed adrenaline autoinjectors had not provided any training for patients and that only 7% of doctors had used a placebo to show patients how to use the device.

Table **1** summarizes all the data exposed on prescription, availability and use of adrenaline autoinjectors.

Reasons for Not Using Adrenaline Autoinjectors

Simons *et al.* [92] found that the reasons why patients did not use their autoinjector were therapy with antihistamines (38%), nonprescription of autoinjector (28%), mild anaphylaxis episodes (13%), use of an inhaler for asthma (8%), nonavailabilty of an autoinjector (8%), uncertainty over when to use the autoinjecctor (8%), no need for treatment in a previous anaphylaxis episode (8%), fear of side effects of adrenaline (6%), fast resolution of symptoms (4%), concern over side effects of adrenaline (4%), assessment of the need for an autoinjector when it is simpler to avoid the trigger (3%), autoinjector out of date (2%), inability to purchase a device (1%), and prescription but no purchase of the device (0.1%).

USE OF ADRENALINE IN THE EMERGENCY DEPARTMENT

Although adrenaline is considered the main treatment for anaphylaxis, its use causes confusion and concern among physicians, and many studies report infrequent use of adrenaline in the emergency department. Different publications show that the use of adrenaline varies widely (Table **2**).

In a retrospective study on the incidence of anaphylaxis in the emergency department of an Italian hospital [45], adrenaline was used in 5.7% of cases among 140 episodes of anaphylaxis recorded over 2 years. Cianferoni *et al.* [98] reported that 15% of 107 anaphylaxis episodes with respiratory and cardiovascular involvement attended in the emergency department were treated with adrenaline. Stewart and Ewan [99] detected 9 cases of severe anaphylaxis during a 1-year period, although only 3 received adrenaline.

In another retrospective series of patients with anaphylaxis from the allergy department of a Portuguese tertiary hospital collected from 2001 to 2009, the authors reported 73 children with anaphylaxis [100]. Most episodes were treated in the emergency department with corticosteroids and antihistamines; adrenaline was only used in one-quarter of the patients during the acute episode.

Rudders *et al.* [101] identified children treated for an acute allergic reaction due to food in a pediatric emergency department and found that the percentage of patients who received adrenaline (both before reaching the emergency department or during their stay in the emergency department) increased after 2000 (40% in 2001-2002 to 59% in 2005-2006), although the frequency of adrenaline use in the emergency department did not change significantly (19% in 2001-2002 to 24% in 2005-2006). Braganza *et al.* [102] performed a study in pediatric population, in which 39% of cases of severe anaphylaxis and 12.3% of all cases of anaphylaxis were treated with adrenaline.

In a retrospective series [103] performed in 2 teaching institutions to estimate the frequency of adrenaline use among adults with food anaphylaxis attending the emergency department of a general hospital from 2001 to 2006, the authors noted that adrenaline was used in 18% of 486 cases of anaphylaxis. Two or more doses were administered during the episode in 17% of patients.

Using the National Electronic Injury Surveillance System in the USA, Ross *et al.* [104] reported that adrenaline was used to treat episodes of food anaphylaxis in 19% of cases. Clark *et al.* [105] conducted a multicenter study of Hymenoptera anaphylaxis treated in the emergency departments of several US hospitals and found that 79% of patients reached the emergency department within 6 hours of the sting, although of those patients who experienced an anaphylactic reaction, only 13% were treated with adrenaline. In a similar study with food, the same authors [75] reported that only 11% of patients with allergic reactions received adrenaline before reaching the emergency department, 16% of patients with generalized allergic reactions or anaphylaxis received adrenaline intramuscularly or intravenously, and only 24% of the total group was treated with adrenaline.

In a national survey to estimate the incidence of acute allergic reactions (including anaphylaxis) in general and short-stay hospitals throughout the United States from 1993 to 2004, Gaeta *et al.* [106] observed that only 11% of patients with acute allergic reactions attended in the emergency department were treated with adrenaline; only 50% of the anaphylaxis episodes (1% of all acute allergic reactions and 0.01% of all visits to emergency departments) were treated with adrenaline. Use of adrenaline fell during the study period (19% to 7%). Moro *et al.* [107] reported that 19% of patients with anaphylaxis were treated with adrenaline in a tertiary hospital of Madrid (Spain) in 2004 and 2005.

Brown AT *et al.* [51] reported an intermediate frequency in the use of adrenaline. In the 142 anaphylaxis episodes identified, adrenaline was only used in 18% of patients before arrival at the hospital and in 27.4% in the emergency department. The findings of Brown SG [108] were similar: 31% of patients with anaphylaxis received adrenaline.

A direct correlation seems to exist between the severity of anaphylaxis and more frequent use of adrenaline [109-112]. In their retrospective 1-year study, Bellou *et al.* [109] found that all 12 patients attended for anaphylactic shock received adrenaline. In a Swiss study [110], the authors analyzed anaphylaxis with circulatory involvement and found 246 episodes of severe anaphylaxis with a risk of death in 226 patients. Adrenaline was used in 47.9% of cases. Another cross-sectional study [111] conducted in children and adolescents in Alabama (USA) showed that 56% of 103 patients who received adrenaline (before or during their stay in the emergency department) had a higher rate of admission and more procedures in the emergency room than patients who were not treated with adrenaline. A recent study on anaphylaxis in patients treated at the emergency department of a hospital in New York between 2004 and 2008 [112] found that adrenaline was administered in 79% of 213 anaphylactic reactions and that 27% of doses were given in the emergency department. The authors also found that the use of 2 doses of adrenaline was associated with an increased risk of admission, while the administration of adrenaline prior to arrival at the emergency room was associated with fewer admissions.

In other series, percentage of use was even higher than that reported by Bellou *et al.* [109]. In a retrospective study performed in Australia in pediatric patients with anaphylaxis attended in a tertiary children's hospital, De Silva *et al.* [113] found that adrenaline was used in 76% of 117 children with anaphylaxis. Several Asian series reported more frequent use of adrenaline: 66.7% in the study by Smit *et al.* [114], 89% in in the study by Poachanukoon and Paopairochanakorn [115] and 77% in the study by Piromrat *et al.* [116].

In a series of 164 deaths by anaphylaxis, Pumphrey [17] reported that adrenaline was used in only 62% of reactions and in only 14% before cardiac arrest or respiratory failure.

In summary, most studies on adrenaline agree that adrenaline is infrequently used in the emergency department; however, this finding is not consistent with those of other studies, namely, Asian studies [115, 116], series of severe anaphylaxis [108-111], series of patients at risk of death [17], and recent works on food anaphylaxis in pediatric populations [111, 113]. The possible reasons for increased use of adrenaline in pediatric series are training for pediatricians [111] and interest in anaphylaxis in this age group, where the risk of experiencing food anaphylaxis is higher than in other age groups.

In contrast, most series of anaphylaxis treated in the emergency department show that corticosteroids and antihistamines were used more frequently than adrenaline (>75%), even in the most severe cases, even though they are considered second-line drugs and evidence of their immediate effectiveness is lacking [3, 4].

Potential reasons for the low frequency of use of adrenaline include poor knowledge of the indications for adrenaline in anaphylaxis, lack of information on when adrenaline should be used [3], different opinions on potential risks, variable interest in anaphylaxis in different emergency services and year of publication.

Table 2: Percentage of adrenaline use in the emergency department.

Studies	Population	% of All Anaphylaxis	% of Severe Anaphylaxis
Low Use			
Pastorello (Italy, 2001)	Adults	5.7%	
Gaeta (USA, 2003)	All acute generalized reactions Anaphylaxis	11% 50%	
Cianferoni (Italy 2001)	Children	15%	
Ross (USA, 2007)	Food anaphylaxis in children	19%	
Clark (USA, 2005)	Acute generalized reactions and anaphylaxis by hymenoptera	12%	
Clark (USA, 2004)	Acute generalized reactions and anaphylaxis by foods	16%	
Rudders (Boston USA 2010)	Children	19% (2001-2) 24% (2005-6)	
Silva (Portugal, 2012)	Children	25%	

Table 2: contd…

Banerji (USA, 2010)	Food anaphylaxis in adults	18%	
Braganza (Australia, 2006)	Children	12.3%	39.3%
Moro (Spain, 2011)	Adults and children	**19.3%**	44.7%
Intermediate Use			
Moro (Spain, 2011)			
Brown (Australia 2001)	Adults	27.4 %	
Brown (Australia 2004)	Adults	31%	
Helbling (Swiss 2004)	Adults(only cases of anaphylactic shock)	47.9%	47.9%
Stewart and Ewan (UK, 1996)	Adults	33% (9 episodes)	33%
High Use			
Smit (Hong-Kong, 2005)	Adults and children	66.7%	
Piromrat (Thailand 2008)	Adults and children	77%	
Poachanukoon (Thailand, 2006)	Adults and children	89%	
De Silva (Australia, 2008)	Children	76%	
Russel (USA, 2010).	Children	56%	
Bellou 2003 (France) Helbling A (Swiss 2004)	Adults and children Only anaphylactic shock		100%
Huang (USA, 2012)	Children	79%	
Pumphrey (UK, 2004)	Only cases of death		62%

SUMMARY

Based on available evidence, the benefit of using appropriate doses of intramuscular adrenaline in anaphylaxis far exceeds the risk. Consensus opinion and anecdotal evidence indicate that adrenaline should be administered sooner rather than later, *i.e.,* when the initial signs and symptoms appear [65].

Patients are at an increased risk of anaphylaxis in the following situations: mastocytosis, previous anaphylactic reactions and comorbid persistent asthma, reaction to trace amounts of allergen, previous mild reaction to peanut or tree nut, and adolescence. Distance from an emergency department should also be considered [30].

No absolute contraindications to the administration of adrenaline to children and adults have been formulated, and the number of devices to be prescribed to a patient remains open to debate.

However, Pumphrey [74] stated that some authors propose that once the trigger had been identified, education about effective avoidance provided, and the management of medical conditions that could make reactions worse optimized [97] (daily management of asthma, hypertension, and any other aggravating conditions), the choice of whether or not to carry an autoinjector should be left to patients after they have been fully informed of benefits and risks. Only patients who wish to use self-treatment are likely to carry the autoinjector [64, 74].

Despite general agreement that anaphylaxis occurring in the community should be treated using adrenaline autoinjectors, prescription rates are low. The percentages for purchase and availability are also low, as is the use of autoinjectors in new episodes of anaphylaxis.

Prescription and use of self-injectable adrenaline are part of a larger, comprehensive approach to the management of anaphylaxis. Education is essential in the prevention of recurrences. Patients need individualized management plans, and regular training programs are required for patients, families, caregivers, and school staff.

Adrenaline is infrequently used in the emergency department, although a trend toward more frequent use has been observed in cases of severe anaphylaxis.

ACKNOWLEDGEMENTS

The authors thank Thomas O'Boyle for proofreading the manuscript.

CONFLICT OF INTEREST

The author(s) confirm that this chapter content has no conflict of interest.

REFERENCES

[1] Lieberman PL Anaphylaxis. In: Adkinson Jr NF, Bochner BS, Busse WW, Holgate ST, Lemmarske RF, Simmons FER, Eds. Middleton´s Allergy. Principles and Practice. 7th Edition. Philadelphia: Mosby Elsevier 2009; pp 1027-49.
[2] Davenport HW. Epinephrin(e). Physiologist 1982; 25(2): 76-82.
[3] Sheikh A, Shehata YA, Brown SGA, Simons FER. Adrenaline for the treatment of anaphylaxis: Cochrane systematic review. Allergy 2009; 64(2): 204-212.
[4] Sheikh A, Ten Broek V, Brown SGA, Simons FER. H1-antihistamines for the treatment of anaphylaxis: Cochrane systematic review. Allergy 2007; 62(6): 830-837.
[5] Sampson HA, Mendelson LM, Rosen JP. Fatal and near-fatal anaphylactic reactions to food in children and adolescents. N Engl J Med 1992; 327(6): 380-384.
[6] Bock SA, Muñoz-Furlong A, Sampson HA. Fatalities due to anaphylactic reactions to foods. J Allergy Clin Immunol 2001; 107(1): 191-193.
[7] Pumphrey RS GM. Further fatal allergic reactions to food in the United Kingdom, 1999–2006 . J Allergy Clin Immunol 2007; 119(4): 1018-1019.
[8] Bock SA, Muñoz-Furlong A, Sampson HA. Further fatalities caused by anaphylactic reactions to food, 2001–2006. J Allergy Clin Immunol 2007; 119(4): 1016-1018.
[9] Camargo CA Jr, Clark S, Kaplan MS *et al.* Regional differences in EpiPen prescriptions in the United States: the potential role of vitamin D. J Allergy Clin Immunol 2007; 120(1): 131-136.
[10] Simons FER, Peterson S, Black CD. Epinephrine dispensing patterns for an out-of-hospital population: a novel approach to studying the epidemiology of anaphylaxis. J Allergy Clin Immunol 2002; 110(4): 647-651.
[11] Westfall TC WD. Adrenergic agonists and antagonists. In: Brunton LL, Lazo JS, Parker KL, editors. Goodman & Gilman's: The pharmacological basis of therapeutics. 11th ed. New York: McGraw-Hill; 2006. pp. 237-247.
[12] Simons FER. First-aid treatment of anaphylaxis to food: focus on epinephrine. J Allergy Clin Immunol 2004; 113(5): 837-844.
[13] Smith PL, Kagey-Sobotka A, Bleecker ER, *et al.* Physiologic manifestations of human anaphylaxis. J Clin Invest 1980; 66(5): 1072-1080.
[14] Sicherer SH, Simons FE, Section on Allergy and Immunology, American Academy of Pediatrics. Self-injectable epinephrine for first-aid management of anaphylaxis. Pediatrics 2007; 119(3): 638-646.
[15] Gold MS SR. First aid anaphylaxis management in children who were prescribed an epinephrine autoinjector device (EpiPen). J Allergy Clin Immunol 2000; 106(1Pt1): 171-176.
[16] Pumphrey RS. Fatal anaphylaxis in the UK, 1992–2001. Novartis Found Symp 2004; 257: 116-128.
[17] Pumphrey RS. Lessons for management of anaphylaxis from a study of fatal reactions. Clin Exp Allergy 2000; 30(8): 1144-1150.
[18] Simons FE. Emergency treatment of anaphylaxis. BMJ 2008; 336(7654): 1141-1142.
[19] Tole JW LP. Biphasic anaphylaxis: review of incidence, clinical predictors, and observation recommendations. Immunol Allergy Clin North Am 2007; 27(2): 309-326, viii.
[20] Simons FER, Roberts JR, Gu X, Simons KJ. Epinephrine absorption in children with a history of anaphylaxis . J Allergy Clin Immunol 1998; 101(1Pt1): 33-37.

[21] Simons FER, Gu X, Simons KJ. Epinephrine absorption in adults: intramuscular *vs.* subcutaneous injection. J Allergy Clin Immunol 2001; 108(5): 871-873.
[22] Simons KJ, Simons FE. Epinephrine and its use in anaphylaxis: current issues. Curr Opin Allergy Clin Immunol 2010; 10(4): 354-361.
[23] American Heart Association in collaboration with International Liaison Committee on Resuscitation. 2005American Heart Association guidelines for cardiopulmonary resuscitation and emergency cardiovascular care. Anaphylaxis. Circulation 2005; 112(Suppl.IV): IV143-IV145.
[24] Lieberman P, Kemp SF, Oppenheimer J, *et al.* Joint Task Force on Practice Parameters. The diagnosis and management of anaphylaxis: an updated practice parameter. J Allergy Clin Immunol 2005; 115(3Suppl2): S483-S523.
[25] Soar J, Deakin CD, Nolan JP, *et al.* European Resuscitation Council guidelines for resuscitation 2005. Section 7. Cardiac arrest in special circumstances. Resuscitation 2005; 67(Suppl1): S135-S170.
[26] Sampson HA, Muñoz-Furlong A, Campbell RL, *et al.* Second symposium on the definition and management of anaphylaxis: summary report – second National Institute of Allergy and Infectious Diseases/Food Allergy and Anaphylaxis Network symposium. J Allergy Clin Immunol 2006; 117(2): 391-397.
[27] Cardona Dahl V, Grupo de trabajo de la Guia GALAXIA de actuacion en anafilaxia. Guideline for the management of anaphylaxis. Med Clin (Barc) 2011; 136(8): 349-355.
[28] Alrasbi M, Sheikh A. Comparison of international guidelines for the emergency medical management of anaphylaxis. Allergy 2007; 62(8): 838-841.
[29] Sicherer SH, Simons FE. Quandaries in prescribing an emergency action plan and self-injectable epinephrine for first-aid management of anaphylaxis in the community. J Allergy Clin Immunol 2005; 115(3): 575-583.
[30] Muraro A, Roberts G, Clark A, *et al.* The management of anaphylaxis in childhood: position paper of the European academy of allergology and clinical immunology. Allergy 2007; 62(8): 857-871.
[31] McLean-Tooke APC, Bethune CA, Fay AC, Spickett GP. Adrenaline in the treatment of anaphylaxis: what is the evidence? BMJ 2003; 327(7427): 1332-1335.
[32] Hourihane J. Controversies in paediatrics? Arch Dis Child 2001; 85(6): 510
[33] Kemp AS. EpiPen epidemic: suggestions for rational prescribing in childhood food allergy. J Paediatr Child Health 2003; 39(5): 372-375.
[34] Dubois AE. The Epipen: panacea or double-edged sword? Curr Opin Allergy Clin Immunol 2006; 6: 278.
[35] Moneret-Vautrin DA, Kanny G, Morisset M *et al.* Food anaphylaxis in schools: evaluation of the management plan and the efficiency of the emergency kit. Allergy 2001; 56(11): 1071-1076.
[36] Hourihane JO, Kilburn SA, Dean P, Warner JO. Clinical characteristics of peanut allergy. Clin Exp Allergy 1997; 27(6): 634-639.
[37] Pumphrey RS. Anaphylaxis: can we tell who is at risk of a fatal reaction? Curr Opin Allergy Clin Immunol 2004; 4(4): 285-290.
[38] Gold MS, Anaphylaxis Working Party, Australasian Society of Clinical Immunology and Allergy. EpiPen epidemic or good clinical practice? J Paediatr Child Health 2003; 39(5): 376-377.

[39] Ewan PW CA. Long term prospective observational study of the outcome of a management plan in patients with peanut and nut allergy referred to a regional allergy centre. Lancet 2001; 357(9250): 111-115.

[40] Moffitt JE, Golden DBK, Reisman RE, *et al.* Stinging insect hypersensitivity: a practice parameter update. J Allergy Clin Immunol 2004; (114): 869-886.

[41] Kagan R, Hayami D, Joseph L, St Pierre Y, Clarke AE. The predictive value of a positive prick skin test to peanut in atopic, peanut-naive children. Ann Allergy Asthma Immunol 2003; 90(6): 640-645.

[42] Van der Leek TK, Liu AH, Stefanski K, Blacker B, Bock SA. The natural history of peanut allergy in young children and its association with serum peanut-specific IgE. J Pediatr 2000; 137(6): 749-755.

[43] Sicherer SH, Furlong TJ, Muñoz-Furlong A, Burks AW, Sampson HA. A voluntary registry for peanut and tree nut allergy: characteristics of the first 5149 registrants. J Allergy Clin Immunol 2001; 108(1): 128-132.

[44] Johnson TL, Parker AL. Rates of retrieval of self-injectable epinephrine prescriptions: a descriptive report. Ann Allergy Asthma Immunol 2006; 97(5): 694-697.

[45] Pastorello EA, Rivolta F, Bianchi M, Mauro M, Pravettoni V. Incidence of anaphylaxis in the emergency department of a general hospital in Milan. J Chromatogr B Biomed Sci Appl 2001; 756(1-2): 11-17.

[46] Ortolani C, Pastorello EA, Farioli L, *et al.* IgE- mediated allergy from vegetable allergens. Ann Allergy 1993; 71(5): 470-476.

[47] Uguz A, Lack G, Pumphrey R, *et al.* Allergic reaction in the community: a questionnaire survey of members of the anaphylaxis campaign. Clin Exp Allergy 2005; 35(6): 746-750.

[48] Mullins RJ. Anaphylaxis : risk factors for recurrence. Clin Exp Allergy 2003; 33(8): 1033-1040.

[49] Cianferoni A, Novembre E, Pucci N, Lombardi E, Bernardini R, Vieruci A. Anaphylaxis: a 7-year follow-up survey of 46 children. Ann Allergy Asthma Immunol 2004; 92(4): 464-468.

[50] Decker WW, Campbell RL, Manivannan V, *et al.* The etiology and incidence of anaphylaxis in Rochester, Minnesota: A report from the Rochester Epidemiology Project. J Allergy Clin Immunol 2008; 122(6): 1161-1165.

[51] Brown AT, McKinnon D, Chu K. Emergency department anaphylaxis: a review of 142 patients in a single year. J Allergy Clin Immunol 2001; 108(5): 861-866.

[52] Yocum MW, Butterfield JH, Klein JS, Volcheck GW, Schroeder DR, Silverstein MD. Epidemiology of anaphylaxis in Olmsted County: a population-based study. J Allergy Clin Immunol 1999; 104(2Pt1): 452-456.

[53] Soar J, Pumphrey R, Cant A, *et al.* Emergency treatment of anaphylactic reactions--guidelines for healthcare providers. Resuscitation 2008; 77(2): 157-169.

[54] Macdougall CF, Cant AJ, Colver AF. How dangerous is food allergy in childhood? The incidence of severe and fatal allergic reactions across the UK and Ireland. Arch Dis Chil 2002; 86(4): 236-239.

[55] Foucard T, Malmheden Yman I. A study on severe food reactions in Sweden – is soy protein an underestimated cause of food anaphylaxis? . Allergy 1999; 54(3): 261-265.

[56] Summers C, Pumphrey RSH, Woods CN, *et al.* Factors predicting anaphylaxisto peanuts and tree nuts in patients referred to a specialist center. J Allergy Clin Immunol 2008; 121(3): 631-638.

[57] Brockow K, Jofer C, Behrendt H, Ring J. Anaphylaxis in patients with mastocytosis: a study on history, clinical features and risk factors in 120 patients. Allergy, 2008: 63(1): 226-232.

[58] Haeberli G, Bronnimann M, Hunziker T, Muller U. Elevated basal serum tryptase and hymenoptera venom allergy: relation to severity of sting reactions and to safety and efficacy of venom immunotherapy. Clin Exp Allergy 2003; 33: 1216–1220.

[59] Ludolph-Hauser D, Rueff F, Fries C, Schopf P, Przybilla B. Constitutively raised serum concentrations of mast-cell tryptase and severe anaphylactic reactions to Hymenoptera stings. Lancet 2001; 357: 361–362.

[60] Vaughan ST, Jones GN. Systemic mastocytosis presenting as profound cardiovascular collapse during anaesthesia. Anaesthesia 1998; 53: 804–807.

[61] Simons FER. Anaphylaxis. J Allergy Clin Immunol 2010; 125(2 Suppl 2): S161-S181.

[62] Mueller UR. Cardiovascular disease and anaphylaxis. Curr Opin Allergy Clin Immunol 2007; 7(4): 337-341.

[63] Rueff F, Przybilla B, Bilo MB, *et al.* Predictors of severe systemic anaphylactic reactions in patients with Hymenoptera venom allergy: importance of baseline serum tryptase – a study of the European Academy of Allergology and Clinical Immunology Interest Group on Insect Venom Hypersensitivity. J Allergy Clin Immunol 2009; 124(5): 1047-1054.

[64] Simons FER, Roberts JR, Gu X, Simons KJ. Anaphylaxis, killer allergy: long-term management in the community. J Allergy Clin Immunol 2006; 117(2): 367-377.

[65] Kemp SF, Lockey RF, Simons FE, World Allergy Organization ad hoc Committee on Epinephrine in Anaphylaxis. Epinephrine: the drug of choice for anaphylaxis. A statement of the World Allergy Organization. Allergy 2008; 63(8): 1061-1070.

[66] American Academy of Allergy Asthma and Immunology Board of Directors. Anaphylaxis in schools and other child-care settings. J Allergy Clin Immunol 1998; 102(2): 173-176.

[67] Cheng A. Emergency treatment of anaphylaxis in infants and children. Paediatr Child Health 2011; 16(1): 35-40.

[68] Liberman DB TS. Management of anaphylaxis in children. Pediatr Emerg Care 2008; 24(12): 861-866.

[69] Yunginger JW, Sweeney KG, Sturner WQ, Giannandrea LA, Teigland JD, Bray M *et al.* Fatal food-induced anaphylaxis. JAMA 1988; 260(10): 1450-1452.

[70] Simons FER, Gu X, Simons KJ. Outdated EpiPenR and Epi Pen Jr.R autoinjectors: past their prime? J Allergy Clin Immunol 2000; 105(5): 1025-1030.

[71] Bautista E, Simons FE, Simons KJ *et al.* Epinephrine fails to hasten the hemodynamic recovery in fully developed canine anaphylactic shock. Int Arch Allergy Immunol 2002; 128(2): 151-164.

[72] Allen CW, Campbell DE, Kemp AS. EpiPen use in children with food allergies. Med J Aust 2007; 187(9): 542.

[73] Ferreira MB AR. Are general practitioners alert to anaphylaxis diagnosis and treatment? European Annals of Allergy and Clinical Immunology 2006; 38(3): 83-86.

[74] Pumphrey RS. When should self-injectible epinephrine be prescribed for food allergy and when should it be used? Curr Opin Allergy Clin Immunol 2008; 8(3): 254-260.

[75] Clark S, Bock SA, Gaeta TJ, Brenner BE, Cydulka RK, Camargo CA. Multicenter study of emergency department visits for food allergies. J Allergy Clin Immunol 2004; 113: 347-353.

[76] Sicherer SH, Forman JA, Noone SA. Use assessment of self-administered epinephrine among food-allergic children and pediatricians. Pediatrics 2000; 105(2): 359-362.
[77] Davis JE. Self-injectable epinephrine for allergic emergencies. J Emerg Med 2009; 37(1): 57-62.
[78] Simons FER. Lack of worldwide availability of epinephrine autoinjectors for outpatients at risk of anaphylaxis. Ann Allergy Asthma Immunol 2005; 94: 534-538.
[79] Simons FE, Chan ES, Gu X, Simons KJ. Epinephrine for the out-of-hospital (first-aid) treatment of anaphylaxis in infants:is the ampule/syringe/needle method practical? J Allergy Clin Immunol 2001; 108(6): 1040-1044.
[80] Singh J, Aszkenasy OM. Prescription of adrenaline auto-injectors for potential anaphylaxis--a population survey. Public Health 2003; 117(4): 256-259.
[81] Järvinen KM, Sicherer SH, Sampson HA, Nowak-Wegrzyn A. Use of multiple doses of epinephrine in food-induced anaphylaxis in children. J Allergy Clin Immunol 2008; 122(1): 133-8.
[82] Kelso JM. A second dose of epinephrine for anaphylaxis: how often needed and how to carry. J Allergy Clin Immunol 2006; 117(2): 464-465.
[83] Oren E, Banerji A, Clark S, Camargo CA. Food-induced anaphylaxis and repeated epinephrine treatments. Ann Allergy Asthma Immunol. 2007; 99(5):429-32.
[84] Skorpinski EW, McGeady SJ, Yousef E. Two cases of accidental epinephrine injection into a finger. J Allergy Clin Immunol 2006; 117(2): 463-464.
[85] Sicherer SH, Munoz-Furlong A, Sampson HA. Prevalence of seafood allergy in the United States determined by a random telephone survey. J Allergy Clin Immunol 2004; 114(1): 159-165.
[86] Sicherer SH, Munoz-Furlong A, Sampson HA. Prevalence of peanut and tree nut allergy in the United States determined by means of a random digit dial telephone survey: a 5-year follow-up study. J Allergy Clin Immunol 2003; 112(6): 1203-1207.
[87] Asero R, Antonicelli L, Arena A, *et al.* Epinephrine autoinjector prescription in food-allergic adults: symptom-based only or allergen-based also? An Italian multi-centre study. Eur Ann Allergy Clin Immunol 2010; 42(1): 25-31.
[88] Mugica MV. Observational study about anaphylaxis recurrence. PhD dissertation. Alcorcón (Madrid). Universidad Rey Juan Carlos, 2011.
[89] Campbell RL, Hagan JB, Li JT, *et al.* Anaphylaxis in emergency department patients 50 or 65 years or older. Ann Allergy Asthma Immunol 2011; 106 (5): 401-406.
[90] Campbell RL, Luke A, Weaver AL, *et al.* Prescriptions for self-injectable epinephrine and follow-up referral in emergency department patients presenting with anaphylaxis. Ann Allergy Asthma Immunol 2008; 121(6): 631-636.
[91] Webb LM, Lieberman P. Anaphylaxis: a review of 601 cases. Ann Allergy Asthma Immunol 2006; 97(1): 39-43.
[92] Simons FE, Clark S, Camargo CA,Jr. Anaphylaxis in the community: learning from the survivors. J Allergy Clin Immunol 2009; 124(2): 301-306.
[93] Huang SW. A survey of Epi-PEN use in patients with a history of anaphylaxis. J Allergy Clin Immunol 1998; 102(3): 525-526.
[94] Kim JS, Sinacore JM, Pongracic JA. Parental use of EpiPen for children with food allergies. J Allergy Clin Immunol 2005; 116(1): 164-168.
[95] Pouessel G, Deschildre A, Castelain C, *et al.* Parental knowledge and use of epinephrine auto-injector for children with food allergy. Pediatr Allergy Immunol 2006; 17(3): 221-226.

[96] Grouhi M, Alshehri M, Hummel D, Roifman CM. Anaphylaxis and epinephrine auto-injector training: who will teach the teachers? J Allergy Clin Immunol 1999; 104(1): 190-193.

[97] Mehr S, Robinson M, Tang M. Doctor: how do I use my EpiPen? Pediatr Allergy Immunol 2007; 18: 448-452.

[98] Cianferoni A, Novembre E, Mugnaini L, *et al.* Clinical features of acute anaphylaxis in patients admitted to a university hospital: an 11-year retrospective review (1985-1996). Ann Allergy Asthma Immunol 2001; 87(1): 27-32.

[99] Stewart AG, Ewan PW. The incidence, aetiology and management of anaphylaxis presenting to an accident and emergency department. QJM 1996; 89(11) 859-864.

[100] Silva R, Gomes E, Cunha L, Falcao H. Anaphylaxis in children: a nine years retrospective study (2001-2009). Allergol Immunopathol (Madr) 2012; 40(1): 31-36.

[101] Rudders SA, Banerji A, Vassallo MF, Clark S, Camargo CA,Jr. Trends in pediatric emergency department visits for food-induced anaphylaxis. J Allergy Clin Immunol 2010; 126(2): 385-388.

[102] Braganza SC, Acworth JP, Mckinnon DR, Peake JE, Brown AF. Paediatric emergency department anaphylaxis: different patterns from adults. Arch Dis Child 2006; 91(2): 159-163.

[103] Banerji A, Rudders SA, Corel B, Garth AM, Clark S, Camargo CA,Jr. Repeat epinephrine treatments for food-related allergic reactions that present to the emergency department. Allergy Asthma Proc 2010; 31(4): 308-316.

[104] Ross MP, Ferguson M, Street D, Klontz K, Schroeder T, Luccioli S. Analysis of food-allergic and anaphylactic events in the National Electronic Injury Surveillance System. J Allergy Clin Immunol 2008; 121(1): 166-171.

[105] Clark S, Long AA, Gaeta TJ, Camargo CA,Jr. Multicenter study of emergency department visits for insect sting allergies. J Allergy Clin Immunol 2005; 116(3): 643-649.

[106] Gaeta TJ, Clark S, Pelletier AJ, Camargo CA. National study of US emergency department visits for acute allergic reactions, 1993 to 2004. Ann Allergy Asthma Immunol 2007; 98(4): 360-365.

[107] Moro-Moro M, Tejedor-Alonso, Esteban-Hernandez J. *et al.* Incidence of Anaphylaxis and Subtypes of Anaphylaxis in a General Hospital Emergency Department Journal of Investigational Allergology And Clinical Immunology, 2011; 21(2): 142-149

[108] Brown SG. Clinical features and severity grading of anaphylaxis. J Allergy Clin Immunol 2004; 114(2): 371-376.

[109] Bellou A, Manel J, Samman-Kaakaji H, *et al.* Spectrum of acute allergic diseases in an emergency department: an evaluation of one years' experience. Emerg Med (Fremantle) 2003; 15(4): 341-347.

[110] Helbling A, Hurni T, Mueller UR, Pichler WJ. Incidence of anaphylaxis with circulatory symptoms: a study over a 3-year period comprising 940,000 inhabitants of the Swiss Canton Bern. Clin Exp Allergy 2004; 34(2): 285-290.

[111] Russell S, Monroe K, Losek JD. Anaphylaxis management in the pediatric emergency department: opportunities for improvement. Pediatr Emerg Care 2010; 26(2): 71-76.

[112] Huang F, Chawla K, Jarvinen KM, Nowak-Wegrzyn A. Anaphylaxis in a New York City pediatric emergency department: triggers, treatments, and outcomes. J Allergy Clin Immunol 2012; 129(1): 162-8.e1-3.

[113] de Silva IL, Mehr SS, Tey D, Tang ML. Paediatric anaphylaxis: a 5 year retrospective review. Allergy 2008; 63(8): 1071-1076.
[114] Smit DV, Cameron PA, Rainer TH. Anaphylaxis presentations to an emergency department in Hong Kong: incidence and predictors of biphasic reactions. J Emerg Med 2005; 28(4): 381-388.
[115] Poachanukoon O, Paopairochanakorn C. Incidence of anaphylaxis in the emergency department: a 1-year study in a university hospital. Asian Pac J Allergy Immunol 2006; 24(2-3): 111-116.
[116] Piromrat K, Chinratanapisit S, Trathong S. Anaphylaxis in an emergency department: a 2-year study in a tertiary-care hospital. Asian Pac J Allergy Immunol 20; 26(2-3): 121-128.

INDEX

A

ABTS Oxidation 251-2, 254-6
Acute allergic reactions 284, 351-2
Acute anaphylaxis 100, 331
Acute asthma 59, 75, 166
Adhesion molecule expression 276, 287, 297-8
Adiponectin deficiency 280-1, 287
Adiponectin levels 271, 280-1
Adiponectin receptor 265, 273, 281
Adiponectin's AMPK 276-7
Adrenal suppression 58-9, 76
Adrenaline 28, 59, 89, 93, 96, 301, 330-1, 333, 335-47, 349, 351-6
Adrenaline autoinjectors 331-2, 336, 340, 343-9, 351
Adverse event reporting system (AERS) 145
Aeroallergens 77, 171, 205
Age-related macular degeneration (AMD) 253
Airway epithelium 55, 294
Airway hyperresponsiveness 125, 284
Airway inflammation 61-2, 121, 126, 173, 283
Airway obstruction 29-30, 51, 296
Airways of athletes 55
Albuterol 61, 97-8
Allergen avoidance 92, 162, 268
Allergen-based vaccines 92, 214
Allergen exposure 40, 138, 162, 229, 270, 281, 286
Allergen extracts 35, 93, 170-1, 210, 215
Allergen immunotherapy 35, 53, 92, 95, 210, 222, 268, 279
Allergen-induced asthma 129
Allergen proteins 25, 192
Allergen tolerance 39, 195-6
Allergen vaccines 268
Allergenic activity 210, 217

Allergenic extracts 37, 210-11
Allergenic sources 36, 203, 205
Allergenicity 204, 215-16, 219
Allergic airway inflammation 126, 154, 172-3, 282
Allergic asthma 27, 35, 94-5, 122, 128, 143, 154, 167, 169, 171, 268, 270, 288
Allergic asthma origin 131
Allergic asthma patients 167, 172
Allergic asthma phenotypes 172
Allergic asthmatics 286
Allergic athletes 50-1
Allergic bronchopulmonary aspergillosis (ABPA) 138
Allergic conjunctivitis 70, 93-5, 99
Allergic contact dermatitis 10, 12, 208
Allergic disease asthma 288
Allergic disease prevalence 162, 302
Allergic disease symptoms 300
Allergic effector cells 123
Allergic eosinophilic atopic disease 294
Allergic flares 283, 286, 295
Allergic inflammatory diseases 267, 292
Allergic inflammatory response 82-3, 268, 281, 291, 295
Allergic patients 34, 202, 204-5, 218, 276, 287, 335
Allergic reactions 140, 163, 183, 190, 194-5, 199, 202, 209, 213, 216, 223, 228, 269, 271, 332
Allergic response 38, 193, 196, 217, 225, 271, 281, 284, 287, 294, 302
Allergic rhinitis 50, 70, 78-9, 84-5, 89-91, 93-5, 99, 118, 122-3, 135-6, 170-2, 212, 265-6, 268-9, 281-2
Allergic sensitization 204, 266
Allergic sources 35, 197
Allergists 186, 337
Allergoids 171, 210
Allergy diagnosis 171, 207
Allergy treatment 212, 265, 300-1
Allergy vaccines 93, 216-17

Alopecia areata 3, 10, 16
Alveolar macrophages 34, 286
Amino acids 197, 217-19
AMPK 275
AMPK-independent 265
Anaphylactic shock 207, 210, 353, 355
Anaphylaxis symptoms 93, 141, 339, 349
Angioedema 85, 133-4, 163, 201
Anisakis anaphylaxis 346-7
Anti-allergic medications 81, 172
Anti allergy agents 162-73, 265-302
Anti-IgE 24, 41, 137, 143, 182, 301
Anti-IgE therapy 126-7, 132-3, 137, 143, 281
Anti-leukotrienes 67-70, 209
Antigen-presenting cells (APCs) 5, 122, 192-3, 195, 286
Antihistamines 50-1, 68, 78-80, 82-90, 99, 133, 136, 206, 301, 351, 354
AntiIgE 118
Antileukotrienes 51, 68, 166
Antioxidant activity 251-3, 257
Apigenin 300-1
Apoptosis 6-7, 245, 249-50, 252, 284, 292
Ascorbate 240-1, 245, 250-3, 257
Asthma attacks 131, 148
Asthma control 52, 57, 63, 98-9, 131, 271
Asthma control test 130, 132
Asthma drugs 97, 100, 145
Asthma exacerbations 62, 93, 128, 130, 166, 173, 278, 281, 284, 298
Asthma medication 95, 145, 147
Asthma patients 168
Asthma phenotypes 72, 166
Asthma symptoms 51, 59, 95, 130, 169
Asthma symptoms risks 164
Asthma treatment 76, 152, 301
Asthmatic airways 55, 285

Asthmatic athletes 54, 57, 97
Asthmatic patients 25, 27-9, 31-4, 39, 41, 54, 166, 276, 281, 284
Asthmatic subjects 168, 171
Asthmatic symptoms 298
Athletes 50-7, 59, 64-8, 71, 75-81, 84-5, 87-90, 92-3, 96-100
Athlete's allergic diseases 50
Athletic performance 52, 77, 80-1, 84
Atopic dermatitis (AD) 3-4, 7-11, 17-20, 72, 82, 84, 87, 118, 123, 135, 163, 172, 253, 269
Atopic dermatitis patients 6, 17
Atopic diseases 56, 191, 267
Atopic patients 12, 119, 334
Atopy 121, 127, 183, 185, 190, 227-8, 284
Autoinjectors 330-4, 336-49, 351, 356
Azelastine 84, 86, 88

B

Basophil stimulation tests 207
Beta 2-agonists 51, 60, 62-3, 71, 97-8
Binding of omalizumab 123
Birch pollen 199-200, 212, 214
Birch pollen allergens 198, 200
Birch pollen allergy 200, 214
Block allergic patients 218
Body mass index (BMI) 266
Bronchial asthma 171, 289
Bronchial hyperresponsiveness 57, 95, 98, 131
Bronchoalveolar lavage 29, 294-5
Bronchoconstriction 65, 70, 164-5
Bronchodilators 60, 67, 99, 162, 164, 209
Budesonide 12, 56, 59, 63, 79, 91

C

Calcineurin inhibitors 3, 5-15, 17, 19-20

Carotene 245, 251, 253, 257
Carotenoids 240, 253-4
Carrier protein 153, 217
Carrot allergy 214
CC-chemokine ligand (CCL) 270
CD4 27, 125-6, 150, 186, 192-3, 196, 226, 285, 296
CD23 34, 122, 152
CD25 195-6, 285
Cell adhesion molecules (CAMs) 271, 286-7
Cell determinants 220-1
Cell epitopes 193, 219-21
Cell epitopes peptides 219, 221
Cell surface 122, 228, 246, 250
Cell survival 255-6
Cells downregulating allergic 279
Cellular stress response 255-6
Chemokines 33, 56, 163, 193, 242, 270-1, 283-4
Chromones 70, 72-4
Chronic asthma 72, 126
Chronic diseases 25, 257
Chronic inflammation 169, 241, 244
Chronic obstructive pulmonary disease (COPD) 34, 64, 241-4, 247
Chronic urticaria 68, 86, 118, 133-4
Churg-Strauss syndrome (CSS) 69-70, 167
Collagen 241-3, 245, 251, 256-7
Combination anti-allergy therapies 269
Component-resolved diagnostics (CRD) 204
Conjugated equine estrogens (CEE) 299
Coronary heart disease 257, 342
Corticosteroids 6-7, 12, 17, 50-1, 56, 63, 70, 72, 75, 80, 91, 138, 164-5, 249-50, 267-8
Cow's milk allergy (CMA) 220
Cromolyn 68, 72-3
Cromolyn sodium 70-4, 91, 99, 301

Cross-reactivity (CR) 182, 190, 197-9, 202, 204, 334
Cutaneous lupus erythematosus 10, 14-15
Cyclosporin 3-4, 6-7, 14
Cysteinyl leukotrienes 55, 66-7, 80, 85, 163
Cytokine production 7, 220

D

Dendritic cells (DC) 6, 27, 38, 60, 74, 83, 118, 122, 125, 163-4, 168-9, 192, 194-6, 223, 226
Dermal fibroblasts 254, 256
Dermatitis 202, 241-3
Dermatomyositis 10, 16
Desensitization 92, 136, 145, 211-13, 223-4
Desloratadine 86-8, 209
Diabetes 150, 184, 257, 270-2, 280-1
Discoid lupus erythematosus (DLE) 14-15
DNA Damage 243-5, 254
Drug allergy 118, 136, 170

E

Effects of adiponectin 272
Effects of adrenaline 343
Effects of omalizumab 125, 139
Efficacy of chromones 72
Efficacy of omalizumab 128, 135, 137, 169
Efficacy of tacrolimus 13-14
Egg allergy 208, 213, 220
EI-anaphylaxis 51-2, 73, 96, 98-100
EI-asthma 51, 54-7, 61, 63, 69-71, 73, 76, 98
EI-bronchoconstriction 51, 54-5, 57, 60-2, 64, 67-8, 71, 97-8
EI-rhinitis 51-2, 80, 82, 98-9
EI-urticaria 51-2, 68, 98, 100
Elastic fibers 246-7
Elastin 240-1, 245-7, 251, 256-7

Elastin fibers 242-3, 246-7
Emphysema 241-3, 247, 296
Endothelial cells 55, 89, 269-71, 275, 283, 287, 289, 293, 298
Endotypes 25-6, 28, 30, 40
Endurance athletes 54, 76-7, 82
Environmental allergens 213, 265, 288
Eosinophilic asthma 151, 168
Eosinophilic esophagitis 138
Eosinophilic syndromes 30
Epidermis 5, 7, 39
Epinephrine 59-60, 206, 208, 301, 330, 343
Estradiol 291-2, 297, 299
Estrogen 252, 265-7, 269, 288-99, 301-2
Estrogen effects 292, 294, 298
Estrogen membrane receptor 265, 291-4
Estrogen receptors (ER) 265, 288-90, 291, 293-8
Estrogen replacement therapy (ERT) 298-9
Estrogens 294-7
Exercise anaphylaxis 334, 346
Extracellular Matrix (ECM) 240-1, 244-5, 247-8, 256-7
Eye symptoms 81-2, 86

F

FAHF-2 225
Fatal anaphylaxis 95, 331, 335
FBNs 246
Fc RI expression 169, 225
FEV1 29, 32, 54, 57-8, 61, 67, 71-2, 128, 132, 152, 168-9, 276
Fibrillar collagens 245, 247
First generation antihistamines 87
Fisetin 300-1
Fish allergic patients 215
Flavonoids 299-300
Fluticasone 58-9, 63

Food allergens pass 192, 194
Food allergic patients 200-1
Food allergic reaction 182, 198
Food allergy mouse model 220-1
Food allergy reaction 202
Food allergy symptoms 201
Food anaphylaxis 137, 333-6, 338, 345-6, 352, 354-5
Food-induced anaphylaxis 183, 338
Formoterol 53, 60-4, 98, 165, 209
Free IgE 74, 124, 205, 223
Fusion proteins 26, 35-6, 153, 218

G

Generation antihistamines 87
Global initiative for asthma (GINA) 126
Glucocorticoid receptor 56, 60, 63
Glucocorticoid response elements (GREs) 164
Glutathione 240, 245, 250-1, 257
Grass pollen 89, 94-5, 281

H

Helminthes 118, 142-3
Helminthic infection 28, 143
Helminths 223, 226-7
High affinity receptor 118, 121
Histamine 18, 55, 66, 70, 82-4, 86, 122, 124, 151, 163, 167, 207, 209, 243, 270
Hormone replacement therapy (HRT) 298-9
House dust mites 93-5, 136, 170-1
Human umbilical vein endothelial cells (HUVECs) 290-1, 293, 297
Hymenoptera anaphylaxis 334, 346, 348, 352
Hypersensitivity 74, 122, 137, 162, 186, 188, 197, 204, 208, 283
Hypersensitivity reactions 30-2, 183, 186, 193, 221, 336, 344
Hypoallergens 182

I

ICAM-1 244, 283, 287, 297-8
ICER 146, 148
ICSs 162, 164, 167-9
Idiopathic anaphylaxis 334, 346-8
IgE 27, 30, 34-5, 74, 82, 118-25, 131-2, 141-2, 182-3, 185-9, 192-3, 200-4, 216-17, 223-4, 279
IgE antibodies 123, 162-3, 170, 183, 186, 188, 192-3, 197, 212, 229
IgE-bearing cells 125
IgE binding 121-3, 173, 215, 218, 271, 276
IgE determinations 202-3
IgE levels 34, 123, 127, 136, 147, 198, 202-3, 205, 213-15, 220
IgE-mediated allergies 92, 186, 204
IgE-mediated food allergy 191, 344
IgE-mediated reactions 182
IgE-mediated responses 190
IgE molecules 122-4, 270
IgE production 35, 120-2, 150, 217, 227, 279
IgE synthesis 34, 119, 122-3, 149, 183, 196-7
IgG antibodies 215-18
IL-1 39, 240-2, 248, 257, 271, 275-6, 291, 297
IL-1Ra 270, 272
IL-4 6, 74, 120-1, 150, 163, 169, 192, 212, 279, 283-5, 296, 298, 300
IL-5 6, 74, 122, 125, 142, 150, 163, 168, 192-3, 212, 225-6, 271, 279, 283-6, 296
IL-6 39, 240-2, 257, 270-2, 275-6, 279-80, 285
IL-8 39, 242, 257, 270-1, 275-6
IL-10 164, 196, 226, 270-2, 279-80, 284-6, 296
IL-12 151, 275-6, 285, 296
IL-13 74, 120, 122, 125, 142, 163, 169, 192, 212, 226, 284-5, 296, 300
IL4 30-2
IL13 30-2
Immune cells 82, 183, 240, 301
Immune response of allergic inflammation 273
Immune responses 4-5, 26, 38, 92, 122, 150, 162, 171, 194-5, 210-11, 216-17, 222, 225-6, 279, 285

Immune system 5, 7, 163, 184, 193-6, 226, 269, 288-90
Immune system cells 192, 194
Immunization 213, 215, 217-18
Immuno solid-phase allergen chip (ISAC) 205
ImmunoCap 202-3
Immunodominant 220-1
Immunoglobulin 24, 27, 119, 153, 192, 196, 265, 272, 286, 296
Immunology of the skin 3
Immunomodulation 18, 24, 225
Immunotherapy 24, 26, 28, 35, 37-9, 51, 78, 92, 132-3, 135-6, 162, 170-1, 182, 210-12, 268-9
Immunotherapy efficacy 36-7, 39, 171
Inflammatory bowel disease 226, 228, 271, 280
Inflammatory cytokines 6, 8, 240-4, 249, 252, 255, 257, 277, 289
Inflammatory skin diseases 3-4, 8
Inhaled allergens 125, 151, 284
Inhaled beta 2-agonists 53-4, 57, 59-62, 70, 76, 97, 100
Inhaled corticosteroids 50, 53-4, 56-60, 62-3, 67, 72, 74, 76, 97-8, 127, 130, 132, 136, 145, 162-4
Inhaled corticosteroids dose 130
Inhaled mast cell stabilizers 73, 99-100
Inhaled steroids 27, 32, 34, 56, 62, 98, 100
Inhibited fish allergic patients 215
Injection immunotherapy 93, 95-6
Interleukin 6, 29-31, 242-3, 270, 272, 274, 281, 284
Interventions 146, 300
Intramuscular adrenaline 96, 99, 330, 332, 341, 355
Intranasal 91, 173
Ipratropium 65-6, 76, 165-6
Ipratropium bromide 64, 66, 91, 166, 209

K

Ketotifen 86, 88, 209

L

Langerhans cells (LCs) 5-8, 122
Late asthmatic responses 151, 169
Latex 198-200, 334, 346
Latex-allergic patients 198
Latex allergies 170, 198
Leukocytes 171-2, 241, 243-4, 249, 256, 287
Leukotriene antagonists 67, 70, 98-9
Leukotriene receptor antagonists 68, 166
Leukotrienes 66-7, 122, 166, 209, 241-2, 256, 270, 283, 285
Lipid mediators 163, 240-2, 255-6, 283
Lipid transfer proteins (LTPs) 198, 200-1, 221
Long-acting beta 2-agonists 59, 62, 67
Lutein 240-1, 250, 253-5, 257
Lymph nodes 5, 39, 163
Lymphocytes 4-5, 26-7, 31, 33-4, 36, 125, 164, 196, 271, 277, 279, 284, 286-7, 289, 296

M

Macrophages 60, 122, 163-5, 244, 250, 272, 276-7, 285-6, 289, 293, 295-6
Major basic protein (MBP) 294
Major histocompatibility complex (MHC) 5, 192-3
Malignancies 19, 144
Mast cell stabilizers 64, 70-1, 91
Mastocytosis 70, 118, 139, 330, 332, 335-6, 339, 355
Matrixmetalloproteinases (MMPs) 242-3, 254, 247-9, 256-7
Mediator antagonists 162, 166
Mediators release 193, 207
Membrane-bound adhesion molecules 298
Mepolizumab 24, 29-30, 168
Meta-analysis 9, 79, 86, 93-5, 99, 188
Metabolite 32, 88
Migration of inflammatory cells 83, 297
Mild allergic asthma 287

Mild asthmatics 287
Milk allergic patients 207
Milk allergy 205, 223
Mitogen activated protein kinase (MAPK) 242-3, 248, 257, 292
MMP-1 247-8, 254
MMP-2 247-8, 254
Moderate asthma 29, 32, 125
Moderate-severe allergic asthma 130
Monoclonal antibodies 24-6, 35, 168
Monotherapy 14-15, 68, 150, 166-7, 224, 287
Montelukast 66-9, 76, 166
Multiple food allergies 138, 182, 225
Murine model 151, 153, 214-15, 225, 227, 285

N

Naive T-cells 163
Nasal congestion 52, 77, 82-4, 86, 88-9, 201
Nasal corticosteroids 53, 77-82, 88
Nasal decongestants 78, 88-90, 99
Nasal mucosa 63, 73, 77, 79, 84, 88, 90, 121, 273, 281
Nasal symptoms 80-1, 90
Natural allergen extracts 171, 210-11
Nedocromil sodium 70-1, 73-4
Neoplasms 28, 140, 144
Netherton syndrome 17, 20
Neutrophils 5, 58, 122, 164-5, 287, 289, 295
NF-kB 242-3, 249, 253, 272
NF-kB activation 249
NFAT 5-6
Nicotinamide 240-1, 250, 255-7
Nitrative stress 275-7, 279, 289, 295
Nitric oxide 56, 249, 274, 277-8, 285, 293-4
Nitric Oxide Synthase (iNOS) 249, 253, 275-6, 278, 294
Non-allergic asthma 154

Non-allergic patients 28
Non-allergic rhinitis treatment 79, 99
Non-atopic patients 203, 284
Non-observed adverse event level (NOAEL) 19
Non-omalizumab-treated patients 131
Non-smokers patients 147-9
Nonallergic patients 66
Nonasthmatic 97
Nongenetic risk factors 184, 190-1
Nongenomic effects 265, 289

O

Occlusive disease 257
Occupational asthma 131-2
OIT 182, 212-13
OIT efficacy 213
Olive pollen-allergic patients 218
Omalizumab 24, 26-8, 41, 74-5, 118, 123-45, 147-9, 154, 162, 168-9, 223-4, 268, 281
Omalizumab anaphylaxis 141
Omalizumab asthma control 131
Omalizumab blocks 125, 168
Omalizumab-induced anaphylaxis 141
Omalizumab labels 144-5
Omalizumab patient 132
Omalizumab-related anaphylaxis 141
Omalizumab Therapy 129-30, 145, 223-4
Omalizumab treatment 124-5, 131, 136, 144
Oral allergy syndrome 200
Oral decongestants 89-90, 92
Oral formulations 60, 88-9
Oral lichen planus 10, 14
Ordinary asthma patient 57
Oxidative damage 244-6, 257

Oxidative stress 172-3, 240-1, 243-5, 247, 250, 252, 255-7, 265, 274-7, 279, 289, 300
Oxidative Stress/Nitrative Stress in Allergic Disease 275
Oxymetazoline 89-90

P

Panallergens 197-8, 221
Parasitic infection 140, 143
Peach-allergic patients 221
Peach allergy 213, 223
Peanut allergen Ara 218, 222
Peanut allergic patients 224
Peanut allergy 137, 182, 190, 205, 212, 214-15, 219, 222, 226-7, 333
Pediatric patients 336, 347, 353
Peptide immunotherapy 162, 215
Perennial aeroallergens 127-8, 136
Perennial allergens 94
Perennial rhinitis 68, 133
Peripheral blood mononuclear cells (PBMCs) 218-20
Peripheral tolerance 195-6
Peroxisome proliferators-activated receptor (PPAR) 40, 150, 273-5
Pimecrolimus 3-4, 6-19
Pimecrolimus cream 9, 11, 13, 16-18
Placebo-treated mice 220
Plasma cell 119, 192-3, 196
Plasma mediators 240-2, 256
Pollen allergies 199
Pollens 81, 170, 172, 189, 198-200, 221, 268-9, 280
Pollinosis 199-200
PPAR gamma activation 150
Prevalence of food allergy 188
Prevention of EI-asthma 63, 73
Prevention of EI-bronchoconstriction 67, 98
Probiotics 223, 227-8

Progesterone 288, 290-1
Prostaglandins 122, 163, 209, 240-2, 244, 249-50, 256, 270
Protein kinase 242-3, 255
Pruritus 18, 82, 86, 89, 139, 201
Pyoderma gangrenosum 3, 10, 15, 17

R

Reactive oxygen species (ROS) 240, 243-5, 252-3, 255, 257, 276, 278, 292
Recombinant allergens 170-1, 210-11, 214
Recombinant fusion proteins 36, 217
Recruitment of inflammatory cells 170, 192
Rhinitis medicamentosa 90-1
Rhinorrhea 52, 66, 79, 81, 99, 201
ROS generation 245, 278, 292

S

Salbutamol 27, 53, 60-1, 63-4, 97-8, 209
Salmeterol 53, 60-4, 68, 97-8, 165, 209
Seafood allergy 339, 346
Seasonal allergic rhinitis 73, 84, 93, 133
Seasonal allergic rhinoconjuntivitis 93, 95
Seborrheic dermatitis 3, 10, 12-13
Secretory leukocyte protease inhibitor (SLPI) 164, 172
Self-injectable adrenaline 332-4, 337, 341-2, 356
Serine protease inhibitors 162, 171-2
Serine proteases 171, 209
Short acting beta 2-agonists 61-2, 71
Side effects of adrenaline 351
Signal-transduction 241
Single dose of omalizumab 134, 138
Skin prick test (SPT) 84, 92, 132, 142, 188, 202, 204, 207
Skin tests 84, 131, 204
Small clinical trial son asthmatic patients 37
Smooth muscle 59-60, 64, 125, 165, 276, 278, 280

Smooth muscle cells 164-5, 270, 294
Sputum 27, 29, 55, 74, 295
Standard therapies 75, 134
STAT 120-1, 242-3, 250
Steroids 24-5, 27, 29-31, 33, 35, 37, 39, 41, 56, 98, 164
Subclinical inflammation 9
Subcutaneous injection 126-8, 170, 220
Sublingual immunotherapy 170, 182, 212-13, 269, 272
Suspected food allergens 198, 204
Symptoms of allergic rhinitis 79, 93
Systemic allergic reactions 93, 135
Systemic corticosteroids 75, 97, 132, 138
Systemic lupus erythematosus (SLE) 14-15, 271, 280

T

T-cell receptor (TCRs) 5, 193
Tacrolimus 3-4, 6-15, 17-20
Tacrolimus ointment 8-13, 17
TCLs 220-1
Terbutaline 60-1, 97, 100, 209
TGF 32, 196, 215, 244, 246, 251, 279, 285
Th-2 cells 192, 196
Th1/Th2 balance 182, 195
Th2 cells 120, 125, 162-3, 192, 226
Th2 responses 173, 192, 225-6, 229, 285, 296
Theophylline-dependent asthma patients 72
TIMP-1 248
TIMP-2 248
TIMPs 248
Tissue architecture 242-3
Tissue inflammatory responses 286
TNF 14, 33, 240, 242-3, 248, 250, 252, 257, 270-2, 274-5, 279, 281, 285, 296-8
Toll-like receptors (TLRs) 37, 225
Topical calcineurin inhibitors 3, 7-10, 12, 14-16, 18-20

Topical corticosteroids 3, 7-8, 10-13, 20, 73, 79, 81
Topical decongestants 89-90
Topical macrolide immunomodulator 3
Topical tacrolimus 10-11, 13-14
Topical therapies 3, 135
Total IgE 32, 123, 128, 131
Total IgE levels 123, 128
Tr1 cells 196
Traditional allergen extracts 210-11
Transcription factors (TF) 6, 149, 249-50, 293
Transcriptional activity 164, 275
Treating allergic disease 267, 277
Treg cells 36, 83, 195-6
Tumor necrosis factor 122, 240-3, 272, 281, 284
Type I hypersensitivity 162, 186, 193

U

Urticaria 51, 82, 84, 86, 93, 96, 133, 140, 163, 172, 201, 288, 339

V

Vascular endothelial cells 282-3
VCAM-1 283, 287, 297-8
Vernal keratoconjunctivitis 72-3, 294
Vitamin B12 257
Vitamin D deficiency (VDD) 191

W

White adipose tissue 270-1

Made in the USA
Las Vegas, NV
03 November 2026

57424456R00233